Biomedical Image Analysis

Statistical and Variational Methods

Ideal for classroom use and self-study, this book explains the implementation of the most effective modern methods in image analysis, covering segmentation, registration, and visualization, and focusing on the key theories, algorithms and applications that have emerged from recent progress in computer vision, imaging, and computational biomedical science.

- Structured around five core building blocks – signals, systems, image formation, and modality; stochastic models; computational geometry; level-set methods; and tools and CAD models – it provides a solid overview of the field.
- Mathematical and statistical topics are presented in a straightforward manner, enabling the reader to gain a deep understanding of the subject without becoming entangled in mathematical complexities.
- Theory is connected to practical examples in X-ray, ultrasound, nuclear medicine, MRI and CT imaging, removing the abstract nature of the models and assisting reader understanding, whilst computer simulations, online course slides, and a solution manual provide a complete instructor package.

Aly A. Farag is Professor of Electrical and Computer Engineering, and the founding Director of the Computer Vision and Image Processing Laboratory, at the University of Louisville. His research interests center around object modeling with biomedical applications, and his more recent biomedical inventions have led to the development of improved methods for tubular object modeling, virtual colonoscopies, lung nodule detection and classification based on CT scans, real-time monitoring of vital signs from thermal imaging, and image-based reconstruction of the human jaw. He is a Fellow of the IEEE.

"This is a comprehensive book on the topic of biomedical image analysis. It covers both statistical and variational approaches as well as some of the foundations of image acquisition. The individual chapters and sections also include practical examples, meaningful exercises, and computer labs. The book is an outstanding and thorough introduction to the field of biomedical image analysis and is suitable both for classroom use and self-study. A well curated bibliography provides starting points for additional study."

Ron Kikinis
Harvard Medical School

Biomedical Image Analysis

Statistical and Variational Methods

ALY A. FARAG
University of Louisville

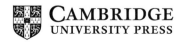

CAMBRIDGE
UNIVERSITY PRESS

University Printing House, Cambridge CB2 8BS, United Kingdom

Cambridge University Press is part of the University of Cambridge.

It furthers the University's mission by disseminating knowledge in the pursuit of education, learning and research at the highest international levels of excellence.

www.cambridge.org
Information on this title: www.cambridge.org/9780521196796

© A. Farag 2014

This publication is in copyright. Subject to statutory exception and to the provisions of relevant collective licensing agreements, no reproduction of any part may take place without the written permission of Cambridge University Press.

First published 2014

Printed in the United Kingdom by TJ International Ltd. Padstow Cornwall

A catalog record for this publication is available from the British Library

Library of Congress Cataloging in Publication data
Farag, Aly A., author.
Biomedical image analysis / Aly A. Farag.
   p. ; cm.
Includes bibliographical references and index.
ISBN 978-0-521-19679-6 (hardback : alk. paper)
I. Title.
[DNLM: 1. Image Interpretation, Computer-Assisted – methods. 2. Biomedical Technology – methods. 3. Image Processing, Computer-Assisted. 4. Information Theory. 5. Signal Processing, Computer-Assisted. WB 141]
R856
610.28–dc23
                                      2014004719

ISBN 978-0-521-19679-6 Hardback

Additional resources for this publication at www.cambridge.org/farag

Cambridge University Press has no responsibility for the persistence or accuracy of URLs for external or third-party internet websites referred to in this publication, and does not guarantee that any content on such websites is, or will remain, accurate or appropriate.

To my dear wife *Salwa* – thank you for love, support and dedication to our blessed family!

Contents

Preface			*page* xvii
Nomenclature			xx

1 Overview of biomedical image analysis — 1

- 1.1 Introduction — 1
- 1.2 The scope of the book — 2
  - 1.2.1 Signals and systems, image formation, and image modality — 2
  - 1.2.2 Stochastic models — 3
  - 1.2.3 Computational geometry — 3
  - 1.2.4 Variational calculus and level-set methods — 3
  - 1.2.5 Image analysis tools — 4
- 1.3 Options for class work — 4
- 1.4 Other references — 4

Part I Signals and systems, image formation, and image modality — 7

2 Overview of two-dimensional signals and systems — 9

- 2.1 Definitions — 9
- 2.2 Signal representations — 10
  - 2.2.1 Special functions — 11
  - 2.2.2 Fourier series — 12
  - 2.2.3 Fourier transform — 13
- 2.3 Basic sampling and quantization — 16
- 2.4 Sequence Fourier series — 18
  - 2.4.1 Sequence Fourier transform — 21
  - 2.4.2 Relationship to the continuous Fourier transform — 22
- 2.5 Discrete Fourier transform — 23
- 2.6 The fast Fourier transform (FFT) algorithm — 25
  - 2.6.1 Effect of periodic shifts — 26
  - 2.6.2 Circular convolution — 27
  - 2.6.3 Linear convolution — 28
- 2.7 The Z-transform — 29

	2.8	Basic 2D digital filter design		31
	2.9	Anisotropic diffusion filtering		33
	2.10	Summary		36
	2.11	Exercises		36
	References			38

3 Biomedical imaging modalities — 39

- 3.1 Introduction — 39
- 3.2 X-rays — 39
  - 3.2.1 Filtration and beam hardening — 41
  - 3.2.2 Simulation of X-ray transmission — 41
- 3.3 Computed tomography — 43
  - 3.3.1 CT scanner generations — 45
  - 3.3.2 Basic CT reconstruction algorithms — 46
  - 3.3.3 Dose — 47
  - 3.3.4 CT image artifacts — 47
- 3.4 Nuclear medicine — 47
  - 3.4.1 Scintillation cameras — 48
  - 3.4.2 Emission computed tomography — 51
- 3.5 Ultrasound — 53
  - 3.5.1 Ultrasound intensity — 54
  - 3.5.2 Attenuation in ultrasound — 54
  - 3.5.3 Reflection in ultrasound — 56
  - 3.5.4 Refraction in ultrasound — 56
  - 3.5.5 Ultrasound transducers — 56
  - 3.5.6 Ultrasound beams — 57
  - 3.5.7 Ultrasound instrumentation — 58
  - 3.5.8 Ultrasound artifacts — 59
  - 3.5.9 Doppler effect — 59
- 3.6 Magnetic resonance imaging — 61
  - 3.6.1 Signal induction — 63
  - 3.6.2 Relaxation processes — 64
  - 3.6.3 Pulse sequences — 65
  - 3.6.4 Spatial encoding — 67
  - 3.6.5 Tissue contrast in MRI — 68
  - 3.6.6 Components of an MRI system — 69
- 3.7 Summary — 71
- 3.8 Exercises — 71
- References — 72
- Appendix 3.1 Parallel beam filtered back-projection algorithm — 72

Part II Stochastic models — 77

4 Random variables — 79

- 4.1 Introduction — 79
- 4.2 Statistical experiments — 79
  - 4.2.1 Sample space Ω — 80
  - 4.2.2 Field (algebra) σ_F — 80
  - 4.2.3 Probability measure P — 80
- 4.3 Random variables — 83
  - 4.3.1 Basic concepts — 83
  - 4.3.2 Properties of the CDF and the PDF of a random variable — 87
  - 4.3.3 The conditional distribution — 88
  - 4.3.4 Statistical expectation — 90
  - 4.3.5 Functions of a random variable — 94
- 4.4 Two random variables — 96
  - 4.4.1 Statistical expectation in two dimensions — 99
  - 4.4.2 Functions of two random variables — 100
  - 4.4.3 Two functions of two random variables — 102
- 4.5 Simulation of random variables — 103
- 4.6 Summary — 104
- 4.7 Computer laboratory — 104
- 4.8 Exercises — 105
- References — 106

5 Random processes — 107

- 5.1 Definition and general concepts — 107
  - 5.1.1 Description of random processes — 109
  - 5.1.2 Classification of a random process — 110
  - 5.1.3 Continuity of a random process — 112
  - 5.1.4 The Kolmogorov consistency conditions — 113
- 5.2 Distribution functions for a random process — 113
  - 5.2.1 Definitions — 113
  - 5.2.2 First- and second-order probability distribution functions — 114
- 5.3 Some properties of a random process — 118
  - 5.3.1 Stationarity — 118
  - 5.3.2 The autocorrelation function — 118
  - 5.3.3 The autocovariance function — 120
  - 5.3.4 The cross-correlation function — 120
  - 5.3.5 Time average — 121
  - 5.3.6 The power spectrum of a random process — 123
  - 5.3.7 Cross-spectral density — 125
  - 5.3.8 Power spectral density of discrete-parameter random process — 125

	5.4	Linear systems with random inputs	126
	5.5	Two-dimensional random processes	128
	5.6	Exercises	128
		References	130
6	**Basics of random fields**	**131**
	6.1	Introduction	131
	6.2	Graphical models	136
	6.3	Markov system	139
	6.4	Hidden Markov model	140
	6.5	Markov random field	141
	6.6	Gibbs model	143
	6.7	Markov–Gibbs random field models	145
		6.7.1 Auto-models	146
		6.7.2 Aura-based GRF model	147
		6.7.3 Other models	148
	6.8	GRF-based image synthesis	149
		6.8.1 Gibbs sampler algorithm	149
		6.8.2 Chen algorithm	149
		6.8.3 Metropolis algorithm	151
	6.9	GRF-based image analysis	153
		6.9.1 Coding estimation	153
		6.9.2 Least square error method	155
		6.9.3 Analytical method for parameter identification	155
	6.10	Summary	159
	6.11	Exercises	159
	6.12	Computer laboratory	161
		References	162
7	**Probability density estimation by linear models**	**163**
	7.1	Introduction	163
	7.2	Nonparametric methods	164
		7.2.1 Kernel-based estimators	166
		7.2.2 Parzen window	167
		7.2.3 k–NN estimator	168
	7.3	Parametric methods	168
		7.3.1 Maximum likelihood estimator (MLE)	169
		7.3.2 Biased versus unbiased estimator	170
		7.3.3 The expectation-maximization (EM) approach	171
	7.4	Linear combination of Gaussians model (LCG1)	172
		7.4.1 Modifications of the linear model (LCG2)	174
	7.5	Modeling the image intensity/appearance through the linear model	175

	7.6	Exercises	176
	7.7	Computer laboratory	177
		References	179

Part III Computational geometry   181

8   Basics of topology and computational geometry   183

	8.1	Introduction	183
	8.2	Shape representation	183
		8.2.1 What is shape?	183
		8.2.2 How should a shape be described?	184
		8.2.3 Criteria for shape representation	184
		8.2.4 Data representation of shape	184
	8.3	Topological equivalence	186
	8.4	Vector spaces	188
	8.5	Surfaces in parameter space	190
		8.5.1 Parametric curves	191
		8.5.2 Parametric surfaces	193
		8.5.3 Surface curvature	196
	8.6	Surfaces as meshes	199
		8.6.1 Manifolds and surfaces	199
		8.6.2 Barycentric coordinates	201
		8.6.3 Triangle local frame	202
		8.6.4 Surface curvature: discrete form	202
	8.7	Summary	204
	8.8	Exercises	205
	8.9	Computer laboratory	207
		References	208

9   Geometric features extraction   213

	9.1	Introduction	213
	9.2	Edges and corners	217
		9.2.1 The Harris detector	217
		9.2.2 The SUSAN corner detector	219
		9.2.3 Harris–Laplace and Harris–affine corner detectors	219
		9.2.4 Blob detectors	221
		9.2.5 Region detectors	223
	9.3	Comparative evaluation of interest points	225
		9.3.1 Multi-scale representations	225
		9.3.2 Scale-space representation	232
		9.3.3 Scale-space and feature detection	233
		9.3.4 Differential singularities and feature detection	234

        9.4 Local descriptors   235
             9.4.1 Scale-invariant feature transform (SIFT)   235
             9.4.2 Case study: Descriptors of small-size lung nodules
                    in chest CT   238
             9.4.3 Extensions to the SIFT algorithms   239
             9.4.4 Speeded-up robust features (SURF)   241
             9.4.5 Multi-resolution local binary pattern (LBP)   241
             9.4.6 Image stitching   245
        9.5 Three-dimensional local invariant feature descriptors   257
             9.5.1 Interest point detection   257
             9.5.2 3D descriptor building   261
             9.5.3 Descriptor matching   264
        9.6 Summary   264
        9.7 Exercises   267
        9.8 Computer laboratory   267
        References   269

Part IV Variational approaches and level sets   273

10 Variational approaches and level sets   275

        10.1 Calculus of variation and Euler equation   275
              10.1.1 Euler–Lagrange equation for one independent variable   276
              10.1.2 Euler–Lagrange equation for multiple independent variables   277
              10.1.3 Euler–Lagrange and the gradient descent flow   278
        10.2 Curve/surface evolution via classical deformable models   279
              10.2.1 Curves and planar differential geometry   279
              10.2.2 Geometry of surfaces   280
              10.2.3 Geodesic curvature   281
              10.2.4 Principal curvatures   281
              10.2.5 Planar curves and surface normal   281
              10.2.6 Curve/surface evolution as a variational problem   282
              10.2.7 Discretization and numerical simulation of snakes   283
        10.3 Level sets   284
              10.3.1 Implicit representation and the evolution PDE   284
              10.3.2 Level-set calculus   286
        10.4 Numerical methods for level sets   287
              10.4.1 Conservation law and weak solutions   287
              10.4.2 Entropy condition and viscosity solutions   288
              10.4.3 Upwind direction and discontinuous solutions   288
              10.4.4 The Eulerian formulation and the hyperbolic conservation law 289
        10.5 Numerical algorithm   290
              10.5.1 Need for reinitialization and the distance function   291
              10.5.2 Front evolution without reinitialization   292

		10.6	Exercises	293
		10.7	Computer laboratory	293
			References	294

Part V Image analysis tools   295

11		**Segmentation: statistical approach**		297
	11.1	Introduction		297
	11.2	Image modelling		299
		11.2.1	Problem formulation and image models	300
	11.3	Experiments and discussion		306
		11.3.1	Ground-truth experiments	307
		11.3.2	Examples of applicability to biomedical images	308
	11.4	Summary		313
	11.5	Exercises		314
		References		314

12		**Segmentation: variational approach**		316
	12.1	Introduction		316
	12.2	Variational segmentation without edges		318
		12.2.1	The Mumford–Shah energy formulation	318
		12.2.2	Chan and Vese variational approach	319
	12.3	Image segmentation using multiple level-set functions		320
	12.4	Implicit shape representation		322
		12.4.1	Shape registration	324
	12.5	Shape-based segmentation		324
	12.6	Curve/surface modeling by level sets		326
	12.7	Variational model for evolution-based region statistics		328
	12.8	Examples and evaluation		329
		12.8.1	Performance on images and volumes	329
		12.8.2	Validation experiment on a real phantom	331
		12.8.3	Blood vessel extraction	332
	12.9	Clinical example: lung nodule segmentation		334
		12.9.1	Variational approach for nodule segmentation	336
		12.9.2	Shape alignment	337
		12.9.3	Level-set segmentation with shape prior	339
		12.9.4	Some results	339
		12.9.5	Extensions	341
	12.10	Summary		342
	12.11	Exercises		342
	12.12	Computer laboratory		342
		References		343

13 Basics of registration — 345

- 13.1 Introduction — 345
- 13.2 Basic concepts and definitions — 346
  - 13.2.1 Components of the registration transformation — 349
  - 13.2.2 Choice of transformation — 352
  - 13.2.3 Similarity measures — 353
- 13.3 Surface registration by the ICP algorithm — 355
  - 13.3.1 Mathematical preliminaries — 355
  - 13.3.2 The ICP algorithm — 359
- 13.4 Global image registration via mutual information — 366
  - 13.4.1 Imaging model — 369
  - 13.4.2 Basics of information theory — 371
  - 13.4.3 Registration metric — 375
  - 13.4.4 Mutual information registration — 377
- 13.5 Applications — 378
- 13.6 Summary — 378
- 13.7 Exercises — 379
- 13.8 Computer laboratory — 380
- References — 380
- Appendix 13.1 MATLAB code implementations — 381

14 Variational methods for shape registration — 387

- 14.1 Introduction — 387
- 14.2 Shape modeling — 389
  - 14.2.1 Parametric representations — 389
  - 14.2.2 Landmark-based representation — 390
  - 14.2.3 Medial axes representation — 391
  - 14.2.4 Implicit representation using the vector distance function — 392
  - 14.2.5 Implicit representation using distance transform — 392
- 14.3 Global registration of shapes in implicit spaces — 394
  - 14.3.1 Global matching of shapes — 394
  - 14.3.2 VDF-based dissimilarity measure — 397
  - 14.3.3 SDF-based dissimilarity measure — 398
  - 14.3.4 Examples — 400
- 14.4 Local shape registration — 403
  - 14.4.1 Local alignment — 405
  - 14.4.2 Gradient descent flows and numerical implementation — 408
- 14.5 Summary — 413
- References — 414

15 Statistical models of shape and appearance — 417

- 15.1 Introduction — 417

15.2	Statistical shape models		417
	15.2.1	Construction of statistical shape model using PCA	419
	15.2.2	Fitting a model to new points	421
	15.2.3	Statistical modeling of structures	422
	15.2.4	Modeling shape variations	424
15.3	Statistical appearance models		428
	15.3.1	Image warping	428
	15.3.2	One-dimensional thin-plate splines	429
	15.3.3	N-dimensional thin-plate splines	429
	15.3.4	Statistical appearance model construction using PCA	431
	15.3.5	Combined appearance models	433
15.4	Analysis of lung nodules in low-dose CT (LDCT) scans		436
	15.4.1	Lung nodules in low-dose CT	437
15.5	Appearance-based approach for complete human jaw reconstruction		441
	15.5.1	Jaw prior models	444
	15.5.2	Model-based shape and albedo recovery	445
	15.5.3	Sample results	446
15.6	Summary		448
References			448
Appendix 15.1	Pseudocodes and MATLAB realizations		450

Index 458

Preface

About two decades ago, I worked with the University of Louisville College of Engineering and the Office of the Vice President for Research to establish the Computer Vision and Image Processing Laboratory (CVIP Lab – www.cvip.uofl.edu) as a multidisciplinary environment for research, teaching, and training in computational image analysis. Over the years, the CVIP Lab has been home to researchers in engineering, medicine, dentistry, mathematics, and psychology who are interested in imaging. The support of the University of Louisville administration and colleagues at various units literally made the CVIP Lab a place that I miss whenever I am away from it, even for an enjoyable vacation.

At the CVIP Lab we pushed agendas for imaging research, from basics to applications, and in the process established immediate and auxiliary but essential infrastructure. Among the auxiliary infrastructure has been high-speed networking to link the University to what has become known as Internet 2, an initiative funded by the National Science Foundation, and to link the main campus (Belknap) to the Health Science Campus (HSC) a few miles away. The auxiliary infrastructure included supercomputers and immersive visualization. The essential hardware included high-end computing and graphics workstations, object scanners, and various laboratory benches for electronic design and testing. The laboratory has been visited by researchers, potential engineering students, faculty candidates in engineering, dentistry and medicine; its research activities have been showcased on national and local media, and the University President (John Shumaker) and the Dean of Engineering (Thomas Hanley) recorded advertisements there as the University pushed to promote biomedical research, and to establish a biomedical engineering department, during 1996–2002. Today the CVIP Lab is well recognized by colleagues elsewhere. Research at the laboratory has been funded by the National Science Foundation (NSF), the National Institutes of Health (NIH), the Department of Defense (DoD), the Department of Homeland Security (DHS), Norton and Jewish Hospitals, and various government and industrial organizations.

At the CVIP Lab I have had the privilege and pleasure of coaching some of the most brilliant students from around the world, and have supervised and hosted a large number of postdoctoral researchers and researchers who have spent sabbaticals and short visits here. The laboratory has three main areas of focus: computer vision, biomedical imaging, and biometrics. Students and researchers at the laboratory have worked on theoretical, algorithmic and practical domains of these three focal areas. A number of courses, seminars, and presentations have been created over the years to train researchers and promote research at the laboratory. This book is one such result of the activities at the

CVIP Lab. It offers both basic background and sample research problems on the subject of biomedical image analysis.

As the CVIP Lab has been the nest of so many brilliant researchers and students with whom I have worked with over the years, I will list only a few who have made an impact on me. First and foremost is Dr. Darrel Chenoweth, the Chairman of the ECE Department from 1994 to 2004. Darrel gave me unconditional support and encouragement; no words are enough to thank him for his impact on me. Thomas Hanley, Dean of J.B. Speed School of Engineering during 1992–2004, was a visionary who gave me freedom to think and never hesitated to provide support. Without him and Darrel, the CVIP Lab would have not been established. Dr. Nancy Martin, Vice President for Research during 1996–2006, kept the CVIP Lab on her radar and provided support whenever asked. Former Dean Mickey Wilhelm and current Dean Neville Pinto have maintained this trend of support, as did Dr. James Graham, ECE Department Chairman during 2006–2013.

More than 50 colleagues have collaborated with me at the CVIP Lab, so I will just mention a few: Dr. Christopher Shields, former Chairman of Neurological Surgery, Dr. Allan Farman, Professor of Dental Radiology, Dr. Thomas Starr, Associate Dean for Research, Dr. Manuel Casanova, Professor of Psychiatry, Dr. Edward Essock, Professor of Psychology and Brain Sciences, and Dr. Robert Falk, Director of Medical Imaging at Jewish Hospital, have been longstanding collaborators and friends with whom I have enjoyed working, and their support has been crucial to whatever I have achieved at the CVIP Lab.

Three scientists and engineers of the highest caliber and professionalism – Charles Sites, Mike Miller and Salwa Elshazly – made me anxious to come to the CVIP Lab; and if I go away, I can trust that it is safe in their hands. Chuck is a visionary; he and I wrote proposals that brought high-speed networking, computing, visualization and autonomous robotics to the University of Louisville. We have worked together since 1996. Salwa agreed to assist me at the Laboratory in 1997 and for 15 years has provided intellectual support and coordination of efforts that have been crucial for success at the laboratory. Mike joined the laboratory in 2006 after two decades of work in the industry. He showed unbounded dedication and rare talent in almost every aspect of computing and circuit design, and has handled the university regulations for biomedical data. Mike has been my right hand in student advising, documentation of research, and communications with the university as well as funding agencies. Many other technical staff have helped the CVIP Lab; too many to list, but I appreciate all their efforts and assistance.

As I mentioned before, I have been privileged to coach some of the most brilliant people from around the world for their Ph.D. and Masters research. They have worked on my funded projects and have excelled in executing the research plans and expanding them to frontiers that I could not imagine, or perform, alone. I owe a great deal of appreciation and thanks to each of them. In this book, I must acknowledge the following: Dr. Mohamed Sabry, Dr. Hossam Abdelmunim, Dr. Asem Ali, Dr. Rachid Fami, Dr. Shireen Elabian, Dr. Amal Farag, Dr. Ham Rara, Dr. Melih Aslan, Mr. Ahmed Shably, Dr. Mostafa Abdelrahman, Ms. Marwa Ismail, and Dr. Aly Abdelrahim. These 12 individuals have had a direct impact on this book and I owe them my deepest appreciation. In particular, Dr. Shireen Elhabian and Dr. Ahmed Shalby have shown tenacity, intelligence and dedication in assisting me throughout the preparation of this book; I remain very grateful to both of them.

Funding from various organizations and support of the University of Louisville are gratefully acknowledged, as is a long stream of local, national and international collaborators with whom I have had the honor and pleasure to collaborate and interact over three decades.

I must state the obvious: all errors and mishaps in the book are mine. I shall be grateful for any hints from readers that might assist in improving the text in revised prints or new editions. Together with Cambridge University Press, I have a website for auxiliary material including teaching aids, newer homework problems and laboratories, solutions to problems, and codes for the implementations in the book.

Michelle Carey and Elizabeth Horne at Cambridge University Press have provided encouragement throughout this project, Lindsay Nightingale provided a most skilled review of the manuscript, and Christina Sarigiannidou managed the book production. They were very patient with me and worked around my schedule, despite my endless obligations to the CVIP Lab and derailment by circumstances, not the least of which has been the engagement of my mind and soul with the events in my beloved home country of Egypt. Since 2011, countless hours of thought have been spent engaging with my compatriots, family members and officials, pushing for the common good and towards peaceful democratic changes in a country that the entire world wishes to see peaceful and prosperous. I thank Michelle, Elizabeth, Lindsay and Christina for their help, and repeat my highest appreciation to the person most deserving of thanks and appreciation, my dear wife, collaborator, and friend, Salwa A. Elshazly.

Aly A. Farag

Nomenclature

The following conventions are used throughout the document.

Symbol	Description
x	Point in 2D or 3D Cartesian space
$\mathbb{R}$	Set of real numbers
Ω	An open bounded subset of $\mathbb{R}$
$\Omega \setminus \Omega_0$	Complement of Ω_0 in Ω
$\in$	Element of
$\subseteq$	Subset of
$\lvert \cdot \rvert$	Absolute value in $\mathbb{R}$
$\lVert \cdot \rVert$	Euclidean norm in a vector space
$\mathcal{C}$	A curve or family of curves in $\mathbb{R}^2$
ϕ	Level set function
Φ_S	Implicit representation of a given shape S
$\tilde{\phi}$	Implicit representation of a shape prior
$L(.)$	Labeling function
$\mathcal{A}$	Rigid or affine transformation in $\mathbb{R}^n$
$\mathcal{S}$	Scale matrix
$\mathcal{R}$	Rotation matrix
θ	Rotation angle
$\mathcal{T}$	Translation vector
$\mathbf{u} = (u_i)_{1 \leq i \leq n}$	Displacement field in $\mathbb{R}^n$
F	Speed function
V	Vector distance function
$div(\cdot)$	Divergence of a vector field
$\mathcal{D}(\cdot)$	Dissimilarity measure
$\mathcal{D}^{MI}(\cdot)$	Mutual information dissimilarity measure
$\mathcal{D}^{SSD}(\cdot)$	Sum of squared differences dissimilarity measure
$\mathcal{R}(\cdot)$	Regularization term
$\mathcal{M}$	Manifold in $\mathbb{R}^n$
$d(\mathbf{x})$	Distance from $\mathbf{x} \in \mathbb{R}^n$ to a manifold $\mathcal{M}$
$\mathbb{D}(\mathbf{x})$	Squared distance from $\mathbf{x} \in \mathbb{R}^n$ to a manifold $\mathcal{M}$

$\delta(\cdot)$	Dirac function
$H(\cdot)$	Heaviside function
α_i	Weight of shape energy
D	Space dimension, degrees of freedom
$W(.)$	Transform on $\mathbb{R}^D$
$\mathbf{t}$	Translation vector
$L(.)$	Linear transform on $\mathbb{R}^D$
$\mathbf{L}$	Matrix form for a linear transform $L(.)$ on $\mathbb{R}^3$ with matrix elements ℓ_{ij}
s	Scaling parameter in the case of uniform scaling
s_x, s_y, s_z	Scaling parameters in the case of non-uniform scaling
$\mathbf{S}$	Matrix form for a scale transform on $\mathbb{R}^3$ with scale parameter(s) $s \in \mathbb{R}$ in the case of uniform scaling and $s_x, s_y, s_z \in \mathbb{R}$ in the case of non-uniform scaling
t_x, t_y, t_z	Translation parameters
$\mathbf{T}$	Matrix form for a translation transform on $\mathbb{R}^3$ with translation parameters $t_x, t_y, t_z \in \mathbb{R}$
$\mathbf{R}_{x,\alpha}$	Matrix form for a rotation transform on $\mathbb{R}^2 \backslash \mathbb{R}^3$ about the x-axis by angle of rotation α
(α, β, γ)	Euler rotation angles
$E(\alpha, \beta, \gamma)$	Euler transform
$\mathbf{v}$	(Eigen)vector in $\mathbb{R}^D$
$\mathbf{A}$	Square transformation matrix defined on $\mathbb{R}^{D \times D}$
λ	Eigenvalue of matrix $\mathbf{A}$
$|\cdot|$	Matrix determinant
$\mathbf{r}, \mathbf{q}$	A quaternion
q_0, q_1, q_2, q_3	Elements of a quaternion $\mathbf{q}$
$\mathbf{V_q}$	An ordinary vector defining the complex part of a quaternion $\mathbf{q}$
q_x, q_y, q_z	The imaginary parts of a quaternion $\mathbf{q}$
i, j, k	Basis defining the imaginary parts of a quaternion
$\mathbf{R}$	Orthogonal matrix defining the multiplication of two quaternions
$\overline{\mathbf{R}}$	Same as $\mathbf{R}$, except that the lower right-hand 3×3 submatrix is transposed
$\mathbf{q}*$	Conjugate of a quaternion $\mathbf{q}$
$\mathbf{I}$	4×4 identity matrix
M	Model shape represented by a set of points $\{\mathbf{m}_i\}$
N_m	Number of points in the model shape
P	Model shape represented by a set of points $\{\mathbf{p}_i\}$
N_p	Number of points in the scene shape
$R(.)$	Rotation operator
$d(\mathbf{p}, \mathbf{m})$	Euclidean distance between two points $\mathbf{p}, \mathbf{m} \in \mathbb{R}^3$
$d(\mathbf{p}_i, M)$	Euclidean distance between a scene point $\mathbf{p}_i$ and the model point set M
Y	Closest point in the model set which yields the minimum distance
C	The closest point operator
e_i	Residual error for each point pair
E	Sum of squares of the residual error for each point pair

$\mathbf{\mu}_P$	Centroids/origins of the shape defined by the point set P
$\mathbf{p}'_i$	Centered (zero-means) points
$\mathbf{t}'$	Translation vector of the centered points
S_y, S_p	Sums of the squares of the distances between points and their centroids
S	The S-matrix whose elements are sums of products of coordinates measured in the scene shape with coordinates measured in the model shape
$p(x_k)$	Probability of the outcome x_k
$I(x_k)$	Information measure of the outcome x_k
$H(X)$	Entropy of the random variable X
$H(X,Y)$	Joint entropy of the random variables X and Y
$p(x_i, y_j)$	Joint probability density function of the two random variables, i.e. the probability of having both outcomes x_i and y_i occur together
$H(X\|Y=y_j)$	Conditional entropy of X given $Y=y_j$
$H(X\|Y)$	Conditional entropy of X given Y
$I(X,Y)$	Mutual information between X and Y
$p_X(x)$	Marginal probability mass function of the random variable X
$p_{XY}(x,y)$	Joint probability mass function of the random variables X and Y
T_Θ	A transformation with registration parameters Θ
R	Random variable denoting the intensities observed in the reference volume
F	Random variable denoting the intensities observed in the floating volume
$T_\Theta F$	Random variable denoting the intensities observed in the transformed floating volume
$h(.)$	Normalized joint histogram

1 Overview of biomedical image analysis

1.1 Introduction

Image analysis is a vibrant field in research, applications, and technologies. Any image is a representation of data gathered by sensors from a physical environment. Biomedical image analysis deals with biological systems; this book focuses on analysis of images that describe the structure or function of the human body. Broadly speaking, biomedical image analysis includes three major components: segmentation, registration, and visualization. Each of these components is a science and art in its own right, with considerable literature spanning over four decades of theory, algorithms, and applications. Each component has been documented in books, conference proceedings, archived journals, technologies, and commercial products.

So a new book on this subject faces two questions: what can it add to the sea of progress, and what distinguishes it from similar books on the subject? The first of these is not a problem per se. This book addresses the common denominator in theory, algorithms and applications that has resulted from this sea of progress, tailored towards a particular audience. To answer the second question, the book covers what is not currently available in textbooks in terms of subjects and educational material. It aims to be a friendly welcome for newcomers to the field, treating it in a rigorous manner, yet without becoming overwhelmed by details. Specifically, the intended audience includes seniors and first-year graduate students in engineering, mathematics, and physics. Those who are experts in the field may also find the book appropriate as a refresher.

The original plan for this book was to focus on statistical methods of biomedical image analysis. However, given current developments in this vibrant field and its multidisciplinary nature, a strictly statistical framework might be too dry. Likewise, the popularity of variational calculus methods in image analysis might make it appealing to have that as the sole focus. But my experience with students taking this subject matter is that they start off very excited about the subject; then their enthusiasm decreases on realizing the prerequisite knowledge of stochastic processes, differential calculus, and algorithms. Hence, a reassessment was necessary, which required a change of plan.

I have therefore added a review of image modalities and the basics of signals and systems, as an overview of the basic information needed for biomedical image analysis. Uncertainties in the imaging process include noise, motion, and occlusion. Hence, some statistical background on random variables, random processes, and random fields has been introduced, as prerequisites to analysis steps such as segmentation, model building, and registration. The same strategy was followed with variational calculus approaches. An introductory chapter on level-set methods has been added, in order to offer the background necessary for deploying elastic deformable models in biomedical image analysis. Statistical and level-set methods may share some shape models, so some basic concepts of topology and shape models have been introduced. With background in statistics, level sets, and computational geometry, the processes of segmentation, registration and visualization become more purposeful, and it becomes possible to extract information and build a hypothesis. Indeed, complete front-end systems for interpreting biomedical imaging data may be established based on this background. For example, computer-assisted diagnosis (CAD) systems, image-guided surgical simulation, and telemedicine require knowledge of statistical, variational, and geometric techniques; they also require an understanding of algorithms and numerical methods.

The risk of this ambitious scope is obvious: the book may become too big and the material may seem too disparate. Every effort has been made to curtail the appetite for comprehensiveness and keep the focus on the fundamentals.

I aim to present the subjects in a standard framework, augmented with examples, computer simulations and exercises, which include computer projects. Advanced seniors and first-year graduates, with basic knowledge of probability, calculus and college algebra, and basic programming skills in a procedural language or MATLAB and Mathematica, should find the book user-friendly and easy to follow. Teachers and educators will appreciate its scope and coverage, and can carve out different strategies for its use based on background and interests. Likewise, researchers will find the book a refresher or a guide to many of the tools in modern biomedical image analysis. Of course, there are chapters that may be skipped by experienced readers and advanced students, who have the requisite background from other classwork.

1.2 The scope of the book

The book contains five basic building blocks: (a) signals and systems, image formation and image modality; (b) stochastic models; (c) computational geometry methods; (d) level-set methods; and (e) tools and CAD models. These blocks are intertwined and are not necessarily in sequence.

1.2.1 Signals and systems, image formation, and image modality

Systems theory has been of great benefit for the development of signal processing and analysis in multiple dimensions. Chapter 2 is an overview of the basics of signals and systems for image representation and processing. I have attempted to make it a succinct briefing on the terminologies, theories and tools of two-dimensional (2D) signal processing, a field that is well established and based on solid theoretical and algorithmic foundation.

Biomedical imaging modalities are numerous. Chapter 3 aims to cover the physics and mathematics of the image formation processes most used in modern medicine, with focus on X-ray, computed tomography (CT), nuclear medicine, ultrasound, and magnetic resonance imaging (MRI). Knowledge of the image formation and its sources of uncertainties serves as a prelude to the mathematical approaches that form the backbone of the image analysis process.

1.2.2 Stochastic models

Statistical models are an essential part of the engineering, mathematics and physics curricula. They are broad and far-reaching. A focused presentation of the essential background for image analysis allows the reader to understand optimal filtering, segmentation, and construction of CAD models. Chapters 4 to 6 are on random variables, random processes, and random fields, respectively. They serve as a rigorous overview of the main topics on which typical statistical models for image analysis are based. Examples, computer projects, and exercises are listed to help crystallize these concepts, which are traditionally hard to appreciate in isolation. Chapter 7 is dedicated to the problem of probability density estimation, which comes into play as we study various image analysis problems, including segmentation, object detection, and classification.

1.2.3 Computational geometry

The shape of objects in a biomedical image may be described by various methods. We are interested in models of shape that are invariant to size, orientation, and translation. To achieve this, proper approaches for definition and extraction of features are needed. Shape models are embedded in segmentation, registration, and recognition methodologies. In Chapter 8, we discuss basics of topology and computational geometry. Chapter 9 deals with object models in the sense of features and their descriptors. There is a rich computer vision literature on this subject matter, which is crucial for object modeling and the intertwined operations of segmentation and registration.

1.2.4 Variational calculus and level-set methods

Deformable models are based on calculus of variations, and partial differential equations govern their mathematical description. They are hard to understand and implement. Application-oriented treatment, for example in the context of image segmentation, is not very beneficial, as it teaches trickery more than fundamentals. While mathematics can be abstract and may seem "over the head" of those interested in applications and "real-world" problem solving, the fact is: mathematics is mathematics. If we do not treat a mathematical concept properly, this only results in ambiguities and inability to interpret the results of an algorithm.

A general framework for deformable models is attempted in Chapter 10. The level-set method (LSM) for implicit object modeling is examined. We also examine the active contours (or "snake") model, which is useful for a class of objects that have distinct boundaries. Energy models for the LSM and active contour models are constructed, and the optimization methods for their solution are discussed.

1.2.5 Image analysis tools

We examine in detail the problems of image segmentation and registration and provide examples of an entire image analysis system used to design CAD models. Chapter 11 examines statistical methods for image segmentation. Chapter 12 examines variational and level-set approaches for segmentation. Chapter 13 examines the problem of image registration, with focus on distance-based rigid registration and image-based mutual information methods. Chapter 14 examines elastic registration with focus on "shape registration." These chapters contain the basic theory and various examples of synthetic as well as real-world images. Chapter 15 examines statistical models for shape and appearance. These models are very popular in various problems in computer vision and biomedical image analysis. Some case studies are considered for analysis of spinal imaging, lung nodules, and reconstruction of the human jaw using images and statistics.

1.3 Options for class work

Image analysis is an art and a science combined. It is impossible to enumerate all the approaches that one may use for analysis of biomedical images. There is no substitute for the talent acquired by experimentation and immersion in a particular biomedical problem; this talent defines the "prior knowledge" which is used in the mathematical framework of segmentation and registration, for example. Typically, the engineering curriculum may contain a series of courses on signals and systems in which image processing, biomedical imaging, and computer vision are taught. Some institutions may have many courses on imaging, computer vision, and machine learning; others only a few. This book is intended for use in both environments.

Depending on the background of the students enrolled in the class, this book may be used for a two-semester or a two-quarter sequence on biomedical imaging. Single-semester coverage may be possible with appropriate prerequisites. Instructors have considerable flexibility based on their circumstances. The review chapters (Chapters 2–5) may be skimmed through for students of engineering who have experience with signals and systems, and the basics of probabilistic modeling. A one-semester course on statistical methods could focus on Chapters 4–9, plus 11, 13, and 15. A one-semester course on variational methods might focus on Chapters 8–10, 12 and 14. A one-semester course for advanced students with appropriate background image processing and statistical modeling might focus on Chapters 3 and 6–15. To assist the reader, a set of homework and computer projects is included, and the website for the book is planned to contain updates and extra material. For instructors, course slides and a solution manual are available.

1.4 Other references

Biomedical imaging is multidisciplinary. It involves three major components: modalities, image analysis, and decision-making. There are many books and periodicals on imaging modalities and imaging sensors. There are also a number of proceedings, annual meetings, and periodicals focused on the analysis and applications of biomedical imaging. Such material is readily available through the World Wide Web. In particular, the following annual meetings promote the basics, research, and technologies of biomedical imaging:

1. Radiological Society of North America (RSNA)
2. Magnetic Resonance Imaging
3. Journal of Radiology
4. IEEE Transactions on Medical Imaging – IEEE-TMI
5. Medical Image Analysis – MedIA
6. Computer-Assisted Radiology and Surgery – CARS
7. International Symposium on Biomedical Imaging – ISBI
8. Medical Imaging, Computing and Computer-Assisted Intervention – MICCAI

There are also a number of books that specialize in particular topics of medical imaging. A listing of these books is also accessible by searching the World Wide Web. In each chapter, I include sample references and make every effort to point to the appropriate follow-up reading material.

Part I
Signals and systems, image formation, and image modality

2 Overview of two-dimensional signals and systems

Signals and systems approaches are based on fundamental theory and form the backbone of various disciplines in engineering and physics. Because of their importance, signals and systems are a well-established component of the engineering curriculum. In this chapter we review some of the basics of signals and systems as they pertain to image representation, processing, and analysis. Specifically, we study Fourier methods, which are fundamental to image reconstruction. We also study some systems methodologies of image processing and analysis. In all, the focus of the chapter is on the basics without plunging into the details of mathematical properties. For the expert reader, the chapter may act as a refresher and a quick overview of some of the well-known results of signals and systems. Otherwise, the intent of the chapter is to form a prelude to generalized model-based approaches of biomedical image analysis.

2.1 Definitions

A signal is a functional representation of a physical phenomenon captured by a sensor. That is, a signal may be defined as a transformation from a physical environment into a mathematical domain. The sensors are assumed to be capable of producing a meaningful description of the physical phenomenon. Signals theory deals, in the abstract sense, with the mathematical characterization of the functional forms of the signal, without regard to the phenomenon that generated it. In this chapter, however, we are interested in using the signal properties to infer information about the physical phenomenon. For example, if the signal is generated from an X-ray sensor directed at biological tissue, we are interested in a representation that describes the characteristics of the tissue. Similarly, in an MRI reconstruction application, we are most interested in signal representations that can describe the process of image formation from MRI. In short, we need to keep the physics of the problem in mind as we discuss signal theory.

We may formally define a signal $x(t)$ as a mapping from a sensor's output to the measurement domain, the N-dimensional space R^N. Figure 2.1 illustrates a basic framework for signal generation and representation.

For numerical manipulation of the representation in the computer, a numerical form (digital) of the signal $x(t)$ is needed. The theory of signals and systems deals with signal representations in analog and digital form, and with its manipulation

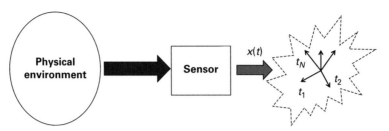

Figure 2.1 Model of signal generation and representation.

to achieve desired characteristics, or to extract particular information. Below we state the basic definitions from signals and systems theory that pertain to biomedical image analysis.

DEFINITION 2.1 *A system is a number of interconnected components, while a system function is a mapping from an input* x(.) $\in R^N$ *to an output* y(.) $\in R^M$, *where the dimensions* N *and* M *need not be the same.*

From the above definition, a system may be a physical entity or a set of steps involved in achieving a particular task. We may consider the process of transforming an *analog* or continuous-time signal (or image) into a *digital* or discrete form as a system. In particular, we are interested in the mapping: $x(t_1,t_2) \rightarrow x[n_1,n_2]$ where the domains of t_1, $t_2, n_1, n_2 \in R$, and so is the range or norm $\|x\|$. The discrete form may be obtained by a sampling and quantization processes which transforms uniformly sampled values of x (t_1,t_2) into a finite form. That is, in the digitization process, both time and amplitude must be sampled. For the case of band-limited signals (i.e., signals with energy within a finite frequency range), time-sampling is governed by the sampling theorem (Nyquist theorem), which requires that the time-sampling be conducted at a rate at least twice the bandwidth. The amplitude-sampling is determined by the desired accuracy and robustness against spurious noise associated with the signal or the time-sampling apparatus. Books on signals and systems are abundant, and the theory of digital signal/image processing is well established in curricula for engineering, physics and computer science. We refer to the classic books of Oppenheim and Shafer [2.1]; Dudgeon and Mersereau [2.2]; and Lim [2.3]. Below we highlight the fundamental equations of signal representations and the process of sampling a band-limited signal. While our focus is on images (i.e., 2D signals), the results also apply to 1D and to higher dimensions.

2.2 Signal representations

Signals take different forms. They may be deterministic or stochastic (random or non-reproducible); and for either case they may be periodic (amplitude repeats every specific period of the indexing parameter) or aperiodic (has no periodic behavior), and they can be of finite length or infinitely long. Signals may be represented by compact mathematical forms. For example, periodic signals may be represented by the Fourier series, while aperiodic signals that are band-limited may be represented by the Fourier transforms. In the following subsections we provide fundamental concepts that are common in signal theory.

2.2.1 Special functions

Special functions that have mathematical appeal and use, although they may be impractical or hard to construct, include the following:

Dirac Delta function $\delta(t_1,t_2)$, defined in terms of three characteristics:

$$\delta(t_1, t_2) = 0; \quad t_1, t_2 \neq 0; \tag{2.1a}$$

$$\int\int_{-\infty}^{\infty} \delta(t_1, t_2) dt_1 dt_1 = 1; \tag{2.1b}$$

$$\int\int_{-\infty}^{\infty} x(t_1 - t'_1, t_2 - t'_2)\delta(t_1, t_2) dt_1 dt_1 = x(t'_1, t'_2) \text{ for a continuous signal } x(t_1, t_2) \tag{2.1c}$$

This last property is known as the *sifting* property.

Unit step function $u(t_1,t_2)$, defined only over the first quadrant; i.e., $u(t_1,t_2) = 1$ for $t_1, t_2 \geq 0$.

The discrete counterparts of the two functions above are defined as follows:

Unit sample (Kronecker delta function):

$$\delta[n_1, n_2] = \begin{cases} 1 \text{ for } n_1, n_2 = 0 \\ 0 \text{ elsewhere} \end{cases} \tag{2.2}$$

Unit step function:

$$u[n_1, n_2] = 1 \text{ for } n_1, n_2 \geq 0, \text{ and vanishes elsewhere.}$$

We note that any discrete sequence $x[n_1,n_2]$ may be represented by weighted shifts of the unit sample function, i.e.,

$$x[n_1, n_2] = \sum_{k_1=-\infty}^{\infty} \sum_{k_2=-\infty}^{\infty} x_{k_1 k_2} \delta[n_1 - k_1, n_2 - k_2], \tag{2.3}$$

where $x_{k_1 k_2}$ is the amplitude of the sequence $x[n_1,n_2]$ at index $n_1 = k_1, n_2 = k_2$. For example, Figure 2.2 illustrates the sequence:

$x[n_1, n_2] =$
$5\delta[n_1 - 4, n_2 - 2] + 3\delta[n_1 - 9, n_2 - 2] + 6\delta[n_1 - 1, n_2 - 4] -$
$5\delta[n_1 - 6, n_2 - 3] + 6\delta[n_1 - 6, n_2 - 7] - 3\delta[n_1 - 4, n_2 - 8] - 6\delta[n_1 - 11, n_2 - 7].$

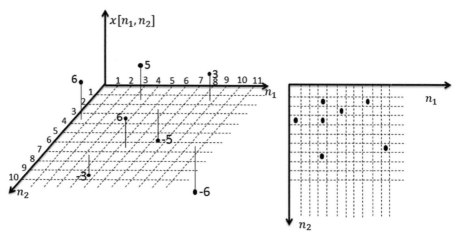

Figure 2.2 Representation of the sequence $x[n_1, n_2] = 5\delta[n_1 - 4, n_2 - 2] + 3\delta[n_1 - 8, n_2 - 2] + 6\delta[n_1 - 1, n_2 - 4] - 5\delta[n_1 - 8, n_2 - 6] + 6\delta[n_1 - 6, n_2 - 7] - 3\delta[n_1 - 5, n_2 - 10] - 6\delta[n_1 - 11, n_2 - 7]$.

2.2.2 Fourier series

A signal $\tilde{x}(t_1, t_2)$ is periodic in t_1, t_2 if $\tilde{x}(t_1, t_2) = \tilde{x}(t_1 - k_1 T_1, t_2 - k_2 T_2)$ for certain values $T_1, T_2 \in R$, known as the periods. For example, $\tilde{x}(t_1, t_2) = A\cos 2\pi(f_1 t_1 + f_2 t_2)$ is a sinusoidal signal with periods $T_1 = 1/f_1$ and $T_2 = 1/f_2$, respectively. Periodic signals may be described in complete and compact form by the Fourier series representation, in which a signal is represented by sinusoidal basis functions. We can also use exponential basis functions (which may be written in terms of sinusoids using the Euler formula), to represent a signal $\tilde{x}(t_1, t_2)$ which is periodic in t_1, t_2 in the following form:

$$\tilde{x}(t_1, t_2) = \tilde{x}(t_1 - k_1 T_1, t_2 - k_2 T_2) = \sum_{k_1=-\infty}^{\infty} \sum_{k_2=-\infty}^{\infty} c_{k_1 k_2} e^{j 2\pi \left(\frac{k_1 t_1}{T_1} + \frac{k_2 t_2}{T_2} \right)} \quad (2.4)$$

where the coefficients $c_{k_1 k_2}$ are obtained by the cross-product of the basis conjugates with the signal over one period, i.e.,

$$c_{k_1 k_2} = \frac{1}{T_1 T_2} \int_{-T_1/2}^{T_1/2} \int_{-T_2/2}^{T_2/2} \tilde{x}(t_1, t_2) e^{-j 2\pi \left(\frac{k_1 t_1}{T_1} + \frac{k_2 t_2}{T_2} \right)} dt_1 dt_2. \quad (2.5)$$

Various interesting characteristics of the Fourier series representation can be extracted from the definitions in Equations (2.4) and (2.5). Table 2.1 lists some of the properties that are straightforward to prove.

Example 2.1 Consider the periodic signal $\tilde{x}(t_1, t_2) = \tilde{x}(t_1 - k_1 T, t_2 - k_2 T) = A; 0 \leq t_1, t_2 \leq T$ and $-\infty < k_1, k_2 < \infty$. The coefficients of the Fourier series would be as follows.

Table 2.1 Some properties of continuous-time Fourier series representation

Signal property	Fourier series correspondence
Linear: $\tilde{y}(t_1,t_2) = a\tilde{x}_1(t_1,t_2) + b\tilde{x}_2(t_1,t_2)$ where $\tilde{x}_1(\cdot,\cdot)$ and $\tilde{x}_2(\cdot,\cdot)$ have the same periods T_1, T_2	$c^{\tilde{y}}_{k_1 k_2} = ac^{\tilde{x}_1}_{k_1 k_2} + bc^{\tilde{x}_2}_{k_1 k_2}$
Even signals: $\tilde{x}(t_1,t_2) = \tilde{x}(-t_1,-t_2)$	$c_{k_1 k_2}$ are defined for even integers $k_1 k_2$ and have zero value for odd integers $k_1 k_2$
Odd signals: $\tilde{x}(t_1,t_2) = -\tilde{x}(-t_1,-t_2)$	$c_{k_1 k_2}$ are defined for odd integers $k_1 k_2$ and have zero value for even integers $k_1 k_2$
Average: $\frac{1}{T_1 T_2} \int_{-T_1/2}^{T_1/2} \int_{-T_2/2}^{T_2/2} \tilde{x}(t_1,t_2) dt_1 dt_2$	c_{00}
Energy: $\frac{1}{T_1 T_2} \int_{-T_1/2}^{T_1/2} \int_{-T_2/2}^{T_2/2} \tilde{x}(t_1,t_2)\overline{\tilde{x}(t_1,t_2)}\, dt_1 dt_2$	$\sum_{k_1=-\infty}^{\infty} \sum_{k_2=-\infty}^{\infty} |c_{k_1 k_2}|^2$

$$c_{k_1 k_2} = \frac{1}{T_1 T_2} \int_{-T_1/2}^{T_1/2} \int_{-T_2/2}^{T_2/2} x(t_1,t_2) e^{-j2\pi\left(\frac{k_1 t_1}{T_1} + \frac{k_2 t_2}{T_2}\right)} dt_1 dt_2$$

$$= \frac{1}{T^2} \int_{-T/2}^{T/2} \int_{-T/2}^{T/2} A e^{-j2\pi\left(\frac{k_1 t_1}{T} + \frac{k_2 t_2}{T}\right)} dt_1 dt_2$$

$$= A \frac{\sin(\pi k_1)}{\pi k_1} \frac{\sin(\pi k_2)}{\pi k_2} \triangleq A\, sinc(\pi k_1) sinc(\pi k_2).$$

From the properties of the $sinc(.)$ function, we can easily conclude that $c_{k_1 k_2}$ will vanish for all coefficients, except the $c_{00} = A$.

2.2.3 Fourier transform

The Fourier transform is an extremely powerful representation for *aperiodic* signals that are absolutely integrable, in general. That is, given $x(t_1,t_2)$ such that $\iint_{-\infty}^{\infty} |x(t_1,t_2)| dt_1 dt_2 < \infty$, the Fourier transform $X(f_1,f_2)$ is defined as:

$$X(f_1,f_2) = \int_{-\infty}^{\infty} \int_{-\infty}^{\infty} x(t_1,t_2) e^{-j2\pi(t_1 f_1 + t_2 f_2)} dt_1 dt_2. \tag{2.6}$$

The inverse Fourier transform is defined as:

$$x(t_1,t_2) = \int_{-\infty}^{\infty} \int_{-\infty}^{\infty} X(f_1,f_2) e^{j2\pi(t_1 f_1 + t_2 f_2)} df_1 df_2. \tag{2.7}$$

The representations in Equations (2.6) and (2.7) are unique and form what is commonly referred to as a Fourier transform pair: $x(t_1,t_2) \leftrightarrow X(f_1,f_2)$. The Fourier transform (or Fourier integral) is well studied in the literature and is a powerful tool for signal

Table 2.2 Some properties of the Fourier transform representation

Signal property	Fourier transform correspondence
Linear: $y(t_1,t_2) = ax_1(t_1,t_2) + bx_2(t_1,t_2)$ where $x_1(\cdot,\cdot)$ and $x_2(\cdot,\cdot)$ are absolutely integrable	$Y(f_1,f_2) = aX_1(f_1,f_2) + bX_2(f_1,f_2)$
Even signals: $x(t_1,t_2) = x(-t_1,-t_2)$	$X(f_1,f_2)$ is real and even
Odd signals: $x(t_1,t_2) = -x(-t_1,-t_2)$	$X(f_1,f_2)$ is imaginary and odd
Average $\int_{-\infty}^{\infty}\int_{-\infty}^{\infty} x(t_1,t_2) dt_1 dt_2$	$X(0,0)$
Energy $\int_{-\infty}^{\infty}\int_{-\infty}^{\infty} x(t_1,t_2)\overline{x(t_1,t_2)}\, dt_1 dt_2$	$\int_{-\infty}^{\infty}\int_{-\infty}^{\infty} X(f_1,f_2)\overline{X(f_1,f_2)}\, df_1 df_2$
Time shift: $y(t_1,t_2) = x(t_1 - t_{10}, t_2 - t_{20})$	$Y(f_1,f_2) = X(f_1,f_2) e^{j2\pi(t_{10}f_1 + t_{20}f_2)}$
Frequency shift: $y(t_1,t_2) = x(t_1,t_2) e^{j2\pi(t_1 f_{10} + t_2 f_{20})}$	$Y(f_1,f_2) = X(f_1 - f_{10}, f_2 - f_{20})$
Time convolution: $y(t_1,t_2) = \int_{-\infty}^{\infty}\int_{-\infty}^{\infty} X_1(\delta_1,\delta_2) X_2(t_1 - \delta_1, t_2 - \delta_2) dt_1 dt_2$	$Y(f_1,f_2) = X_1(f_1,f_2) \times X_2(f_1,f_2)$
Time product: $y(t_1,t_2) = x_1(t_1,t_2) \times x_2(t_1,t_2)$	$Y(f_1,f_2) = \int_{-\infty}^{\infty}\int_{-\infty}^{\infty} X_1(\gamma_1,\gamma_2) X_2(f_1 - \gamma_1, f_2 - \gamma_2) df_1 df_2$

imaging. It forms the basis for CT reconstruction, and for K-space representation in MRI and various other signal processing tasks. Table 2.2 lists a few of the common properties of the Fourier transform. All the properties can be derived in a straightforward manner using the definitions above.

Example 2.2 The Fourier transform of a unit impulse $\delta(t_1,t_2)=1$. This follows easily from the definition and the properties of the Dirac delta function.

$$X(f_1, f_2) = \int_{-\infty}^{\infty}\int_{-\infty}^{\infty} x(t_1, t_2) e^{-j2\pi(t_1 f_1 + t_2 f_2)} dt_1 dt_2$$

$$= \int_{-\infty}^{\infty}\int_{-\infty}^{\infty} \delta(t_1, t_2) e^{-j2\pi(t_1 f_1 + t_2 f_2)} dt_1 dt_1 \equiv 1.$$

Example 2.3 The Fourier transform of an impulse train. Consider the impulse train $p(t_1,t_2)$:

$$p(t_1,t_2) = \sum_{k_1=-\infty}^{\infty} \sum_{k_2=-\infty}^{\infty} \delta(t_1 - k_1 T_1, t_2 - k_2 T_2)$$

2.2 Signal representations

Its Fourier transform would be:

$$P(f_1,f_2) = \int_{-\infty}^{\infty}\int_{-\infty}^{\infty} p(t_1,t_2)e^{-j2\pi(t_1f_1+t_2f_2)}dt_1dt_2$$

$$= \int_{-\infty}^{\infty}\int_{-\infty}^{\infty} \sum_{k_1=-\infty}^{\infty}\sum_{k_2=-\infty}^{\infty} \delta(t_1-k_1T_1,t_2-k_2T_2)e^{-j2\pi(t_1f_1+t_2f_2)}dt_1dt_2$$

$$= \sum_{k_1=-\infty}^{\infty}\sum_{k_2=-\infty}^{\infty} \int_{-\infty}^{\infty}\int_{-\infty}^{\infty} \delta(t_1-k_1T_1,t_2-k_2T_2)e^{-j2\pi(t_1f_1+t_2f_2)}dt_1dt_2$$

$$\equiv \sum_{k_1=-\infty}^{\infty}\sum_{k_2=-\infty}^{\infty} e^{-j2\pi(k_1T_1f_1+k_2T_2f_2)} \tag{2.8}$$

We may also look at the impulse train as a periodic signal with fundamental $\delta(t_1,t_2)$ and periods T_1 and T_2. That is, we may write as in Eq. (2.4):

$$p(t_1,t_2) = \sum_{k_1=-\infty}^{\infty}\sum_{k_2=-\infty}^{\infty} c_{k_1k_2} e^{j2\pi\left(\frac{k_1t_1}{T_1}+\frac{k_2t_2}{T_2}\right)},$$

where $c_{k_1k_2}$ is given by

$$c_{k_1k_2} = \frac{1}{T_1T_2}\int_{-T_1/2}^{T_1/2}\int_{-T_2/2}^{T_2/2} x(t_1,t_2)e^{-j2\pi\left(\frac{k_1t_1}{T_1}+\frac{k_2t_2}{T_2}\right)}dt_1dt_2$$

$$= \frac{1}{T_1T_2}\int_{-T_1/2}^{T_1/2}\int_{-T_2/2}^{T_2/2} \delta(t_1,t_2)e^{-j2\pi\left(\frac{k_1t_1}{T_1}+\frac{k_2t_2}{T_2}\right)}dt_1dt_2 \equiv \frac{1}{T_1T_2},$$

(the equivalence comes from the *sifting* property of the Dirac delta function). Hence, we may express the impulse train as:

$$p(t_1,t_2) = \sum_{k_1=-\infty}^{\infty}\sum_{k_2=-\infty}^{\infty} \delta(t_1-k_1T_1,t_2-k_2T_2)$$

$$= \frac{1}{T_1T_2}\sum_{k_1=-\infty}^{\infty}\sum_{k_2=-\infty}^{\infty} e^{j2\pi\left(\frac{k_1t_1}{T_1}+\frac{k_2t_2}{T_2}\right)}$$

Therefore, the Fourier transform $P(f_1,f_2) = \frac{1}{T_1T_2}\sum_{k_1=-\infty}^{\infty}\sum_{k_2=-\infty}^{\infty} \delta\left(f_1-\frac{k_1}{T_1},f_2-\frac{k_2}{T_2}\right)$ by the *frequency-shifting* property of the Fourier transform (see Table 2.2). Symbolically, we may write:

$$\sum_{k_1=-\infty}^{\infty}\sum_{k_2=-\infty}^{\infty} \delta(t_1 - k_1 T_1, t_2 - k_2 T_2) \longleftrightarrow \frac{1}{T_1 T_2} \sum_{k_1=-\infty}^{\infty}\sum_{k_2=-\infty}^{\infty}$$
$$\delta\left(f_1 - \frac{k_1}{T_1}, f_2 - \frac{k_2}{T_2}\right) \tag{2.9}$$

Equation (2.9) will simplify the representation of the sampling process, as we shall see later.

Example 2.4 Consider a finite-length signal $x(t_1,t_2) = A$; $0 \leq t_1, t_2 \leq T$. The Fourier transform

$$\begin{aligned} X(f_1,f_2) &= \int_{-\infty}^{\infty}\int_{-\infty}^{\infty} x(t_1,t_2) e^{-j2\pi(t_1 f_1 + t_2 f_2)} dt_1 dt_2 = \int_{0}^{T}\int_{0}^{T} A e^{-j2\pi(t_1 f_1 + t_2 f_2)} dt_1 dt_2 \\ &= \frac{A}{j2\pi f_1 \times j2\pi f_2}(1 - e^{-j2\pi f_1 T})(1 - e^{-j2\pi f_2 T}) \\ &= T^2 A e^{-j2\pi(f_1 T/2 + f_1 T/2)} \, \text{sinc}(\pi f_1 T)\, \text{sinc}(\pi f_2 T). \end{aligned}$$

We note that if the signal is symmetric, i.e. if $x(t_1, t_2) = A$; $0 \leq |t_1, t_2| \leq T/2$, then the exponential term of the last integral will disappear and the resulting transform will be real and even, i.e. $X(f_1, f_2) = T^2 A \,\text{sinc}(\pi f_1 T)\, \text{sinc}(\pi f_2 T)$. We also note that for the symmetric case, the Fourier transform may be related to the Fourier coefficients in the Fourier series in Example 2.1, which has $x(t_1, t_2)$ as its fundamental. That is, we have $x(t_1, t_2) = \tilde{x}(t_1, t_2)$ over one period. In this case,

$$c_{k_1 k_2} = \frac{1}{T^2} X(f_1, f_2)\Big|_{f_1 = \frac{k_1}{T}, f_2 = \frac{k_2}{T}}.$$

We shall return to the relationship between various Fourier representations after we have discussed the sequence Fourier transform. Understanding this relationship is crucial to proper interpretation of numerical computations of the discrete Fourier transform (DFT) using the fast Fourier transform (FFT) algorithm.

2.3 Basic sampling and quantization

The golden era of analog signal processing was in the 1930s to 1960s, when an enormous body of literature was generated for signal analysis based on calculus. As computation moved from analog to hybrid, and then to digital, the theory of digital signal processing and number theory took off. When the capabilities of computing engines and storage media were limited, due attention was paid to proper sampling (digitization in the time domain) and quantization (digitization in the spatial domain).

2.3 Basic sampling and quantization

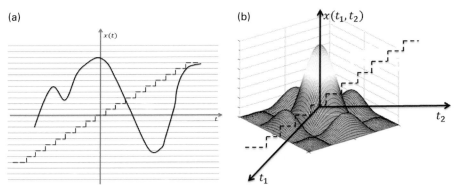

Figure 2.3 Illustration of (a) one- and (b) two-dimensional signal sampling and quantization.

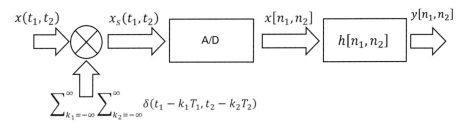

Figure 2.4 A generic 2D signal/image processing system.

As illustrated in Figure 2.3, in one and two dimensions, sampling in time is governed by the frequency spectrum of the signal, while sampling in amplitude is governed by the desired bit resolution of the signal. Modern computing and storage have made concerns over quantization less severe than they were before 2000. However, portable electronics and applications in telemedicine restrict the size of files that can be uploaded and disseminated over broadband shared networks. Hence, adequate quantization is still desired. With color coding for video and standard file formats for medical images (e.g. DICOM), the state-of-the-art of image capturing and dissemination has come a very long way. We shall not dwell on this appealing and fascinating history of evolution of signal theory; instead, we shall restrict attention to the basics of sampling in time. Below, we consider impulse sampling.

The process of generating a discrete representation $x[n_1,n_2]$, for a continuous signal $x(t_1,t_2)$, starts by multiplying this signal by an impulse train, as shown in Figure 2.4 (a pulse train of finite width may be used instead).

We may define a signal $x(t_1,t_2) = x(t_1,t_2) \cdot p(t_1,t_2)$; i.e.

$$x_s(t_1,t_2) = x(t_1,t_2) \cdot \sum_{k_1=-\infty}^{\infty} \sum_{k_2=-\infty}^{\infty} \delta(t_1 - k_1 T_1, t_2 - k_2 T_2) \qquad (2.10)$$

is the sampled signal resulting from multiplication of the input signal by an impulse train. The Fourier transform of the sampled signal may be derived as follows:

$$X_s(f_1,f_2) = \iint_{-\infty}^{\infty} x_s(t_1,t_2)\, e^{-j2\pi(f_1 t_1 + f_2 t_2)} dt_1 dt_2$$

$$= \iint_{-\infty}^{\infty} x(t_1,t_2) \cdot \sum_{k_1=-\infty}^{\infty} \sum_{k_2=-\infty}^{\infty} \delta(t_1 - k_1 T_1, t_2 - k_2 T_2) e^{-j2\pi(f_1 t_1 + f_2 t_2)} dt_1 dt_2$$

$$= \iint_{-\infty}^{\infty} x(t_1,t_2) \cdot \frac{1}{T_1 T_2} \sum_{k_1=-\infty}^{\infty} \sum_{k_2=-\infty}^{\infty} e^{j2\pi\left(\frac{k_1 t_1}{T_1} + \frac{k_2 t_2}{T_2}\right)} e^{-j2\pi(f_1 t_1 + f_2 t_2)} dt_1 dt_2$$

$$= \frac{1}{T_1 T_2} \sum_{k_1=-\infty}^{\infty} \sum_{k_2=-\infty}^{\infty} \iint_{-\infty}^{\infty} x(t_1,t_2) e^{-j2\pi\left(t_1\left(f_1 - \frac{k_1}{T_1}\right) + t_2\left(f_2 - \frac{k_2}{T_2}\right)\right)} dt_1 dt_2$$

$$\triangleq \frac{1}{T_1 T_2} \sum_{k_1=-\infty}^{\infty} \sum_{k_2=-\infty}^{\infty} X\left(f_1 - \frac{k_1}{T_1}, f_2 - \frac{k_2}{T_2}\right) \quad (2.11)$$

which is the famous impulse sampling formula. If the signal is band-limited, with bandwidth $f_1 = w_1$ and $f_2 = w_2$, then a proper sampling rate can be achieved such that $\frac{1}{T_1} - w_1 \geq w_1$ and $\frac{1}{T_2} - w_2 \geq w_2$; or equivalently, $f_{s1} = \frac{1}{T_1} \geq 2w_1$ and $f_{s2} = \frac{1}{T_2} \geq 2w_2$, which is known as the Nyquist rate. Hence, the sampling theorem for band-limited signals may be stated as follows:

THEOREM 2.1 *Given a signal $x(t_1,t_2)$ that is band-limited, with bandwidth $f_1 = w_1$ and $f_2 = w_2$ Hz, a faithful reconstruction of the signal is possible from samples taken at a rate least twice the bandwidth, using an ideal low-pass filter of cutoff frequency $w_1 \leq f_{c1} \leq \frac{1}{T_1} - w_1$ and $w_2 \leq f_{c2} \leq \frac{1}{T_2} - w_2$. The amplitude of the ideal low-pass filter is $T_1 T_2$.*

Figure 2.5 illustrates the sampling theorem, showing a 2D signal with bandwidth $|f_1| \leq w_1, |f_2| \leq w_2$. The signal may be reconstructed from the sampled version by an ideal low-pass filter, shown by dashed lines, with bandwidth $w_1 \leq f_{c1} \leq \frac{1}{T_1} - w_1$ and $w_2 \leq f_{c2} \leq \frac{1}{T_2} - w_2$.

From a numerical perspective, the sampled and quantized signal $x[n_1,n_2] \equiv x(t_1,t_2)|_{t_1 = n_1 T_1, t_2 = n_2 T_2}$. We may study the properties of sampled-data systems keeping in mind how the discrete signals were obtained, or, alternatively, devise a complete and independent theory for discrete-time signals and systems. We will take the latter route, yet we can always relate the two representations if necessary. We therefore focus on sequences $x[n_1,n_2]$ which may be periodic or aperiodic, infinitely long or with finite physical domain.

2.4 Sequence Fourier series

A periodic sequence $\tilde{x}[n_1,n_2]$ with periods N_1, N_2 is such that $\tilde{x}[n_1,n_2] = \tilde{x}[n_1 - k_1 N_1, n_2 - k_2 N_2]$, for $-\infty < k_1, k_2 < \infty$. Such sequences may be uniquely represented by the sequence Fourier series (SFS) defined as follows:

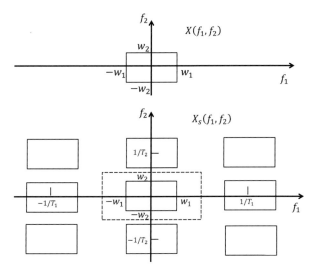

Figure 2.5 Illustration of the sampling process of a band-limited signal. The dashed rectangle in the middle represents the frequency domain of an ideal low-pass filter that can be used to extract the original signal from its sampled version.

$$\tilde{X}[k_1, k_2] = \sum_{N_1=0}^{N_1-1} \sum_{N2=0}^{N_2-1} \tilde{x}[n_1, n_2] e^{-j2\pi\left(\frac{n_1 k_1}{N_1} + \frac{n_2 k_2}{N_2}\right)}, \ k_1 \in [0, N_1 - 1], \ k_2 \in [0, N_2 - 1],$$
(2.12a)

where

$$\tilde{x}[n_1, n_2] = \frac{1}{N_1 N_2} \sum_{k_1=0}^{N_1-1} \sum_{k_2=0}^{N_2-1} \tilde{X}[k_1, k_2] e^{j2\pi\left(\frac{n_1 k_1}{N_1} + \frac{n_2 k_2}{N_2}\right)}, \ n_1 \in [0, N_1 - 1],$$

$$n_2 \in [0, N_2 - 1].$$
(2.12b)

The representations in Eq. (2.12a) and (2.12b) are unique and as such form a transform pair. This is expressed symbolically as $\tilde{x}[n_1, n_2] \leftrightarrow \tilde{X}[k_1, k_2]$, and both sequences are periodic with the same periods. We can derive various interesting characteristics of the SFS representations using the definitions in Eq. (2.12). Table 2.3 lists a few common properties which are straightforward to prove.

Example 2.5 Derive the SFS representation for the periodic sequence with constant value

$$\tilde{x}[n_1, n_2] = \tilde{x}[n_1 - l_1 N_1, n_2 - l_2 N_2] = A,$$

for

$$n_1 \in [0, N_1 - 1], \ n_2 \in [0, N_2 - 1], \ -\infty < l_1, l_2 < \infty.$$

Table 2.3 Basic properties of the sequence Fourier series

Sequence property	Sequence Fourier series (SFS)
Linear: $\tilde{y}[n_1,n_2] = a\tilde{x}_1[n_1,n_2] + b\tilde{x}_2[n_1,n_2]$ where $\tilde{x}_1[\cdot,\cdot]$ and $\tilde{x}_2[(\cdot,\cdot)]$ have same periods N_1, N_2	$\tilde{Y}[k_1,k_2] = a\tilde{X}_1[k_1,k_2] + b\tilde{X}_2[k_1,k_2]$
Even signals: $\tilde{x}[n_1,n_2] = \tilde{x}[-n_1,-n_2]$	$\tilde{X}[k_1,k_2]$ are defined for even integers $k_1 k_2$ and have zero value for odd integers $k_1 k_2$
Odd signals: $\tilde{x}[n_1,n_2] = -\tilde{x}[-n_1,-n_2]$	$\tilde{X}[k_1,k_2]$ are defined for odd integers $k_1 k_2$ and have zero value for even integers $k_1 k_2$
Time-shift: $\tilde{x}_1[n_1 - m_1, n_2 - m_2]$	$e^{-j2\pi\left(\frac{m_1 k_1}{N_1} + \frac{m_2 k_2}{N_2}\right)} \tilde{X}[k_1,k_2]$
Duality $\tilde{X}[n_1,n_2]$	$N_1 N_2 \tilde{x}[-n_1,-n_2]$
Complex conjugate: $\overline{\tilde{x}}[n_1,n_2]$	$\overline{\tilde{X}}[-k_1,-k_2]$
Periodic convolution: $\tilde{y}[n_1,n_2] = \tilde{x}_1[n_1,n_2] \oplus \tilde{x}_2[n_1,n_2]$ $\sum_{m_1=0}^{N_1-1} \sum_{m_2=0}^{N_2-1} \tilde{x}_1[m_1,m_2]\tilde{x}_2[m_1-n_1,m_2-n_2]$	$\tilde{Y}[k_1,k_2] = \tilde{X}_1[k_1,k_2] \cdot \tilde{X}_2[k_1,k_2]$
Product: $\tilde{y}[n_1,n_2] = \tilde{x}_1[n_1,n_2] \cdot \tilde{x}_2[n_1,n_2]$	$\tilde{Y}[k_1,k_2] = \frac{1}{N_1 N_2} \tilde{X}_1[k_1,k_2] \oplus \tilde{X}_2[k_1,k_2]$

Solution: From the definition, we have

$$\tilde{X}[k_1,k_2] = \sum_{n_1=0}^{N_1-1} \sum_{n_2=0}^{N_2-1} \tilde{x}[n_1,n_2] e^{-j2\pi\left(\frac{n_1 k_1}{N_1} + \frac{n_2 k_2}{N_2}\right)}, \quad k_1 \in [0, N_1-1], \; k_2 \in [0, N_2-1]$$

Therefore,

$$\tilde{X}[k_1,k_2] = \sum_{n_1=0}^{N_1-1} \sum_{n_2=0}^{N_2-1} A e^{-j2\pi\left(\frac{n_1 k_1}{N_1} + \frac{n_2 k_2}{N_2}\right)}$$

which, using the geometric series summation, has the following form:

$$\tilde{X}[k_1,k_2] = A \frac{\left(1 - e^{-j2\pi\left(\frac{N_1 k_1}{N_1}\right)}\right)\left(1 - e^{-j2\pi\left(\frac{N_2 k_2}{N_2}\right)}\right)}{\left(1 - e^{-j2\pi\left(\frac{k_1}{N_1}\right)}\right)\left(1 - e^{-j2\pi\left(\frac{k_2}{N_2}\right)}\right)} = 0; \text{ for } k_1, k_2 \neq 0.$$

By **l'Hospital's** rule we have $\tilde{X}[0,0] = A$.

Figure 2.6 illustrates these results.

2.4 Sequence Fourier series

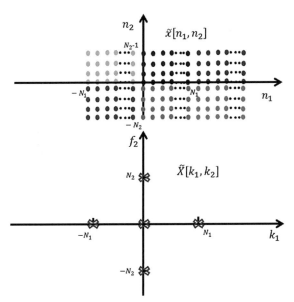

Figure 2.6 The SFS of a fixed sequence $\tilde{x}[n_1, n_2] = A$.

2.4.1 Sequence Fourier transform

As with continuous-time functions that are aperiodic, aperiodic sequences $x[n_1, n_2]$, $-\infty < n_1, n_2 < \infty$, may also have a unique Fourier representation defined as follows:

$$X(\tilde{f}_1, \tilde{f}_2) = \sum_{n_1=-\infty}^{\infty} \sum_{n_2=-\infty}^{\infty} x[n_1, n_2] \, e^{-j2\pi(n_1\tilde{f}_1 + n_2\tilde{f}_2)} \qquad (2.13)$$

The quantities $\tilde{f}_1, \tilde{f}_2$ have dimensions of *cycles*. The superscript ~ has been chosen to flag a distinct property of the representation in Eq. (2.13) which we now discuss. If the series is absolutely convergent; i.e. $\sum_{n_1=-\infty}^{\infty} \sum_{n_1=-\infty}^{\infty} |x[n_1, n_2]|$, then the representation in Eq. (2.13) exists and is unique for a given sequence $x[n_1, n_2]$, $-\infty < n_1, n_2 < \infty$. Now we note that $X(\tilde{f}_1 + 1, \tilde{f}_2 + 1) = X(\tilde{f}_1, \tilde{f}_2)$. That is, the Fourier representation is periodic with period equal to 1 in both $\tilde{f}_1$ and $\tilde{f}_2$. We note also that basis functions in Eq. (2.13) are continuous; hence $X(\tilde{f}_1, \tilde{f}_2)$ is a continuous function. The periodicity and continuity of $X(\tilde{f}_1, \tilde{f}_2)$ invites a Fourier series representation as in Equations (2.4)–(2.5). That is, we may define:

$$x[n_1, n_2] = \int_{-1/2}^{1/2} \int_{-1/2}^{1/2} X(\tilde{f}_1, \tilde{f}_2) e^{j2\pi(n_1\tilde{f}_1 + n_2\tilde{f}_2)} d\tilde{f}_1 d\tilde{f}_2 \qquad (2.14)$$

We note that if $x[n_1, n_2] \equiv x(t_1, t_2)|t_1 = n_1 T_1, t_2 = n_2 T_2$, then we may relate the frequency expressions in the continuous and sequence Fourier series representations by setting $\tilde{f}_1 = \frac{k_1}{T_1}$ and $\tilde{f}_2 = \frac{k_2}{T_2}$.

The representation in Eq. (2.13) and (2.14) is unique and defines a sequence Fourier transform (SFT) pair, which may be expressed as $x[n_1, n_2] \leftrightarrow X(\tilde{f}_1, \tilde{f}_2)$. The SFT

Table 2.4 Sequence properties and Fourier transforms

Sequence property	Sequence Fourier transform (SFT)
Linear: $y[n_1,n_2] = ax_1[n_1,n_2] + bx_2[n_1,n_2]$ where $x_1[\cdot,\cdot]$ and $x_2[(\cdot,\cdot)]$ are aperiodic sequences, not necessarily of the same length	$Y(\tilde{f}_1,\tilde{f}_2) = aX_1(\tilde{f}_1,\tilde{f}_2) + bX_2(\tilde{f}_1,\tilde{f}_2)$
Even signals: $x[n_1,n_2] = x[-n_1,-n_2]$	$X(\tilde{f}_1,\tilde{f}_2)$ is even function in $\tilde{f}_1$ and $\tilde{f}_2$
Odd signals: $x[n_1,n_2] = -x[-n_1,-n_2]$	$X(\tilde{f}_1,\tilde{f}_2)$ is odd function in $\tilde{f}_1$ and $\tilde{f}_2$
Time-shift: $x_1[n_1-m_1, n_2-m_2]$	$e^{-j2\pi(m_1\tilde{f}_1+m_2\tilde{f}_2)}X(\tilde{f}_1,\tilde{f}_2)$
Linear convolution: $y[n_1,n_2] = x_1[n_1,n_2] * x_2[n_1,n_2]$ $\sum_{m_1=-\infty}^{\infty}\sum_{m_2=-\infty}^{\infty} x_1[m_1,m_2]x_2[n_1-m_1,n_2-m_2]$	$Y(\tilde{f}_1,\tilde{f}_2) = \tilde{X}_1(\tilde{f}_1,\tilde{f}_2) \cdot \tilde{X}_2(\tilde{f}_1,\tilde{f}_2)$
Product: $y[n_1,n_2] = x_1[n_1,n_2] \cdot x_2[n_1,n_2]$	$Y(\tilde{f}_1,\tilde{f}_2) = \tilde{X}_1(\tilde{f}_1,\tilde{f}_2) \oplus \tilde{X}_2(\tilde{f}_1,\tilde{f}_2)$; i.e., convolution over one period

possesses a great many interesting properties. Table 2.4 lists some of the common properties, all of which may be derived using the definitions.

Example 2.6 Evaluate the sequence Fourier transform of an exponential sequence: $x[n_1,n_2] = e^{-0.5(n_1+n_1)}u[n_1,n_2]$.

Solution:

$$X(\tilde{f}_1,\tilde{f}_2) \triangleq \sum_{n_1=-\infty}^{\infty}\sum_{n_2=-\infty}^{\infty} x[n_1,n_2] e^{-j2\pi(n_1\tilde{f}_1+n_2\tilde{f}_2)}$$

$$= \sum_{n_1=0}^{\infty}\sum_{n_2=0}^{\infty} e^{-0.5(n_1+n_1)} e^{-j2\pi(n_1\tilde{f}_1+n_2\tilde{f}_2)} = \left(\frac{1}{1-e^{-(0.5+j2\pi)\tilde{f}_1}}\right)\left(\frac{1}{1-e^{-(0.5+j2\pi)\tilde{f}_2}}\right)$$

which is a low-pass signal, as $|X(\tilde{f}_1,\tilde{f}_2)|$ vanishes quickly past $|\tilde{f}_1|, |\tilde{f}_2| \leq 0.2$.

Example 2.7 The sequence Fourier transform of the unit sample $x[n_1,n_2] = \delta[n_1,n_2]$ is $X(\tilde{f}_1,\tilde{f}_2) \triangleq \sum_{n_1=-\infty}^{\infty}\sum_{n_2=-\infty}^{\infty} x[n_1,n_2] e^{-j2\pi(n_1\tilde{f}_1+n_2\tilde{f}_2)} = 1$, for all values of $\tilde{f}_1, \tilde{f}_2$.

2.4.2 Relationship to the continuous Fourier transform

We may relate the continuous-time Fourier transform in Eq. (2.6)–(2.7) to the discrete-time (sequence) Fourier transform in Eq. (2.13)–(2.14) by considering the sequence $x[n_1,n_2]$ to be a properly sampled version of the continuous signal $x_c(t_1,t_2)$. Let $x[n_1,n_2] = x_c[n_1T_1,n_2T_2] \equiv x_c(t_1,t_2)|t_1 = n_1T_1, t_2 = n_2T_2$. We note that:

$$x_c[n_1T_1, n_2T_2] = \int_{-\infty}^{\infty}\int_{-\infty}^{\infty} X_c(f_1,f_2) e^{j2\pi(t_1f_1+t_1f_2)} df_1 df_2 \big|_{t_1=n_1T_1, t_2=n_2T_2} \quad (2.15)$$

Substituting in Eq. (2.13), we can write

$$X(\tilde{f}_1,\tilde{f}_2) = \sum_{n_1=-\infty}^{\infty}\sum_{n_2=-\infty}^{\infty} x[n_1,n_2] e^{-j2\pi(n_1\tilde{f}_1+n_2\tilde{f}_2)}$$

$$= \sum_{n_1=-\infty}^{\infty}\sum_{n_2=-\infty}^{\infty} \left(\int_{-\infty}^{\infty}\int_{-\infty}^{\infty} X_c(f_1,f_2) e^{j2\pi(n_1T_1f_1+n_2T_2f_2)} df_1 df_2\right) e^{-j2\pi(n_1\tilde{f}_1+n_2\tilde{f}_2)}$$

which, after some mathematical manipulation, provides the desired relationship between $X(\tilde{f}_1,\tilde{f}_2)$ and $X_c(f_1,f_2)$:

$$X(\tilde{f}_1,\tilde{f}_2) = \frac{1}{T_1T_2}\sum_{n_1=-\infty}^{\infty}\sum_{n_2=-\infty}^{\infty} X_c(f_1T_1-n_1, f_2T_2-n_2) \quad (2.16)$$

where $\tilde{f}_1 = f_1T_1$ and $\tilde{f}_2 = f_2T_2$. The relationship in Eq. (2.16) will help in interpreting the numerical computation of the Fourier transform, as we shall see in the next section.

2.5 Discrete Fourier transform

Symbolic computing has advanced enormously in the past two decades, and various Fourier integral properties may be obtained numerically without being overly conscious of the discretization process. In the past half century, clever implementations of the DFT (which attempts to approximate the continuous Fourier transform) have evolved. These developments and their evolution not only help in efficient computation but in interpretation of the results, especially for finite length sequences, i.e. $x[n_1, n_2]$, $n_1 \in [0, N_1-1]$, $n_2 \in [0, N_2-1]$. For these sequences, we would like to use summations instead of integrations in both analysis, Eq. (2.13), and synthesis, Eq. (2.14). That is, we define the following formulations, known as the discrete Fourier transform (DFT):

$$X(k_1, k_2) = \sum_{N_1=0}^{N_1-1}\sum_{N_2=0}^{N_2-1} x[n_1,n_2] e^{-j2\pi\left(\frac{n_1k_1}{N_1}+\frac{n_2k_2}{N_2}\right)}, \quad k_1\in[0, N_1-1], k_2\in[0, N_2-1] \quad (2.17)$$

$$x[n_1,n_2] = \sum_{k_1=0}^{N_1-1}\sum_{k_2=0}^{N_2-1} X(k_1,k_2) e^{j2\pi\left(\frac{n_1k_1}{N_1}+\frac{n_2k_2}{N_2}\right)} \quad n_1\in[0, N_1-1], n_2\in[0, N_2-1] \quad (2.18)$$

which form a unique representation for finite-length sequences. We may write the DFT pair symbolically as: $x[n_1, n_2] \longleftrightarrow X(k_1, k_2)$.

Careful examination of the analysis and synthesis formulas above reveals a contradiction. While we start with a finite-length sequence $x[n_1,n_2]$, $n_1 \in [0,N_1-1]$, $n_2 \in [0,N_2-1]$, the synthesis formula Eq. (2.18) defines a periodic sequence, i.e. $x[n_1, n_2] = x[n_1 - l_1 N_1, n_2 - l_2 N_2]$, where l_1 and l_2 are integers. Similarly, $X[k_1, k_2] = X[k_1 - m_1 N_1, k_2 - m_2 N_2]$, where m_1 and m_2 are integers. These apparent contradictions can be resolved by considering the finite-length sequences as the *fundamental period* of a *periodic sequence*, governed by the discrete Fourier series (DFS) in Eq. (2.12a) and (2.12b). The results of the DFT, however, will be captured only within the fundamental period; $n_1 \in [0, N_1 - 1]$, $n_2 \in [0, N_2 - 1]$. As the formulas (2.17) and (2.18) possess a clear numerical convenience, the DFS is used only to interpret the results properly. The DFT formulation received considerable intelligent attention in the signal analysis literature during 1960–1990, in which the fast Fourier transform (FFT) algorithms was developed and ingenious methods were established for efficient use of memory and computation time (see for example [2.1]). We note from Eq. (2.13) and (2.17) that the relationship between the DFT and sequence Fourier transform (SFT) for finite-length sequence is immediate, i.e. $X(\tilde{f}_1, \tilde{f}_2) = X[k_1, k_2]|_{\tilde{f}_1 = \frac{k_1}{N_1}, \tilde{f}_2 = \frac{k_2}{N_2}}$. We also note that Eq. (2.16) enables the continuous Fourier transform to be linked to the DFT. For example, the fundamental period of $X(\tilde{f}_1, \tilde{f}_2)$ and $X[k_1, k_2]$ can be related to $X(f_1, f_2)$ using the formulas $\tilde{f}_1 = \frac{k_1}{N_1} = f_1 T_1$ and $\tilde{f}_2 = \frac{k_2}{N_2} = f_2 T_2$. We discuss a complete example below.

Example 2.6 Consider the low-pass signal $x(t_1, t_2) = 10 \, e^{-\alpha(t_1+t_2)} u(t_1, t_2)$. Suppose we sample it at a convenient rate; perhaps we can use the 3 dB bandwidth as a measure of the frequency span of $X(f_1, f_2)$ and select a sampling frequency based on that bandwidth. Develop the relationship between $X(f_1, f_2)$, $X(\tilde{f}_1, \tilde{f}_2)$ and $X[k_1, k_2]$ using an adequate number of samples.

Solution:

$$X(f_1, f_2) = \int_{-\infty}^{\infty}\int_{-\infty}^{\infty} x(t_1, t_2) e^{-j2\pi(t_1 f_1 + t_2 f_2)} dt_1 dt_2 = \int_{0}^{\infty}\int_{0}^{\infty} 10 \, e^{-\alpha(t_1+t_2)} e^{-j2\pi(t_1 f_1 + t_2 f_2)} dt_1 dt_2$$

$$= \frac{10}{(\alpha + j2\pi f_1)(\alpha + j2\pi f_2)} = \frac{10(\alpha^2 - 4\pi^2 f_1 f_2) - j2\pi\alpha(f_1 + f_2)}{\left(\alpha^2 + (2\pi f_1)^2\right)\left((\alpha^2 + (2\pi f_1)^2\right)}$$

$$= X_r(f_1, f_2) + j X_i(f_1, f_2)$$

(where i and r stand for real and imaginary)

$$|X(f_1, f_2)| = \frac{10}{\sqrt{[\alpha^2 + (2\pi f_1)^2][\alpha^2 + (2\pi f_2)^2]}} \qquad (2.19)$$

Let us consider the case of $\alpha = 0.5$; the 3 dB bandwidth is about 1 Hz. We may take the sampling rate $f_s = \frac{1}{T} = 2Hz$ for both the t_1 and t_2 axis. We can get exact formulas for $X(\tilde{f}_1, \tilde{f}_2)$ and $X[k_1, k_2]$, and we can also obtain a numerical evaluation using the FFT algorithm. Let $x[n_1, n_2] = x_c[n_1 T, n_2 T] = 10\, e^{-\alpha(n_1 T + n_2 T)} u(n_1 T, n_2 T)$. Hence,

$$X(\tilde{f}_1, \tilde{f}_2) = \sum_{n_1=0}^{\infty} \sum_{n_2=0}^{\infty} 10\, e^{-\alpha(n_1 T + n_2 T)} e^{-j2\pi(n_1 \tilde{f}_1 + n_2 \tilde{f}_2)}$$

$$= 10 \sum_{n_1=0}^{\infty} \sum_{n_2=0}^{\infty} e^{-(\alpha T + j2\pi \tilde{f}_1) n_1} e^{-(\alpha T + j2\pi \tilde{f}_2) n_2} = \frac{10}{(\alpha T + j2\pi \tilde{f}_1)(\alpha T + j2\pi \tilde{f}_2)}$$

$$= \frac{10/T^2}{\left(\alpha + \frac{j2\pi \tilde{f}_1}{T}\right)\left(\alpha + \frac{j2\pi \tilde{f}_2}{T}\right)} = \frac{1}{T^2} X(f_1, f_2)|_{\tilde{f}_1 = f_1 T, \tilde{f}_2 = f_2 T}$$

(2.20)

On the other hand, if we force the signal $x(t_1, t_2)$ to be finite length, then we may consider only $t_1 = t_2 = \Delta$ (in seconds). Hence,

$$X(f_1, f_2) = \int_0^\Delta \int_0^\Delta 10\, e^{-\alpha(t_1 + t_2)} e^{-j2\pi(t_1 f_1 + t_2 f_2)} dt_1 dt_2$$

$$= \int_0^\Delta \int_0^\Delta 10\, e^{-(\alpha + j2\pi f_1) t_1} e^{-(\alpha + j2\pi f_2) t_2} dt_1 dt_2 = \frac{10(1 - e^{-(\alpha + j2\pi f_1)\Delta})(1 - e^{-(\alpha + j2\pi f_2)\Delta})}{(\alpha + j2\pi f_1)(\alpha + j2\pi f_2)}$$

(2.21)

Suppose we have $\Delta = N_1 T = N_2 T$, where $T = 1/f_s$ is the sampling rate and $N_1 = N_2 =$ number of samples on the t_1 and t_2 axes. Then we can relate $X(f_1, f_2)$, $X(\tilde{f}_1, \tilde{f}_2)$ and $X[k_1, k_2]$ as follows:

$$X(\tilde{f}_1, \tilde{f}_2) = \frac{1}{T^2} X(f_1, f_2)|_{\tilde{f}_1 = f_1 T, \tilde{f}_2 = f_2 T}$$

$$X[k_1, k_2] = X(\tilde{f}_1, \tilde{f}_2)|_{\tilde{f}_1 = \frac{k_1}{N_1}, \tilde{f}_2 = \frac{k_2}{N_2}}.$$

Figure 2.7 illustrates these results. Of course, we are interested in relating $X(f_1, f_2)$, $X(\tilde{f}_1, \tilde{f}_2)$ to $X[k_1, k_2]$, which will be calculated using the FFT algorithm.

2.6 The fast Fourier transform (FFT) algorithm

The FFT algorithm is among the best developed and studied algorithms in the signal processing literature. The idea of the algorithm stems from the insight that the basis function $e^{\pm j2\pi\left(\frac{n_1 k_1}{N_1} + \frac{n_2 k_2}{N_2}\right)}$ in Eq. (2–16) and (2.17) need not be calculated for all values of N_1 and N_2 because they are related to each other. Likewise, smart usage of the data structure can store the results of the FFT algorithm in the memory space occupied by the original

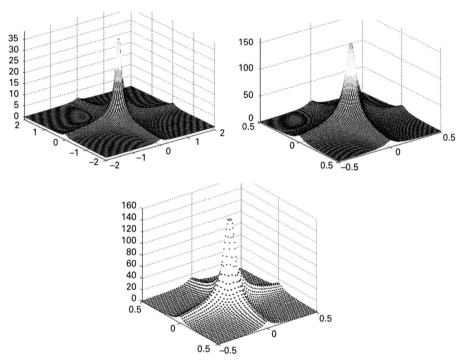

Figure 2.7 Left to right, $X(f_1, f_2)$, $X(\tilde{f}_1, \tilde{f}_2)$ and $X[k_1, k_2]$, $\tilde{f}_1 = k_1/N_1, \tilde{f}_2 = k_2/N_2$, for the exponentially decaying sequence.

sequence itself. We shall study the output of a common implementation of the FFT algorithm using some signals with known Fourier transform.

2.6.1 Effect of periodic shifts

Example 2.7 Consider the sequence $x[n_1, n_2] = 1$, $|n_1| \leq M_1 - 1$, $|n_2| \leq M_2 - 1$. For this sequence we have

$$X(\tilde{f}_1, \tilde{f}_2) = \sum_{n_1=-(M_1-1)}^{M_1-1} \sum_{n_2=-(M_2-1)}^{M_2-1} e^{-j2\pi(n_1\tilde{f}_1 + n_2\tilde{f}_2)}$$

$$= \left(\frac{(1 - e^{j\pi M_1 \tilde{f}_1})}{(1 - e^{j2\pi \tilde{f}_1})} + \frac{(1 - e^{-j\pi M_1 \tilde{f}_1})}{(1 - e^{-j2\pi \tilde{f}_1})} - 1\right) \left(\frac{(1 - e^{j\pi M_2 \tilde{f}_2})}{(1 - e^{j2\pi \tilde{f}_2})} + \frac{(1 - e^{-j\pi M_2 \tilde{f}_2})}{(1 - e^{-j2\pi \tilde{f}_2})} - 1\right)$$

(2.22)

Let us consider the sequence $y[n_1, n_2] = 1$, $n_1, n_2 \leq 20$, i.e. $y[n_1, n_2] = x[n_1 - 10, n_2 - 10]$. Hence, $Y(\tilde{f}_1, \tilde{f}_2) = e^{-j2\pi(10\tilde{f}_1 + 10\tilde{f}_2)} X(\tilde{f}_1, \tilde{f}_2)$. We know that $X[k_1, k_2] = X(\tilde{f}_1, \tilde{f}_2)|_{\tilde{f}_1 = \frac{k_1}{N_1}, \tilde{f}_2 = \frac{k_2}{N_2}}$. In order to avoid confusion, we may calculate

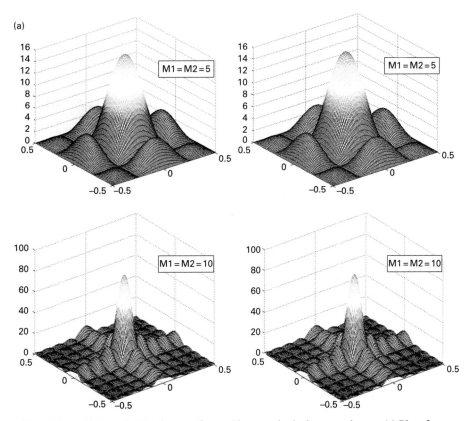

Figure 2.8 Effect of time-shifts on the Fourier transforms. The magnitude does not change. (a) Plots for $X(\tilde{f}_1,\tilde{f}_2)$, left column, and $Y(\tilde{f}_1,\tilde{f}_2)$, right column, for various lengths of the moving average sequence; (b) plots for $X[k_1,k_2]$ (left) and $Y[k_1,k_2]$ (right) for various lengths of the moving average sequence.

$$Y[k_1,k_2] = Y(\tilde{f}_1,\tilde{f}_2)|_{\tilde{f}_1=\frac{k_1}{N'_1},\tilde{f}_2=\frac{k_2}{N'_2}}, \text{ where } N'_1 = N'_2 = 20. \text{ We can then obtain}$$

$$X[k_1,k_2] = e^{j2\pi\left(10\frac{k_1}{N'_1} + 10\frac{k_2}{N'_2}\right)} Y[k_1,k_2] = e^{j\pi(k_1+k_2)} Y[k_1,k_2].$$

Figure 2.8(a) shows the plots for $X(\tilde{f}_1,\tilde{f}_2)$ (left) and $Y(\tilde{f}_1,\tilde{f}_2)$ (right), while Figure 2.8(b) shows the plots for the magnitudes $X[k_1,k_2]$ and $Y[k_1,k_2]$ on the same scale. The magnitude does not change, only the phase is affected.

2.6.2 Circular convolution

The circular (or periodic) convolution of two sequences $x_1[n_1,n_2]$ and $x_2[n_1,n_2]$; $0 \leq n_1 \leq N_1 - 1, 0 \leq n_2 \leq N_2 - 1$; $x_3[n_1,n_2] = x_1[n_1,n_2] \oplus x_2[n_1,n_2]$ is defined as follows (Table 2.3): $x_3[n_1,n_2] = \sum_{m_1=0}^{N_1-1} \sum_{m_2=0}^{N_2-1} x_1[m_1,m_2] x_2[n_1 - m_1, n_2 - m_2]$.

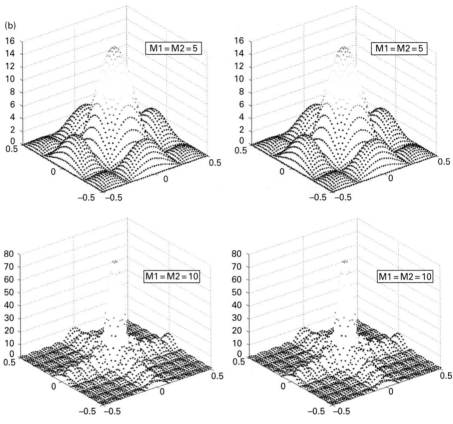

Figure 2.8 (cont.)

Example 2.8 Evaluate the circular convolution of the sequence $x[n_1,n_2]$ in Example 2.7 with itself, i.e. $x_1[n_1,n_2] = x_2[n_1,n_2] = 1$; $|n_1,n_2| \leq 10$. It is straightforward to show that the output will be: $x_3[n_1,n_2] = \sum_{m_1=-10}^{10} \sum_{m_2=-10}^{10} x_1[m_1,m_2]x_2[n_1-m_1,n_2-m_2]$

The same calculation using the FFT algorithm is shown in Figure 2.9.

2.6.3 Linear convolution

The linear convolution may be evaluated by "going around" the circular convolution formula, manipulating it so that the circular convolution of two sequences will provide the linear convolution results. Given two sequences $x_1[n_1,n_2]$, $0 \leq n_1 \leq N_1 - 1, 0 \leq n_2 \leq N_2 - 1$ and $x_2[n_1,n_2]$, $0 \leq n_1 \leq M_1 - 1, 0 \leq n_2 \leq M_2 - 1$, the linear convolution $x_3[n_1,n_2] = \sum_{m_1=-\infty}^{\infty} \sum_{m_2=-\infty}^{\infty} x_1[m_1,m_2]x_2[m_1-n_1,m_2-n_2]$ will have a range of values

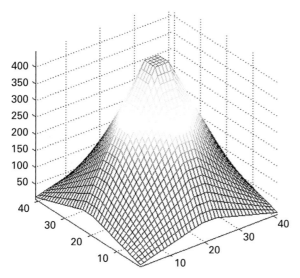

Figure 2.9 Results of Example 2.8 using the FFT algorithm.

$0 \leq n_1 \leq N_1 + M_1 - 1, 0 \leq n_2 \leq N_2 + M_2 - 1$. Therefore, we may calculate the linear convolution as a circular convolution of the two sequences $x_1[n_1, n_2]$ and $x_2[n_1, n_2]$, $0 \leq n_1 \leq N_1 + M_1 - 1, 0 \leq n_2 \leq N_2 + M_2 - 1$, where we have augmented (or padded) them with zeros. Linear convolution of the original sequences will have the same formulation as the circular convolution of the extended sequences, which may be calculated faster using the FFT algorithm.

Example 2.9 The linear convolution of the two sequences in the previous example can be obtained from the linear convolution equation:

$$x_3[n_1, n_2] = \sum_{m_1=-\infty}^{\infty} \sum_{m_2=-\infty}^{\infty} x_1[m_1, m_2] x_2[n_1 - m_1, n_2 - m_2].$$

The calculations using the FFT algorithm are shown in Figure 2.10.

2.7 The Z-transform

Given a sequence $x[n_1, n_2]$, the Z-transform $X(z_1, z_2)$ is defined as:

$$X(z_1, z_2) = \sum_{n_1=-\infty}^{\infty} \sum_{n_2=-\infty}^{\infty} x[n_1, n_2] z_1^{-n_1} z_2^{-n_2} \qquad (2.23)$$

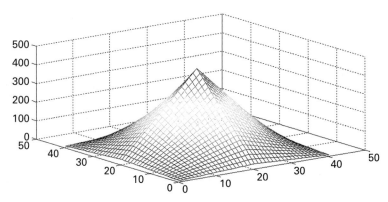

Figure 2.10 Results of the FFT algorithm for Example 2.9.

If we set $z_1 = e^{j2\pi \tilde{f}_1}$ and $z_2 = e^{j2\pi \tilde{f}_2}$, i.e. $X(z_1, z_2) = X(\tilde{f}_1, \tilde{f}_2)|_{z_1 = e^{j2\pi \tilde{f}_1}, z_2 = e^{j2\pi \tilde{f}_2}}$, then $X(z_1, z_2)$ exists if $|X(z_1, z_2)| \leq \sum_{n_1=-\infty}^{\infty} \sum_{n_2=-\infty}^{\infty} |x[n_1, n_2]| < \infty$; that is, $x[n_1, n_2]$ is absolutely summable. The *region of convergence* (ROC) is the region over which the $X(z_1, z_2)$ uniformly converges. The ROC contains no poles and is continuous, and it must be satisfied for complete description of the Z-transform as sequences may have similar description but be defined over different ranges, which results in a different ROC. In 1D, the ROC is a ring which in 2D is a complicated surface in 4D space. It can be easier to illustrate the ROC, as in Example 2.10 below, if we express the Z-transform in terms of the magnitude of $|z|$ (in 1D) or $|z_1|, |z_2|$ (in 2D) (e.g. [2.3]).

Example 2.10 Evaluate the Z-transform of $x[n_1, n_2] = a^{n_1} b^{n_2} u(n_1, n_2)$.

$$X(z_1, z_2) = \sum_{n_1=-\infty}^{\infty} \sum_{n_2=-\infty}^{\infty} x[n_1, n_2] z_1^{-n_1} z_2^{-n_2} = \sum_{n_1=0}^{\infty} \sum_{n_2=0}^{\infty} a^{n_1} b^{n_2} z_1^{-n_1} z_2^{-n_2}$$

$$= \sum_{n_1=0}^{\infty} a^{n_1} z_1^{-n_1} \cdot \sum_{n_2=0}^{\infty} b^{n_2} z_1^{-n_2}$$

$$= \frac{1}{1 - az_1^{-1}} \frac{1}{1 - bz_2^{-1}}, \; |z_1| > |a| \text{ and } |z_2| > |b|.$$

Example 2.11 Evaluate the Z-transform $x[n_1, n_2] = \dfrac{(n_1 + n_2)!}{n_1! n_2!} a^{n_1} b^{n_2} u(n_1, n_2)$.

$$X(z_1, z_2) = \sum_{n_1=-\infty}^{\infty} \sum_{n_2=-\infty}^{\infty} x[n_1, n_2] z_1^{-n_1} z_2^{-n_2} = \sum_{n_1=0}^{\infty} \sum_{n_2=0}^{\infty} \frac{(n_1 + n_2)!}{n_1! n_2!} a^{n_1} b^{n_2} z_1^{-n_1} z_2^{-n_2}$$

Let $m = n_1 + n_2$, then

$$X(z_1, z_2) = \sum_{n_1=0}^{\infty} \sum_{m=n_1}^{\infty} \frac{m!}{n_1!(m-n_1)!} (az_1^{-1})^{n_1} (bz_2^{-1})^{m-n_1}$$

$$= \sum_{m=0}^{\infty} \sum_{n_1}^{m} \frac{m!}{n_1!(m-n_1)!} (az_1^{-1})^{n_1} (bz_2^{-1})^{m-n_1}$$

Since summation expansion may be expressed as $(x+y)^m = \sum_{n_1=0}^{m} \frac{m!}{n_1!(m-n_1)!} x^{n_1} y^{m-n_1}$

then $X(z_1, z_2) = \sum_{m=0}^{\infty} (az_1^{-1} + bz_2^{-1})^m = \frac{1}{1-(az_1^{-1}+bz_2^{-1})}$, $|az_1^{-1} + bz_2^{-1}| < 1$
ROC: $|az_1^{-1} + bz_2^{-1}| < 1 \rightarrow |a||z_1|^{-1} + |b||z_2|^{-1} < 1$. (See Figure 2.6 of Lim [2.3] p. 72.)

Properties of the Z-transform
The definition of the Z-transform provides clues to various properties that may be proved in a straightforward fashion as in the 1D case. For example, linearity, convolution, separability, shifting, differentiation, and symmetry properties follow in a similar fashion to the sequence Fourier transform. However, devising the appropriate ROC may not be straightforward. See Lim [2.3] for details.

The inverse Z-transform
The Cauchy integral theorem may be used to obtain the inverse Z-transform, i.e.

$$x[n_1, n_2] = \frac{1}{(2\pi j)^2} \oint \oint X(z_1, z_2) z_1^{n_1-1} z_2^{n_2-1} dz_1 dz_2, \qquad (2.24)$$

where the integrals are carried out over closed contours in the ROC of $X(z_1, z_2)$. The interpretation of complex integration requires knowledge of complex analysis and the Cauchy theorem. As we did in the 1D case, special (though important) cases of sequences representing impulse responses of linear shift-invariant (LSI) systems may be obtained from tabulated elementary Z-transform pairs. The Z-transform enables synthesis as well as analysis of LSI systems. (The Fourier transform is superior in analysis, but offers very little help in synthesis.) Therefore, properties such as causality, stability, and realizations of finite-impulse response (FIR) and infinite-impulse response (IIR) systems may also be studied from the 2D Z-transform. Rigorous treatment of these characteristics exists elsewhere: see for example Lim [2.3] or Dudgeon and Mersereau [2.2].

2.8 Basic 2D digital filter design

Digital filters are good examples of systems that are based on Fourier transform methods. We examine a few basics of digital filter design in this section. The ideal low-pass filter equation is

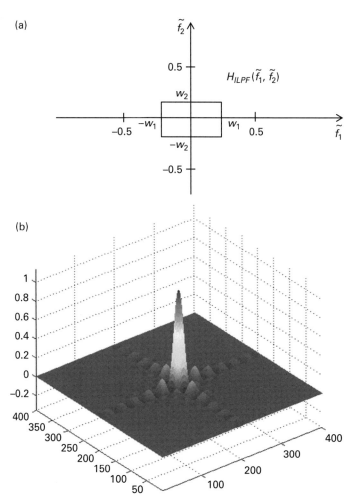

Figure 2.11 The frequency and time-domain representations of the ideal low-pass filter function. (a) Ideal low-pass filter $H_{\text{ILPF}}(\tilde{f}_1,\tilde{f}_2)$. (b) Ideal low-pass filter $h_{\text{ILPF}}[n_1,n_2]$ (sinc function).

$$H_{\text{ILPF}}(\tilde{f}_1,\tilde{f}_2) = \begin{cases} 1, & |\tilde{f}_1| \leq W_1,\ |\tilde{f}_2| \leq W_2 \\ 0, & W_1 < |\tilde{f}_1| \leq 0.5,\ W_2 < |\tilde{f}_2| \leq 0.5, \end{cases} \quad (2.25)$$

where W_1 and W_2 are the cutoff frequencies in *cycles*. The impulse response $h_{\text{ILPF}}[n_1,n_2]$ is:

$$h_{\text{ILPF}}[n_1,n_2] = \int_{-0.5}^{0.5}\int_{-0.5}^{0.5} H_{\text{ILPF}}(\tilde{f}_1,\tilde{f}_2) e^{j2\pi(n_1\tilde{f}_1+n_2\tilde{f}_2)} \quad (2.26)$$

$$= \frac{\sin 2\pi W_1 n_1}{\pi n_1} \frac{\sin 2\pi W_2 n_2}{\pi n_2} = 4W_1 W_2 \text{sinc}(2\pi W_1 n_1) \cdot \text{sinc}(2\pi W_2 n_2)$$

Figure 2.11 shows plots of $H_{\text{ILPF}}(\tilde{f}_1,\tilde{f}_2)$ and $h_{\text{ILPF}}[n_1,n_2]$.

Equation (2.26) shows that the ideal low-pass filter has infinite length, i.e. it is non-realizable. We can approximate the filter using finite number of samples; equivalent to multiplying $h_{\text{ILPF}}[n_1, n_2]$ by a window function. The practical low-pass filter may be expressed as follows:

$$h_{\text{LPF}}[n_1, n_2] = h_{\text{ILPF}}[n_1, n_2] \cdot w[n_1, n_2] \qquad (2.27)$$

If we choose $(2M_1 - 1) \times (2M_2 - 1)$ points from $h_{\text{ILPF}}[n_1, n_2]$, where M_1, M_2 are even integers, then the window function may be written as:

$$w[n_1, n_2] = \begin{cases} 1, & |n_1| \leq (M_1 - 1);\ |n_2| \leq (M_2 - 1) \\ 0, & \text{otherwise} \end{cases} \qquad (2.28)$$

Hence, $H_{\text{LPF}}(\tilde{f}_1, \tilde{f}_2) = H_{\text{ILPF}}(\tilde{f}_1, \tilde{f}_2) \oplus W(\tilde{f}_1, \tilde{f}_2)$; or equivalently, from Eq. (2.22)

$$\begin{aligned} H_{\text{LPF}}(\tilde{f}_1, \tilde{f}_2) &= \sum_{n_1=-(M_1-1)}^{M_1-1} \sum_{n_2=-(M_2-1)}^{M_2-1} e^{-j2\pi(n_1\tilde{f}_1 + n_2\tilde{f}_2)} \\ &= \left(\frac{(1 - e^{j\pi M_1 \tilde{f}_1})}{(1 - e^{j2\pi \tilde{f}_1})} + \frac{(1 - e^{-j\pi M_1 \tilde{f}_1})}{(1 - e^{-j2\pi \tilde{f}_1})} - 1 \right) \\ &\quad \times \left(\frac{(1 - e^{j\pi M_2 \tilde{f}_2})}{(1 - e^{j2\pi \tilde{f}_2})} + \frac{(1 - e^{-j\pi M_2 \tilde{f}_2})}{(1 - e^{-j2\pi \tilde{f}_2})} - 1 \right) \end{aligned}$$

From Figure 2.8 we see the ripple effects (caused by making the filter finite) in the finite-length low-pass filter expression. Various window functions may be deployed to reduce the ripples and provide a better compromise between the width of the main lobe (pass band) and the transition period of the stop band – see [2.1].

It is straightforward to define the functions for high-pass, band-pass and band-reject filters. These filters are straight modifications of the low-pass filter functions (see Section 2.2).

2.9 Anisotropic diffusion filtering

Anisotropic diffusion filtering is a variational approach to filtering which reduces image noise while maintaining edge information. The derivation is involved and is beyond the focus of this book. It suffices for our purpose that it is a well-proven approach in various image analysis applications. The following requirements should ideally be fulfilled (e.g. [2.5][2.6]):

(a) Minimize information loss by preserving object boundaries and detailed structures;
(b) Efficiently remove noise in regions of homogeneous physical properties;
(c) Enhance morphological definition by sharpening discontinuities.

In general, smoothness (regularization) is introduced into the filter function to make a discrete signal/image continuous, in order for it to be differentiable, and to reduce noise, while keeping edges unsmoothed. Smoothness is formulated as a diffusive process:

$$\frac{\partial}{\partial t} u(X,t) = \text{div}(c(X,t)\nabla u(X,t)) \tag{2.29}$$

where $X=(x,y)$, $u(X,t)$ is the diffusion strength, and div is the divergence operator. $C(X,t)$ is the diffusion function, which can be chosen from the following:

$$c_1 = \exp\left(-\frac{|\nabla I(X,t)|}{\kappa}\right) \tag{2.30}$$

$$c_2 = \frac{1}{1 + \frac{|\nabla I(X,t)|}{\kappa}} \tag{2.31}$$

where $I(.)$ is the image and the parameter κ is chosen to control the noise level and the edge strength.

$$\frac{\partial}{\partial t} I(X,t) = \text{div}(c(X,t)*\text{grad}\, I(X,t))$$

$$= \nabla^T(c(X,t)*\nabla I(X,t))$$

$$= \frac{\partial}{\partial x}\left(c(X,t)*\frac{\partial}{\partial x} I(X,t)\right) + \frac{\partial}{\partial y}\left(c(X,t)*\frac{\partial}{\partial x} I(X,t)\right)$$

$$= \frac{1}{\Delta x^2}\left(c\left(x+\frac{\Delta x}{2},y,t\right)*(I(x+\Delta x,y,t) - I(x,y,t))\right.$$

$$\left. - c\left(x-\frac{\Delta x}{2},y,t\right)*(I(x,y,t) - I(x-\Delta x,y,t))\right)$$

$$+ \frac{1}{\Delta y^2}\left(c\left(x,y+\frac{\Delta y}{2},t\right)*(I(x,y+\Delta y,t) - I(x,y,t))\right.$$

$$\left. - c\left(x,y-\frac{\Delta y}{2},t\right)*(I(x,y,t) - I(x,y-\Delta y,t))\right)$$

$$= \phi_{east} - \phi_{west} + \phi_{north} - \phi_{south} \tag{2.32}$$

where ∇ is the divergence operator.

In the 2D case, the pixel intensities are updated by the local sum of the flow contributions:

$$I(t+\Delta t) \approx I(t) + \Delta t \times \frac{\partial}{\partial t} I(t) = I(t) + \Delta t \times (\phi_{east} - \phi_{west} + \phi_{north} - \phi_{south}) \tag{2.33}$$

Figure 2.12 shows the performance of anisotropic diffusion filtering in CT imaging.

2.9 Anisotropic diffusion filtering

> **Box 2.1** Algorithm for anisotropic diffusion filtering [2.6]
>
> (1) Load in the original image;
> (2) Choose the integration constant (time interval) Δt based on the different neighborhood structures, e.g. for 2D case, four neighboring pixels, $0 < \Delta t < 1/5$;
> (3) Determine the diffusion function kernels by choosing either Equation (2.30) or (2.20);
> (4) Follow Equation (2.32) to compute ϕ_{east}, ϕ_{west}, ϕ_{north}, and ϕ_{south};
> (5) Follow Equation (2.33) to update the value at each pixel;
> (6) Iteration stops if the value difference at each pixel for two consecutive iterations is less than 0.5.

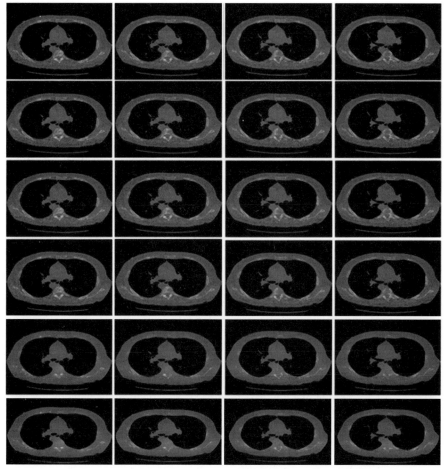

Figure 2.12 Anisotropic filter for different κ values. The first row shows the four original images; second row shows the filtered image with $\kappa = $ (std of a slice)/511, where std = standard deviation of intensity values; third row $\kappa = $ (std of slice)/21; fourth row $\kappa = $ (std of slice)/11; fifth row $\kappa = $ (std of slice)/9; and the last row $\kappa = $ (std of slice)/3.

2.10 Summary

This chapter has provided a brief overview of the main concepts of signals and systems for deterministic image modeling. Using these concepts we can study other important tools such wavelets, diffusion filters, or edge enhancement filters.

2.11 Exercises

2.1 Relationship between continuous and sequence Fourier transforms in one dimension. Consider a signal $x(t) = 10\, e^{-5t} u(t)$.

(a) Evaluate the Fourier transform $X(f) = \int_{-\infty}^{\infty} x(t) e^{-j2\pi ft} dt$.

(b) Create a properly sampled version $x[n]$, $n \in [0, 1000]$. Assume that $x(t)$ is band-limited and estimate the bandwidth in terms of the 3 dB value of $X(f)$.

(c) Evaluate the sequence Fourier transform $X(\tilde{f}) = \sum_{n=0}^{N-1} x[n]\, e^{-j2\pi n \tilde{f}} =$

$$|X(\tilde{f})| e^{j\theta_x(\tilde{f})} = X_R(\tilde{f}) + X_I(\tilde{f})$$

(d) Plot the magnitude $|X(\tilde{f})|$ and phase $e^{j\theta_x(\tilde{f})}$. Note that $X(\tilde{f})$ is periodic with period 1.

(e) Relate $X(\tilde{f})$ to $X(f)$ if we know the sampling frequency of $x(t)$.

(f) Evaluate the discrete Fourier transform $X[k] = \sum_{n=0}^{N-1} x[n] e^{-j2\pi kn/N}$. Use variable values of N.

(g) Find an expression relating $X[k]$ to $X(\tilde{f})$.

(h) Evaluate $X[k] = \sum_{n=0}^{N-1} x[n] e^{-j2\pi kn/N}$ using the FFT algorithm and plot the results. Compare with the results in (f).

(i) Repeat (a)–(g) for the two-dimensional signal $x(t_1, t_2) = 10\, e^{-5(t_1+t_2)} u(t_1, t_2)$ Note:

$$X(\tilde{f}_1, \tilde{f}_2) = \sum_{n_1=0}^{N_1-1} \sum_{n_2=0}^{N_2-1} x[n_1, n_2]\, e^{-j2\pi(n_1 \tilde{f}_1 + n_2 \tilde{f}_2)}$$

$$= |X(\tilde{f}_1, \tilde{f}_2)| e^{j\theta_x(\tilde{f}_1, \tilde{f}_2)} = X_R(\tilde{f}_1, \tilde{f}_2) + X_I(\tilde{f}_1, \tilde{f}_2)$$

2.2 Design of a low-pass filter in 1D and 2D using the windowing method. Use the following steps:

(a) Evaluate the sequence $x[n]$ of the *ideal* LPF $H_{\text{ILPF}}(\tilde{f}) = \begin{cases} 1, \tilde{f} \leq |f_c| < 0.5 \\ 0. \end{cases}$

(b) Plot $h_{\text{ILPF}}[n]$, $n \in [-N-1, N-1]$ for $N = 100$.

(c) Limiting the number of samples is equivalent to using a sequence $h_{\text{LPF}}[n] = h_{\text{ILPF}}[n] \times w[n]$, where $w[n]$ is a *rectangular window function*. Evaluate $H_{\text{LPF}}(\tilde{f}) = H_{\text{ILPF}}(\tilde{f}) * W(\tilde{f})$ for various window lengths. Explain the Gibbs phenomenon (the introduction of "ripples" in the Fourier transform of finite-length signals or sequences).

(d) Repeat part (c) using *cosine* and *triangular* windows (see [2.1]) instead of the rectangular window. Plot the results for the three windows in dB. Compare the ripples in the pass- and stop-bands, and the width of the transition bands for the filters designed using the three windows.

(e) Repeat (a) to (d) for the 2D LPF case.

(f) Repeat (a) to (e) for high-pass filters.

2.3 Use the 1D and 2D filters in Exercise 2 to smooth the signal in Exercise 1 using convolution. Apply the results to:

(a) The signal in Exercise 1 corrupted with white Gaussian noise in 1D and 2D.

(b) Images having edges of different sizes and slopes; e.g. an image of optic nerves.

2.4 Reconstruction of a 2D signal from phase. Given a 2D finite range sequence $x[n_1, n_2]$ such that $n_1 \in [0, N_1 - 1]$, $n_2 \in [0, N_2 - 1]$, we define the following quantities. The sequence Fourier transform is:

$$X(\tilde{f}_1, \tilde{f}_2) = \sum_{n_1=0}^{N_1-1} \sum_{n_2=0}^{N_2-1} x[n_1, n_2] e^{-j2\pi(n_1\tilde{f}_1 + n_2\tilde{f}_2)}$$

$$= |X(\tilde{f}_1, \tilde{f}_2)| e^{j\theta_x(\tilde{f}_1, \tilde{f}_2)} = X_r(\tilde{f}_1, \tilde{f}_2) + X_i(\tilde{f}_1, \tilde{f}_2)$$

The phase-only reconstruction is defined as:

$$x_p[n_1, n_2] = F^{-1}\{1 e^{j\theta_x(\tilde{f}_1, \tilde{f}_2)}\}$$

The magnitude-only reconstruction is defined as:

$$x_m[n_1, n_2] = F^{-1}\{|X(\tilde{f}_1, \tilde{f}_2)| e^{j0}\}$$

We can reconstruct the signal by following one of two approaches.

- Reconstruction from phase, approach 1: closed form

$$\tan \theta_x(\tilde{f}_1, \tilde{f}_2) = \frac{X_I(\tilde{f}_1, \tilde{f}_2)}{X_R(\tilde{f}_1, \tilde{f}_2)} = -\frac{\sum_{n_1=0}^{N_1-1} \sum_{n_2=0}^{N_2-1} x[n_1, n_2] \sin 2\pi(n_1\tilde{f}_1 + n_2\tilde{f}_2)}{\sum_{n_1=0}^{N_1-1} \sum_{n_2=0}^{N_2-1} x[n_1, n_2] \cos 2\pi(n_1\tilde{f}_1 + n_2\tilde{f}_2)}$$

By cross-multiplication, we get

$$\sum_{n_1=0}^{N_1-1} \sum_{n_2=0}^{N_2-1} x[n_1, n_2] \cos 2\pi(n_1\tilde{f}_1 + n_2\tilde{f}_2) \tan \theta_x(\tilde{f}_1, \tilde{f}_2)$$

$$= -\sum_{n_1=0}^{N_1-1} \sum_{n_2=0}^{N_2-1} x[n_1, n_2] \sin 2\pi(n_1\tilde{f}_1 + n_2\tilde{f}_2)$$

At every value of $\tilde{f}_1, \tilde{f}_2$, we can rewrite the above equation as a set of linear equations in $x[n_1, n_2]$, giving us $N_1 \times N_2$ equations for every value of $\tilde{f}_1, \tilde{f}_2$. Note: $\theta_x(\tilde{f}_1, \tilde{f}_2)$ is an odd function, periodic with period (-0.5 to 0.5) in both directions. Proper choice of the samples of $\tilde{f}_1,\tilde{f}_2$ can be shown to result in a solution to $x[n_1,n_2]$ within a scale factor. The above approach is suitable only for small-sized images, owing to the number of equations that must be solved for each sample of $\tilde{f}_1,\tilde{f}_2$.

- Reconstruction from phase, approach 2: iterative approach
  The reconstructed $x[n_1,n_2]$ must be:

  (a) Real;
  (b) Zero outside $n_1 \in [0, N_1 - 1]$, $n_2 \in [0, N_2 - 1]$; and
  (c) The phase of the Fourier transform of the reconstructed image must be similar to the given phase $\theta_x(f_{d_1}, f_{d_2})$

  Algorithm: Given $\theta_x(\tilde{f}_1,\tilde{f}_2)$, over the period $-0.5 \leq \tilde{f}_1,\tilde{f}_2 \leq 0.5$

  i. Start with an initial image $x_0[n_1, n_2]$ such that $n_1 \in [0, N_1 - 1]$, $n_2 \in [0, N_2 - 1]$
  ii. Obtain the sequence Fourier transform $X_0(\tilde{f}_1,\tilde{f}_2)$
  iii. Replace the phase of $X_0(\tilde{f}_1,\tilde{f}_2)$ by $\theta_x(\tilde{f}_1,\tilde{f}_2)$, over the period $-0.5 \leq \tilde{f}_1,\tilde{f}_2 \leq 0.5$; i.e. obtain $\hat{X}(\tilde{f}_1,\tilde{f}_2)$
  iv. Obtain the inverse Fourier transform $\hat{x}[n_1, n_2]$ and apply the constraints (a)–(c)
  v. Repeat steps ii–iv until convergence (i.e. a certain criterion is obtained, perhaps that the sum square error reaches a certain threshold). Of course, the best criterion is always to check whether $\hat{\theta}_x(\tilde{f}_1,\tilde{f}_2) = \theta_x(\tilde{f}_1,\tilde{f}_2)$.

Note: The above algorithm may be implemented by FFT, which provides a fast computation of the DFT (see Figure 1.30 of Lim [2.3], p. 37). Note the change in notation, $\omega = 2\pi \tilde{f}$.

References

[2.1] A. V. Oppenheim and R. W. Schafer, *Discrete-Time Signal Processing*. New Jersey: Prentice-Hall (2010).
[2.2] D. E. Dudgeon and R. M. Mersereau, *Multidimensional Digital Signal Processing*. New Jersey: Prentice-Hall (1984).
[2.3] J. S. Lim, *Two-dimensional Signal and Image Processing*. New Jersey: Prentice-Hall (1990).
[2.4] R. C. Gonzalez and R. E. Woods, *Digital Image Processing*, 3rd Edition. New Jersey: Prentice-Hall (2008).
[2.5] P. Perona and J. Malik, Scale-space and edge detection using anisotropic diffusion. *IEEE Trans. Pattern Anal. Machine Intel.* **12**(7) (1990) 629–639.
[2.6] G. Grieg, O. Kubler, , R. Kikinis and F. A. Jolesz, Nonlinear anisotropic filtering of MRI data, *IEEE Trans. Med. Imaging* **11**(2) (1992) 221–232.

3 Biomedical imaging modalities

3.1 Introduction

Methods of examining the anatomy and function of living organisms have advanced immensely over the past century. Biomedical imaging has evolved in terms of types of imaging system (modalities) and capabilities, and has improved our understanding of biological systems. It has affected the quality of our lives by transforming various medical practices from arts to science, enabling better healthcare administration, and leading on average to longer and healthier lives. The technology also has an economic impact: vast numbers of technical professionals (chemists, mathematicians, physicists, engineers, and computer scientists) work in companies making biomedical imaging devices, or in research laboratories and hospitals. One chapter cannot hope to cover a vibrant and ever-dynamic field; we will merely scratch the surface in understanding the process of image formation in some of the common imaging modalities. There are more specialized books, periodicals, and manufacturers' reports that should be consulted by readers interested in delving into the field of biomedical imaging.

This chapter serves as a brief tour of a field of ever-expanding diversity and capabilities. The focus, however, will be on the imaging *modalities* that have guided the development of the basic theories and approaches to image analysis covered in the subsequent chapters of this book. We concentrate on image analysis approaches that have been well-studied for images from two broad categories of imaging sensors: those based on ionizing radiations (e.g. X-rays and computed tomography) and those based on magnetization (e.g. magnetic resonance imaging). Positron emission tomography (PET), ultrasound imaging, laser imaging, thermal infrared imaging and other modalities are also important, but this chapter will not cover all of these.

3.2 X-rays

Wilhelm C. Röntgen, a physicist at the University of Würzburg in Germany, is accredited with discovering X-rays in 1895, an invention for which he received the first Nobel Prize in Physics in 1901. However, Röntgen was not the first to acquire an X-ray photograph. In 1890, Alexander Goodspeed of the University of Pennsylvania, and the photographer William Jennings, accidentally exposed some photographic plates to X-rays, although they were only able to explain the images produced on the developed plates after Röntgen announced his discovery of X-rays.

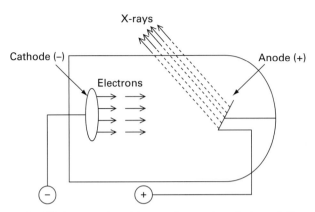

Figure 3.1 A simplified X-ray tube with a rotating anode and a heated filament.

The majority of the material on X-rays in this section comes from Hendee and Ritenour [3.1].

Figure 3.1 shows the basic components of an X-ray tube. A heated filament releases electrons that are accelerated across a high voltage onto the target. X-rays are produced as the electrons interact with the target. The rays emerge from the target in all directions but are restricted by collimators to form a useful beam. A vacuum is maintained inside the glass envelope of the X-ray tube to prevent the electrons from interacting with gas molecules. X-ray production is most efficient (i.e. more X-rays are produced per second) if the potential of the target is always positive, and if the voltage between the filament and target is kept at its maximum value. During the interaction between the electrons and the target, the electron may be slowed or stopped and a *bremsstrahlung* ('braking ray') photon released. The maximum energy of this photon is equal to the maximum kinetic energy of the electrons produced at that tube voltage. Photons with maximum energy in the X-ray beam have maximum frequency and minimum wavelength such that

$$E_{max} = h\upsilon_{max} = \frac{hc}{\lambda_{min}} \qquad (3.1)$$

and the minimum wavelength for an X-ray beam is

$$\lambda_{min} = \frac{hc}{E_{max}} = \frac{hc}{kVp} \qquad (3.2)$$

where h is Planck's constant, kVp is the maximum voltage applied across an X-ray tube (peak kilovoltage), and c is the speed of light. With known values of h and c, we can show that λ_{min} would be equal to 1.24/kVp.

For example, for an X-ray beam generated at 200 kVp, the maximum energy numerically equals the maximum tube voltage; thus, the maximum energy is 200 keV (kiloelectronvolt), and the minimum wavelength is λ_{min} = 1.24/200kVp = 0.0062 nm.

In order to prevent collisions between air molecules as electrons accelerate between the filament and target, X-ray tubes are evacuated to pressures less than 10^{-5} mmHg. Removal of air also reduces deterioration of the hot filament by oxidation. During the manufacture of X-ray tubes, evacuation is accomplished by "outgassing" procedures that employ repeated heating cycles to remove gas occluded in components of the X-ray tube.

The useful beam of an X-ray tube is composed of photons with an energy distribution that depends on many factors. (i) The energy of the bombarding electrons changes with tube voltage. (ii) *Bremsstrahlung* X-rays are produced with a wide energy range. (iii) X-rays released as characteristic K-shell radiation from the target atoms have energies independent of that of the bombarding electrons (so long as the energy of the bombarding electrons exceeds the threshold energy for characteristic X-ray emission). (iv) X-rays are produced at a range of depths in the target of the X-ray tube. They travel through different thicknesses of target, and may lose energy through one or more interactions.

Other variables such as filtration, target material, peak tube voltage, current, and exposure time may affect the range and intensity of X-ray energies in the useful beam.

3.2.1 Filtration and beam hardening

An X-ray beam traverses several attenuating materials before it reaches the object (or patient). These include the glass envelope of the X-ray tube, the oil surrounding the tube, and the exit window in the tube housing. These attenuators are referred to collectively as the inherent filtration of the X-ray tube. The "aluminum equivalent" for each component of inherent filtration is the thickness of aluminum that would reduce the exposure rate by an amount equal to that provided by the component. In any medium, the probability that incident X-rays interact photoelectrically varies roughly as $1/E^3$, where E is the energy of the incident photons. That is, low-energy X-rays are attenuated more than those of high energy (Ter-Pogossian [3.2]).

After passing through a material, an X-ray beam has a higher average energy per photon (that is, it is "harder") even though the total number of photons in the beam has been reduced, because more low-energy photons than high-energy photons have been removed from the beam. The inherent filtration of an X-ray tube "hardens" the X-ray beam. Further hardening may be achieved by adding filters of various materials to the beam. The total filtration in the X-ray beam is the sum of the inherent and added filtration. Usually, additional hardening is included to remove low-energy X-rays that, if left in the beam, would increase the radiation dose to the patient without significant contribution to image formation.

3.2.2 Simulation of X-ray transmission

The transmission of X-rays in a homogeneous medium may be expressed as follows:

$$I = I_0 e^{-\mu x} \tag{3.3}$$

where I_0 is the initial intensity of the beam, μ is the attenuation coefficient, and x is the distance traveled. If the X-ray beam is intercepted by two regions with different attenuation coefficients μ_1 and μ_2, and thicknesses x_1 and x_2, the X-ray transmission will be as follows:

$$I = I_0 e^{-(\mu_1 x_1 + \mu_2 x_2)} \tag{3.4}$$

The transmission across n regions with different linear attenuation coefficients may be expressed as follows:

$$I = I_0 e^{-\sum_{i=1}^{n} \mu_i x_i} \qquad (3.5)$$

where μ_1 is the attenuation of the region i in the path of the X-ray beam.

The basic system of X-ray imaging works as follows: the X-ray source is collimated and directed towards the plane of interest, where the rays travel through the tissues and are attenuated. Detectors, which are positioned opposite to the X-ray source, record the projections.

Example 3.1 Consider an ellipsoid filled with water with height 20 cm and spatial domain 30 × 20 cm. A square-based prism made of copper is inscribed in the ellipsoid with the base of the prism centered at the maximum square contained in the ellipsoid. Consider a slice of this volume containing both water and copper. Show how a single X-ray passes through the object and is attenuated until it emerges to form the projection.

Solution Figure 3.2 shows a sample slice containing both water and copper. Consider the single ray shown on the right side of Figure 3.2. Assume the full intensity of the X-ray is I_0. At the beginning, there is no object in the path (i.e. there is a vacuum), so the ray is not attenuated, and $I_1 = I_0 e^{-0 \times (1/7)}$. The ray then passes through a water voxel with attenuation factor 0.002; the intensity will be $I_2 = I_1 e^{-(0.002) \times (2/7)}$. Then the ray passes through a copper voxel with attenuation factor 0.5253; the intensity will be $I_3 = I_2 e^{-(0.5253) \times (3/7)}$. Similarly, the two other copper voxels lead to $I_4 = I_3 e^{-(0.5253) \times (4/7)}$ and $I_5 = I_4 e^{-(0.5253) \times (5/7)}$. Then we have a water voxel, hence $I_6 = I_5 e^{-(0.002) \times (6/7)}$. As the X-ray exits, no attenuation occurs; hence, $I_7 = I_6$.

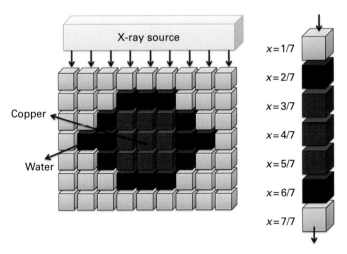

Figure 3.2 Sample slice, with water in dark gray and copper in light gray. On the right is a zoom view of a single X-ray entering and exiting the slice.

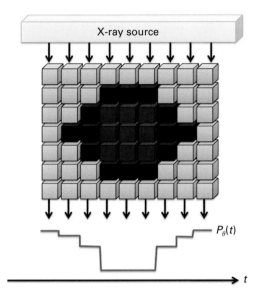

Figure 3.3 X-ray projection resulting from the setup in Figure 3.2. P_θ stands for projections at angle θ.

Figure 3.3 shows the resulting projection of all the rays of the slice shown in Figure 3.2.

3.3 Computed tomography

Tomography is the process of collecting data about an object from multiple views, and using these data to construct an image of a slice through the object. In computed tomography (CT), a computer is used to reconstruct an image of the patient from multiple views.

X-rays provide a composite image of the tissues in the path of the X-ray beam; hence tissue specificity is hard to decipher, and the exact dimensions of anatomy in the path of the rays cannot be inferred. Nevertheless, X-ray imaging is a very powerful imaging modality for gross examination, bone assessment and surgeries, and various chest examinations. It is fast and relatively inexpensive to perform, and is often used in a first attempt at diagnosis. In order to obtain an estimate of 3D anatomy (and some functions), computed tomography (CT) was invented. This provides cross-sectional images which may be combined to form a 3D object. Although various attempts were made in the 1940s to 1950s to produce cross-sectional imaging using X-rays, modern CT is credited to the pioneering work of Godfrey Hounsfield, an engineer with EMI Ltd., and Allen Cormack, a South African medical physicist; they shared the Nobel Prize for Medicine in 1970. Figure 3.4 illustrates the basic components of a CT scan setup.

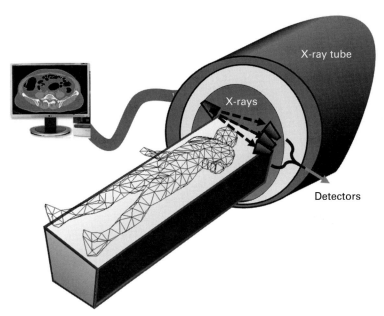

Figure 3.4 A simple CT scan setup with an X-ray tube, patient, detector, and image reconstruction computer and display monitor.

Here we summarize the main components of a typical CT machine (see Hendee and Ritenour [3.1]).

Tube: CT machines use fast rotating-anode X-ray tubes, with a pulsed X-ray beam; tubes with ratings greater than 6 million heat units are standard. With 1 BTU = 1055 joules, 6 M heat units would be 6.33×10^9 J.

Collimators: Collimation helps to reduce scattered radiation to less than 1% of the primary beam intensity. CT units contain two types of collimators: source collimators to shape the X-ray beam and limit patient dose, and a detector collimator to control the slice thickness. The width of the detector collimator defines the thickness of the CT slice, and when combined with the area of a pixel defines the voxel corresponding to the 2D pixel of the display.

Detectors: All detectors used in CT are operated in current rather than pulse mode. Detectors for CT scanning, either gas-filled ionization chambers or solid-state detectors, are chosen for their detection efficiency, short response time, and stability of operation. Solid-state detectors include NaI (Tl) (i.e. sodium iodide activated with tantalum), CaF, and CsI scintillation crystals. Gas-filled ionization chambers contain xenon pressurized up to 25 atmospheres (atm) to improve their X-ray detection efficiency.

What is detected is energy due to X-rays projected on to a material. This generates the function P_θ (standing for projections at angle θ), which is used for reconstruction of an image. The numbers computed by the reconstruction algorithm are not exact values of attenuation coefficients. Instead, they are integers termed CT numbers that

3.3 Computed tomography

are related to attenuation coefficients. The CT numbers range from −1000 for air to +1000 for bone, with the CT number for water set at 0. The relationship between CT number and linear attenuation coefficient μ of a material is:

$$\text{CT number} = 1000 \frac{(\mu - u_w)}{u_w} \quad (3.6)$$

where u_w is the linear attenuation coefficient of water. A monitor is used to portray CT numbers as a grayscale display. The viewing device has a contrast enhancement feature, which is essential because the X-ray attenuation is similar for most tissues of diagnostic interest.

3.3.1 CT scanner generations

Figure 3.5 summarizes the scan motions in different generations of CT scanners. Early scanners used a pencil-like beam with a combination of translational and rotational motion to accumulate the transmission measurements needed for reconstruction. This was inefficient with respect to time (~5 minutes per scan), and blurring was inevitable because of patient movement and physiological functions. The second generation introduced fan-shaped beams, where multiple measures of X-ray transmission were made simultaneously. This reduced the scan time to 20 to 60 seconds, and also greatly reduced the effects of motion. Translational motion was then eliminated in subsequent generations. Third-generation CT relies only on the rotational motion of both the tube and the detector array, whereas the array of detectors is stationary in the fourth generation and only the tube rotates. With the last two generations, data accumulation time can be as little as 1 second per scan. The third generation uses a large number of detectors (512–768), and two collimators that restrict both the angular width and the beam. Ring artifacts were prevalent in the early days of this generation, as the rotate/rotate geometry leads to a situation in which each detector is responsible for data corresponding to a ring in the image, but this is better now with improved detectors. The fourth generation does not suffer from such artifacts, since detectors are located 360° around the patient. Unlike the

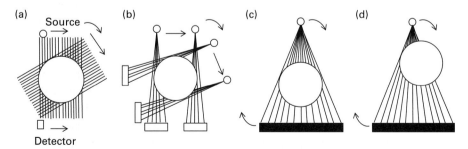

Figure 3.5 Scan motions in CT (from left). (a) First-generation scanner using a combination of rotational and translational motions and a pencil X-ray beam. (b) Second generation, with a fan X-ray beam, multiple detectors, and translational and rotational motions. (c) Third-generation scanner using a fan X-ray beam and smooth rotational motion of the tube and detector array. (d) Fourth-generation scanner with rotational motion of the tube and a stationary circular array of detectors. Circle = source, box = detector.

third-generation systems, detectors in the fourth generation are shallow because rays need be able to strike a given detector at different angles.

3.3.2 Basic CT reconstruction algorithms

There are four types of reconstruction algorithms for CT images (e.g. [3.3]; [3.4]):

Simple back-projection: Each X-ray transmission path through the body is divided into equally spaced elements. By summing the attenuation for each element over all X-ray paths that intersect the element at different angles, a final summed attenuation coefficient is determined for each element. When this coefficient is combined with the summed coefficients for all other elements in the anatomic section scanned by the X-ray beam, a composite image of attenuation coefficients is obtained. Consider the area of interest as a number of scan lines with N elements per line; f_{ij} is the calculated attenuation of each element, and g_{ij} is the measured projection along each line (the measurement obtained for each individual scan line or ray). An iterative process is done to calculate the attenuation as follows:

$$f_{ij}^{q+1} = f_{ij}^q + \frac{g_{ij} - \sum_{i=1}^{N} f_{ij}^q}{N} \qquad (3.7)$$

Although the simple back-projection approach to reconstruction algorithms is straightforward, it produces blurred images of sharp features in the object.

Filtered back-projection: This reconstruction algorithm uses a 1D integral equation for the reconstruction of a 2D image. A "deblurring" function is convolved with the X-ray transmission data to remove most of the blurring before the data are back-projected. The most common deblurring function is a filter that removes the frequency components of the X-ray transmission data that are responsible for most of the blurring in the image.

Fourier transform: In this approach, X-ray attenuation at each angular orientation is separated into frequency components of various amplitudes from which the entire image is assembled into a spatially correct image and then reconstructed by an inverse Fourier transform process. Note that for each orientation the detector takes a specific angle increment.

Series expansion: In this technique, variations of which are known as *algebraic reconstruction technique* (ART), *iterative least-squares technique* (ILST), and *simultaneous iterative reconstruction technique* (SIRT), X-ray attenuation data at one angular orientation are divided into equally spaced elements along each of several rays. These data are compared with similar data at different angular orientations, and differences in X-ray attenuation at the two orientations are added equally to the appropriate elements. This process is repeated for all angular orientations.

Kak and Slaney [3.4] offer a detailed treatment of various computed tomography techniques with straightforward algorithmic description. Appendix 3.1 shows implementation of the parallel beam reconstruction algorithm. It also provides the mathematical details of the filtered back-projection technique.

3.3.3 Dose

Increasing the X-ray dose improves the contrast of CT images. The relationship between resolution and dose can be expressed as follows:

$$\eta = a\left(\frac{s^2}{e^3 b}\right) \tag{3.8}$$

where η is the patient dose, s is the signal to noise ratio, e is the spatial resolution, b is the slice thickness, and a is a constant. From Eq. (3.8), we can conclude the following. (1) A twofold improvement in the signal-to-noise ratio (contrast resolution) requires a fourfold increase in patient dose. (2) A twofold reduction in slice thickness means a twofold increase in patient dose. (3) A twofold improvement in spatial resolution requires an eightfold increase in patient dose.

It is worth mentioning that in projection radiography, the dose is greatest where the beam enters the patient, yet in CT it is relatively uniform across the section of the tissue exposed to the beam, because the tube rotates around the patient during exposure. See Cacak [3.5] for detailed description of the measurement of CT dose parameters.

3.3.4 CT image artifacts

Other than the ring artifact mentioned earlier, artifacts in CT images include the following. (1) *Metal artifacts* caused by implants in patients. Such implants usually have higher atomic numbers that cause far more photoelectric interaction than adjacent tissues. (2) *Incomplete projections* from large objects. (3) *Patient motion*. (4) *Respiratory motion*. (5) *Aliasing* caused by insufficient number of detectors. (6) *Beam hardening*; filtering of low-energy X-rays from the beam as it penetrates the patient yields a beam of higher energy in the center of the patient, which results in reduced attenuation coefficients in the center compared with the periphery, and this is known as the beam hardening effect.

3.4 Nuclear medicine

Nuclear medicine studies can be categorized into studies of : (1) localization, (2) dilution, (3) flow or diffusion, and (4) biochemical and metabolic properties. Many of the properties of radioactive tracers were first demonstrated by the Hungarian physicist George de Hevesy, leading to his Nobel Prize in Chemistry in 1943. The first application of radioactive tracers to experimental medicine was by Blumgart, Weiss, and Yens in 1926, when they used a decay product of radium to measure the circulation time of blood. Most nuclear medicine studies use detectors outside the body to measure the rate of distribution of radioactivity in regions of interest inside it. The rate of accumulation of radioactivity may be measured with one or more detectors, usually NaI(Tl) scintillation crystals, positioned at fixed locations outside the body. Images of the distribution of radioactivity usually are obtained with a stationary imaging device known as a scintillation camera.

Measurement of the accumulation of radioactive iodine in the thyroid gland was the first routine clinical use of a radioactive nuclide. Since then, many diagnostic applications of radioactive nuclides have been developed. Often, these applications require measurement of the change in radioactivity in a selected region of the body as a function of time. The rate of accumulation (uptake) of iodine in the thyroid gland may be estimated from measurements of the radioactivity in the thyroid at specified times (usually 6 and 24 hours) after a selected amount of radioactive iodine is administered.

Dilution measurements with radioactive nuclides are used for a variety of diagnostic tests in clinical medicine. If a solution of volume v_i that contains a known concentration $(cpm/ml)_i$ of radioactive material is thoroughly mixed with a large volume of non-radioactive solution, then the volume v_f of the final solution may be estimated by measuring the specific count rate $(cpm/ml)_f$ of the final solution:

$$v_f = \frac{(cpm/ml)_i}{(cpm/ml)_f} v_i \tag{3.9}$$

During some applications of the dilution technique, the specific count rate $(cpm/ml)_f$ of the final solution must be corrected for activity that escapes (by decay) from the volume to be measured.

Static images display the spatial distribution of radioactivity in an organ in order to demonstrate structural abnormalities, reveal physiologic defects, or estimate relative mass. Some nuclear medicine studies measure the radioactivity in an organ over time after administration of a radioactive compound. These studies are termed dynamic studies. Examples are renal studies to evaluate blood flow and studies to determine kidney function. Dynamic and static studies often involve different radiopharmaceuticals.

3.4.1 Scintillation cameras

Scintillation cameras (Figure 3.6), often referred to as gamma- or γ-cameras, were first assembled by Anger in 1956 at the University of California [3.6]. This was a major advance in static imaging, as they allowed simultaneous collection of γ-rays from all regions of small organs. The camera contained a 6-mm-thick sodium iodide [NaI (TI)] crystal 10 cm in diameter, and viewed by seven photomultiplier (PM) tubes, each 3.8 cm in diameter. Six PM tubes were hexagonally arranged about the central seventh tube. A larger camera was built in 1963, where the crystal was 28 cm in diameter, along with 19 PM tubes arranged hexagonally.

In early models, the PM tubes were optically coupled to the scintillation crystal with mineral oil to provide efficient transmission of light from the crystal, but this restricted the position of the detector to an overhead view of the patient. The later replacement of

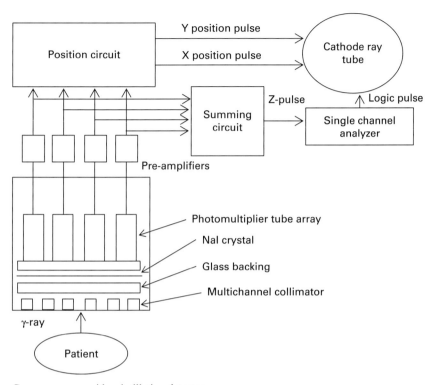

Figure 3.6 Gamma camera with scintillation detector.

mineral oil by a solid plastic light guide and optical coupling grease permitted the rotation of the detector head to any desired position.

Improvements to the basic design of the scintillation camera increased its speed and usefulness in clinical medicine. Some of these improvements include:

- Replacement of vacuum tubes by integrated circuits.
- The use of precision electronic components to obtain a more reliable signal that is less sensitive to power fluctuations.
- Crystal diameters up to 0.5 m, and coupled to as many as 91 PM tubes.
- Interfacing of cameras to data storage and processing systems.
- Use of digital computers for image acquisition and display network.
- The availability of the metastable radionuclide technetium-99, or ^{99m}Tc. This has contributed greatly to the field of nuclear medicine because of the following properties: (a) Short half-life (6 hours). (b) Readily detectable γ-ray energy of 140 keV. (c) because of the short half-life, it permits the administration of large amounts of radioactive material without excessive radiation doses to patients. This means that more rays will be emitted over a shorter period of time, which helps the scintillation camera to operate at its full capacity.

Scintillation cameras are separated into four main components: collimator, detector, data processing section, and display unit.

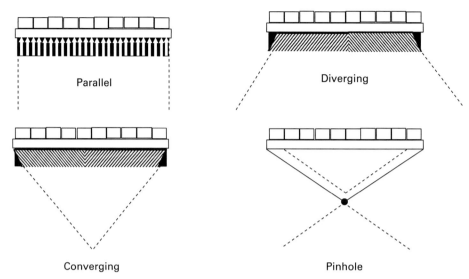

Figure 3.7 Collimator types.

Collimator: This is placed between the crystal and the patient, in order to relate the absorption sites of γ-rays in the crystal to their origin within the patient. There are four types of collimator (see Figure 3.7).

- *The parallel multihole collimator:* The most commonly used collimator, this consists of small, straight cylinders separated by lead septa. A collimator with many cylinders of small diameter is termed a high-resolution collimator, whereas a collimator with fewer cylinders of larger diameter allows more photons to reach the collimator and is called a high-sensitivity collimator. From this it can be concluded that a gain in sensitivity is accompanied by a loss of resolution and vice versa.
- *The pinhole collimator:* This consists of a pinhole aperture in a lead or tungsten absorber. It is mainly used to obtain high-resolution images from small organs such as the thyroid. The main drawback of this type of collimators is its low sensitivity, as only a few photons emitted by the patient are collected to form the image.
- *The diverging collimator:* This allows the camera to image regions larger than the dimensions of the crystal itself. Its resolution is lower than that of a parallel multihole collimator.
- *The converging collimator:* Resolution is better with this collimator, as the region of interest is projected over the entire crystal face rather than onto a limited region of it.

Scintillation crystal: NaI (Tl) is the detector used today in almost all clinical applications. Other detectors investigated recently include bismuth germanate (BGO) and barium fluoride (BaF_2). The periphery of the crystal is always masked to prevent image distortion caused by inefficient collection of the light there. Thicker crystals provide more detection efficiency, but greater thickness also increases multiple scattering within the crystal.

Detectors may also have a light guide that transmits and distributes light from the primary interaction site in the crystal to the PM tubes, but this is not required in digital scintillation cameras.

The light transmitted to a PM tube strikes the photocathode element of the tube. In response, electrons are ejected from the photocathode and acelerated towards the first of a series of dynodes (positively charged electrodes), where it generates additional electrons. These in turn cause more electrons to be released from the remaining dynodes, and this cascade effect means that 10^6 to 10^8 electrons are collected at the final electrode or anode for each electron released at the photocathode. The number of electrons finally collected at the anode is proportional to the amount of light striking the photocathode.

Data processing: Each PM tube transmits its output electrical signal to its own pre-amplifier. This circuit is used primarily to match the PM tube impedance to that of the succeeding electronic circuits. The PM tubes are positioned in a hexagonal array above the scintillation crystal, with the spacing and separation from the crystal selected to provide an optimum combination of spatial uniformity and resolution. The signal from each preamplifier enters the array and is applied across four precision resistors to produce four separate electrical signals for each PM tube. The position signals for each PM tube are transmitted to four summation amplifiers. The product of the summation operation is four electrical signals, one for each of the four deflection plates in the cathode-ray tube (CRT). Normally, the electron beam is prevented from flowing across the CRT. Only when the signal is received at the CRT is the electron beam permitted to flow and produce a light flash on the screen. During this brief interval, the position signals are applied to the deflection plates so that the light flashes on the screen at a position corresponding to the site of γ-ray absorption in the crystal.

Processing and display: The image of a radionuclide distribution created in the scintillation camera is digitized and stored in computer memory. The analog signals from the camera's electronics are converted to digital signals by analog-to-digital (ADC) converters.

3.4.2 Emission computed tomography

As described in Section 3.3, in computed tomography (CT), an image of a patient is reconstructed from multiple views. CT using X-rays transmitted through the patient is termed transmission CT. A similar type of study can be performed in nuclear medicine by detecting photons emitted from a radiopharmaceutical distributed within the body. The term emission computed tomography (ECT) refers to this procedure. Positron emission tomography (PET) is the process of producing tomographic images by detection of annihilation photons released during positron decay. Single-photon emission computed tomography (SPECT) is the process of creating tomographic images computed from the registration of interactions of individual γ-rays in a crystal acting as detector.

3.4.2.1 Single-photon emission computed tomography

In earlier SPECT units, the detectors rotated in a circular orbit around the body. In newer units, the detectors follow an elliptical path so that they remain close to the skin surface during the entire scan. Reconstruction of a SPECT image is similar to that performed in X-ray CT. The most common algorithm is convolution (filtered) back-projection.

Longitudinal-section SPECT

This involves the use of multiple views to provide a coronal, sagittal, or oblique slice of information within the patient. Superposition of data from the multiple views leads to multiple images and therefore blurring of all objects except those at the plane defined by the junction of the viewing areas of the detector. In order to obtain multiple views for focal-plane SPECT, special collimators are used for this purpose. Some of these systems include multiple pinhole techniques [3.7].

Transverse-section SPECT

Most transverse-section SPECT systems have a rotating detector (a scintillation camera) and a stationary source of γ-rays (the patient). One, two, or three scintillation cameras are mounted on a rotating gantry. This technique has many features in common with X-ray CT, but one major difference between them is that a SPECT image represents the distribution of radioactivity in the patient, whereas an X-ray CT image reflects the attenuation of X-rays within the tissue. SPECT needs attenuation correction for the fact that fewer photons are recorded from voxels at greater depths in the patient. One possible solution is to estimate the body contour, sample the patient from both sides, and then construct a correction matrix to adjust the scan data for attenuation. Transverse-section SPECT is useful in several clinical applications including cardiac imaging, liver/spleen studies, and chest–thorax procedures [3.8] [3.9] [3.10].

3.4.2.2 Positron emission tomography

In PET, the radiation detected is annihilation radiation released as positrons interact with electrons. The directionality of the annihilation photons (two 511-keV annihilation photons emitted in opposite directions) provides a mechanism for localizing the origin of the photons and hence the radioactive decay process that resulted in their emission. Hence collimators are of no use in PET imaging.

The PET scanner was devised in the early 1950s by Brownell, Sweet, and Aronow at Massachusetts General Hospital. In a PET system, the patient is surrounded by a ring of detectors. Detectors opposite to each other register annihilation photons simultaneously, and the decay process that created the photons is assumed to have occurred along a line between the detectors (see Figure 3.8). The PET image reveals the number of counts that occurred in each of the voxels represented by pixels in the image.

PET uses short-lived radionuclides such as ^{11}C, ^{13}N, and ^{15}O, which have physiological potential because they can replace atoms in molecules that are essential for metabolism. Clinical applications use the ^{18}F-labeled fluorodeoxyglucose [^{18}FDG]. These positron emitters are produced in a cyclotron.

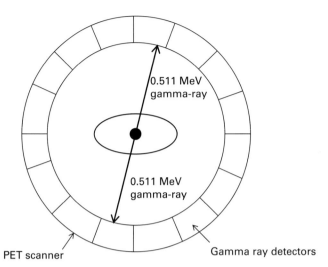

Figure 3.8 In PET, two detectors opposite each other record the interaction of 0.511-MeV photons, which is an indicator of the positron decay process that occurred somewhere along a line connecting the two detectors within the patient.

One of the major challenges of PET system design is the detector sensitivity. The detector is manufactured from bismuth germanate (BGO) which has high intrinsic efficiency for the high-energy photons.

Integration of a PET unit with a CT unit in one machine has recently become a common procedure for the purpose of tumor identification and localization in oncology.

3.5 Ultrasound

Ultrasound, or very high-frequency sound, is a mechanical disturbance that moves as a pressure wave through a medium and can be detected for use in imaging. French physicist Paul Langevin developed ultrasonic technology to detect submarines during the first world war. Ultrasound was introduced to industry in 1928 by Soviet physicist Sokolov who proposed its use for detecting flaws in materials. Ultrasound was then used in medical applications in the 1930s, although it was limited to therapeutic applications such as cancer treatment. It was not until the late 1940s that ultrasound began to be used for diagnostic applications.

Figure 3.9 illustrates the generation and propagation of sound waves. A force (represented here by the piston) is applied to a fluid medium. This results in a higher concentration of molecules in front of the piston, leading to an increased pressure at that location. This region is termed the "zone of compression" which then begins to migrate away from the piston. If the piston is withdrawn, this creates a region of reduced pressure, the "zone of refraction." The propagation of these zones establishes a wave disturbance in the medium (termed a longitudinal wave, because the motion of the molecules in the medium is parallel to the direction of wave propagation).

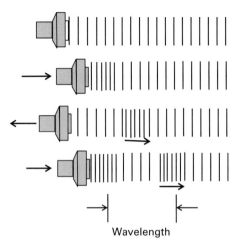

Figure 3.9 Uniform distribution of molecules in the medium, then alternating movement of the piston to establish the longitudinal wave.

3.5.1 Ultrasound intensity

Medical ultrasound is produced in beams that are described in terms of the power per unit area, also known as the beam's "intensity" and described relative to some reference intensity. A logarithmic scale is the most appropriate one used for recording data over a range of many orders of magnitude. In acoustics the decibel scale is widely used, which is defined as:

$$\text{dB} = 10 \, \log(I/I_0) \tag{3.10}$$

where I_0 is the reference intensity.

3.5.2 Attenuation in ultrasound

Attenuation refers to any process that contributes to the loss of the ultrasound beam energy. When the beam enters a medium, energy is lost by the processes of absorption, scattering, refraction, diffraction, interference, and reflection. In absorption, part of the energy of the beam is converted into other forms of energy, such as increase in the molecules' motion. Reflection means that there is a deflection of all or part of the beam. Scattering means that the beam changes direction in a less orderly fashion.

When an ultrasound beam encounters obstacles, its behavior depends on the size of these obstacles compared with the wavelength of the sound. For example, if the obstacle size is large compared with the wavelength, then the beam retains its integrity as it changes direction. This type of reflection is termed "specular." Part of the beam is reflected and the remainder is transmitted through the obstacle as a beam of lower intensity. If the size of the obstacle is the same as or smaller than the ultrasound wavelength, then the obstacle will scatter energy in various directions. Some of the energy may return to its original source after "non-specular" scatter. When the scattering objects are much smaller in size than the wavelength, the process is termed "Rayleigh scattering." This occurs, for example, with red blood cells.

The energy that remains in the beam as it encounters obstacles decreases exponentially with the depth of penetration of the beam into the medium. The attenuation of ultrasound in a material is described by the attenuation coefficient α in units of decibels per centimeter. This is the sum of all of the individual coefficients for scatter and absorption. Table 3.1 shows the attenuation coefficients of ultrasound in different materials. We can see that the attenuation is very high in bone, which makes it difficult to visualize structures that lie behind it. The table also shows that very little attenuation occurs in water, which means that it is a very good transmitter of ultrasound energy. In general, the attenuation of ultrasound energy increases with frequency in biological tissues, meaning that higher-frequency ultrasound is attenuated more readily and is less penetrating than ultrasound of lower frequency.

An example of the attenuation in ultrasound is shown in Figure 3.10, where there is a block of tissue with multiple layers of different materials, each with a different attenuation coefficient (see Table 3.1). The beam traverses to the first layer (fat), where part of its energy is lost and reflected back to the transducer. The remainder of the beam is transmitted to the subsequent layers, where the process is repeated.

Table 3.1 Attenuation coefficients for 1-MHz ultrasound

Material	Blood	Fat	Muscle (across fibers)	Muscle (along fibers)	Skull bone	Lung	Liver	Brain	Kidney	Spinal cord	Water
α (dB/cm)	0.18	0.6	3.3	1.2	20	40	0.9	0.85	1.0	1.0	0.0022

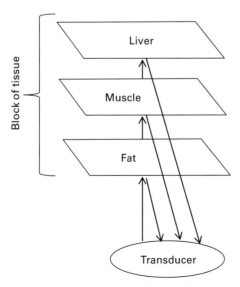

Figure 3.10 Attenuation of an ultrasound beam as it traverses tissue with multiple layers of materials.

To calculate the total energy loss in Figure 3.10, suppose that this block of tissue is made up of 3 cm fat, 4 cm muscle, and 3 cm liver. The total energy loss is then:

Energy loss in fat + energy loss in muscle + energy loss in liver

$$= \left(0.6\frac{dB}{cm}\right)(3\text{ cm}) + \left(1.2\frac{dB}{cm}\right)(4\text{ cm}) + \left(0.9\frac{dB}{cm}\right)(3\text{ cm}) = 9.3\text{ dB}.$$

After reflection, i.e. when the beam returns to the transducer through the tissue block, the total attenuation is doubled and thus is 18.6 dB.

3.5.3 Reflection in ultrasound

The fraction of energy reflected from an interface depends on the difference in impedance of the media on opposite sides of the interface. The acoustic impedance of a medium is:

$$Z = \rho C \tag{3.11}$$

The fraction α_R of the incident energy that is reflected is:

$$\alpha_R = \left(\frac{z_2 - z_1}{z_2 + z_1}\right)^2 \tag{3.12}$$

where z_1 and z_2 are the acoustic impedances of the two media. The transmission coefficient, which describes the fraction of the incident energy that is transmitted, is:

$$\alpha_T = \frac{4 z_1 z_2}{(z_1 + z_2)^2} \tag{3.13}$$

$$\alpha_R + \alpha_T = 1 \tag{3.14}$$

3.5.4 Refraction in ultrasound

An ultrasound beam will be bent as it crosses an interface obliquely between two media. The relationship between incident and refraction angles is described by Snell's law:

$$\frac{\sin \theta_i}{\sin \theta_r} = \frac{c_i}{c_r} \tag{3.15}$$

where θ_i and θ_r are the incident and refracted angles, and c_i and c_r are the velocities in incidence and refractive media respectively.

Refraction is one of the major causes of artifacts in clinical ultrasound images. It adds spatial distortion to images and contributes to resolution loss.

3.5.5 Ultrasound transducers

Ultrasound transducers convert electrical energy into ultrasound energy and vice versa. The piezoelectric effect, discovered in 1880 by French physicists Pierre and Jacques

Curie [3.11], is exhibited by certain crystals: they develop a voltage across opposite surfaces in response to pressure applied [3.12]. This can be used to produce an electrical signal from ultrasound waves. Many crystals show this effect at low temperatures. The temperature above which a crystal's piezoelectric properties disappear is known as the Curie point of the crystal. The most frequently used man-made crystals are barium titanate, lead metaniobate, and lead zirconate titanate (PZT).

The crystal exhibits its greatest response at its resonance frequency, which is determined by the crystal thickness. Thin crystals yield high resonance frequencies. The Q value of the transducer describes the sharpness of the frequency response curve. Transducers in ultrasound must have short pulses and be responsive to a wide range of frequencies.

3.5.6 Ultrasound beams

Ultrasound waves generated from a source of large dimensions are represented as equally spaced straight lines, and are termed planar wavefronts. In contrast, a wave originating from a source of very small dimensions can be represented by spheres of increasing diameter at increasing distance from the source, and such waves are termed spherical wavefronts. With many spherical wavelets radiating from a transducer, regions of constructive and destructive interference are established in the medium. The region near the source where the interference of wavelets is most apparent is termed the Fresnel zone, near zone or near field; see Figure 3.11. For a disk-shaped transducer of radius r, the length L of the Fresnel zone is:

$$L_{Fresnel} = r^2/\lambda \tag{3.16}$$

Beyond the Fresnel zone, some of the energy escapes along the beam periphery, resulting in divergence of the beam that is described by:

$$\sin\theta = 0.6\lambda/r \tag{3.17}$$

where θ is the Fraunhofer divergence angle. The region beyond the Fresnel zone is termed the Fraunhofer or far zone. Long Fresnel zones are preferred in medical

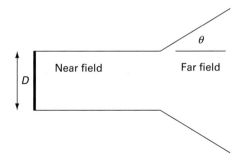

Figure 3.11   Near and far field of an ultrasound transducer.

applications of ultrasound. This can be achieved by using ultrasound of short wavelengths, which means employing high frequencies; as mentioned before, however, absorption of ultrasound energy increases at high frequencies.

Example 3.2 Compute the length of the Fresnel zone for a 20-mm diameter, 1-MHz ultrasound transducer.

Solution

$$\lambda = \frac{1540 \text{ m/sec}}{1 \times 10^6/\text{sec}} = 1540 \times 10^{-6} \text{ m} = 1.54 \text{ mm}$$

$$L_{\text{Fresnel}} = \frac{(10 \text{ mm})^2}{1.54 \text{ mm}} = 65 \text{ mm}$$

3.5.7 Ultrasound instrumentation

For displaying the echo-range information, there are several modes used. Three modes discussed here are: amplitude (A), brightness (B) and motion (M).

A-mode: In this mode, echoes returning from the body are displayed as signals on an oscilloscope. This presents a graph of voltage representing echo amplitude on the ordinate as a function of time on the abscissa. A-mode displays are no longer widely used.

B-mode: In this mode, the location of echo-producing interfaces is displayed in two dimensions (x and y) on a video screen. The amplitude of each echo is represented by the brightness value at the xy location. B-mode images may be displayed as either "static" or "real-time" images. In static imaging the image is compiled as the sound beam is scanned across the patient, and the image presents a snapshot averaged over the time required to sweep the sound beam. In real-time imaging, images follow one another in quick succession. At image frequencies greater than approximately 24 per second, the motion of moving structures seems continuous, even though it may appear that the images are flickering. Images that are refreshed at frequencies greater than approximately 48 per second are free of flicker. The real-time mode is useful in the display of moving structures such as heart valves.

M-mode: This depicts moving structures. In an M-mode display, the position of each echo-producing interface is presented as a function of time. The most important application of M-mode scanning is echocardiography, where the motion of various interfaces in the heart is depicted graphically on a cathode-ray tube (CRT) display.

In order to create ultrasound images, echo information must be received along discrete paths called scan lines. The time required to complete each line is determined by the speed of sound. In order to obtain a line of information, an ultrasound pulse is sent. The transducer is then quiescent for the remainder of the pulse repetition period (PRP), defined as the time from the beginning of one pulse to the next. During the quiescent time, echoes returning from interfaces within the patient excite the transducer and cause voltage pulses to be transmitted to the imaging device. These echoes are processed by the device and added to the image only if they fall within a preselected "listen time." Acquisition of echoes during the listen time provides information about reflecting interfaces along a single path in the object, which is the scan line.

The PRP determines the maximum field of view (FOV), which is the length of the scan lines:

$$\text{PRP} = \text{FOV (cm)} \times 13 \times 10^{-6} \text{ sec/cm} \tag{3.18}$$

The frame time (τ) is the time required to obtain a complete frame consisting of N scan lines:

$$\tau = \text{PRP} \times N \tag{3.19}$$

This time can be reduced by obtaining two or more scan lines simultaneously. The ratio of the largest to the smallest echo processed by an ultrasound device is known as the dynamic range of that device. This value decreases as signals pass through the imaging system.

Example 3.3 Compute the length of a scan line from ultrasound with PRP of 200 μs.

Solution

$$\text{Length of the scan line} = \frac{\text{PRP}}{13 \text{ μsec/cm}} = \frac{200}{13} = 15.38 \text{ cm}.$$

3.5.8 Ultrasound artifacts

Some artifacts which appear in ultrasound images include the following.

Multiple pathways: When an echo returns to a transducer, the imaging device assumes that the sound traveled in a straight line following a single reflection from some interface in the patient. The scan converter then places the brightness value at an appropriate location in the image. If the actual path of the echo involves multiple reflections, the echo will take longer to return, and the scan converter will place the interface at too great a depth in the image.

Refraction: Refraction sometimes causes displacement of the sound beam as it crosses tissue boundaries. Because the scan converter assumes that the ultrasound travels in straight lines, refraction causes displacement errors in positioning reflective interfaces in the image.

3.5.9 Doppler effect

The Doppler effect is used along with real-time pulse-echo imaging and motion mode (M-mode) for identification of moving structures. It has applications in clinical medicine,

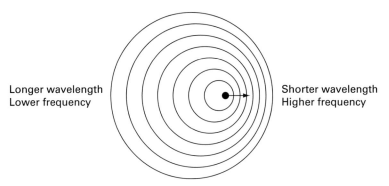

Figure 3.12 The Doppler effect.

such as detection of fetal heartbeat, blood pressure monitoring, detection of blood flow, and localization of blood vessel occlusions [3.13]. The principle of Doppler shift measurements is as follows: when there is relative motion between a source and a detector of ultrasound, the frequency of the detected ultrasound differs from that emitted by the source (see Figure 3.12). Consider an ultrasound source moving with velocity v_s towards a detector. After time t, the distance between the wavefront and the source is $(c - v_s)t$, where c is the velocity of the ultrasound in the medium. The wavelength λ of ultrasound in the direction of motion then becomes:

$$\lambda = (c - v_s)/v_0 \qquad (3.20)$$

where v_0 is the frequency of the ultrasound from the source. What is needed then is to calculate the frequency of the ultrasound that reached the detector:

$$v = c/\lambda = v_0\, c/(c - v_s) \qquad (3.21)$$

This means that the frequency of detected ultrasound shifts to a higher value when the source is moving towards the detector. The shift in frequency is Δv and is given by:

$$\Delta v = v - v_0 = [v_0 c/(c - v_s)] - v_0 = v_0\, v_s/(c - v_s) \qquad (3.22)$$

If the ultrasound source is moving away from the detector, then the wavelength of the ultrasound is:

$$\lambda - (c + v_s)/v_0 \qquad (3.23)$$

So the frequency shifts to a lower value, and the shift in frequency Δv is:

$$\Delta v = v - v_0 = v_0 c/(c + v_s) - v_0 = -v_0\, v_s/(c + v_s) \qquad (3.24)$$

If the velocity c of ultrasound is much greater than that of the source, then $c + v_s \cong c$. If the source and detector are at the same location, and an object is moving towards them at velocity v, then the frequency shift is:

$$\Delta v = 2\, v_0\ v/c \qquad (3.25)$$

where $c \gg v$; and for an object moving away from the source and the detector, the Doppler shift is:

$$\Delta v = 2 v_0 \ (-v/c) \tag{3.26}$$

This all assumes that the beam is parallel to the motion of the object. For the general case, where the beam strikes a moving object at an angle θ, the Doppler shift is:

$$\Delta v = 2 v_0 \ (v/c) \cos \theta \tag{3.27}$$

This angle between the beam and the direction of motion of the object is called the sonation angle.

Example 3.4 A 1.5-kHz Doppler shift is detected by a 5-MHz ultrasound transducer at a sonation angle of 45°. Compute the estimated velocity of blood flow.

Solution

$$v = \frac{\Delta vc}{2 v_0 \cos \theta} = \frac{(1.5 \times 10^3)(1.54 \times 10^5)}{2 \times 5 \times 10^6 \times 0.707} = 32.67 \ \text{cm/sec}$$

Note: 1540 m/sec is the speed of ultrasound in soft tissue [3.13].

3.6 Magnetic resonance imaging

In order to understand the principles of magnetic resonance imaging, we need to consider the properties of nuclei. Each proton in a nucleus has a property known as "spin." This means that it acts as a small magnet with a magnetic moment that has magnitude and direction. The magnetic moments of protons in a sample are initially oriented randomly, i.e. they are not aligned (see Figure 3.13). If a strong external magnetic field is applied to

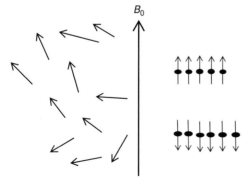

Figure 3.13 (Left) nuclear magnetic moments before applying external magnetic field, where they are oriented in random directions. (Right) Magnetic moments aligned after applying the external field: some of them are parallel to the static main field, while others are antiparallel.

the sample, the magnetic moments become aligned with the direction of the applied field (see Figure 3.13, right). The Earth's magnetic field (0.5 gauss) is not strong enough to produce this effect; hence MRI systems use a much stronger magnetic field (for example 20 000 gauss) to align all nuclear magnetic moments. Protons with spin parallel to the static main field are in a lower energy state than protons that are antiparallel, so this is the preferred state, and the net moment is parallel to the external field.

If there exists a photon with energy equal to the energy difference between the two states, then it can change a proton from the low-energy state to the high-energy state.

Rotating objects have the property of angular momentum that causes them to behave as gyroscopes. Nuclei react to forces just as objects with angular momentum respond to forces. Protons and other subatomic particles are assumed to rotate about their axes and are described as having spin. This kind of motion is known as precession. So the magnetic moments not only align with the field, but they also precess about it. Precession, illustrated in Figure 3.14, is a second order motion, as it is the rotation of the axis of a rotating object. A good example is the spinning top, which precesses about a vertical axis defined by the Earth's gravitational field. The frequency of precession f of a proton (in megahertz per tesla) depends mainly on the gyromagnetic ratio γ and the strength of the magnetic field B in tesla. This relationship is called the Larmor equation:

$$f = \gamma B \tag{3.28}$$

Example 3.5 Find the frequency of precession for protons in a 1.5 tesla magnetic field.

Solution

$$f = 42.6 \frac{\text{MHz}}{\text{tesla}} \times 1.5 = 63.9 \text{ MHz}. \tag{3.29}$$

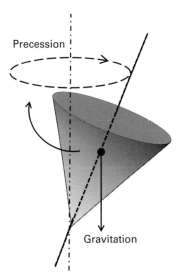

Figure 3.14 Precession of the magnetic moments around the main magnetic field.

3.6.1 Signal induction

Faraday's law states that a changing magnetic field can induce a current in a loop of conducting wire. Precessing protons act like small rotating magnets. Their magnetic fields intersecting a nearby coil will induce an electrical current inside that coil, and this forms the magnetic resonance (MR) signal.

The component of magnetization in the transverse plane (M_y) is responsible for the magnetization, and the induced MR signal is greatest when magnetic moments are tipped 90 degrees from M_z (axis parallel to the static main field) to the transverse plane. If the magnetization component is still parallel to M_z, there is no signal as it is parallel to the main field. From this, it is concluded that the component of magnetization in the transverse plane is responsible for MR signal induction.

The nuclei all precess at nearly the same frequency, but out of phase with each other. This means that their transverse components tend to cancel each other out. It is important that those individual magnetic moments are working together or pointing in the same direction, and thus an RF pulse is applied (see Figure 3.15) to bring the protons into phase. It does this by applying a force that acts in resonance with the physical system: when the RF frequency is equal to the Larmor frequency of the protons, the magnetic moments resonate and absorb a maximum amount of energy from the pulse. When the nuclear magnetic moments are brought into synchrony, they reinforce each other to produce a strong magnetic moment.

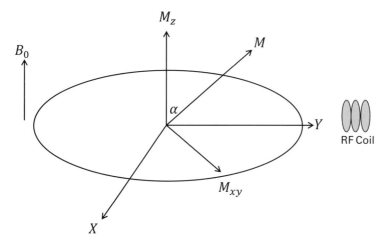

Figure 3.15 Applying the RF pulse nutates (flips) the net magnetization vector by the flip angle α from the longitudinal plane to the transverse plane. M refers to the magnetization tipped by this flip angle. M_z: component parallel to the external main field. M_{xy}: magnetization in the transverse xy plane, responsible for inducing MR signal. When $\alpha = 90$ degrees, this means the magnetization component will be perpendicular to M_z, and this is the greatest MR signal that can be induced. If the tip angle α is zero, this means there is no induced MR signal, as the magnetization component is parallel to M_z or the static main field. The RF coil collects the MRI signal.

3.6.2 Relaxation processes

When the RF pulse is applied to a sample, magnetization is nutated (flipped) into the transverse plane and an MRI signal is induced in the coil. When the radio wave is switched off, the signal decays away as the protons return to their original state. This is known as relaxation. There are two basic relaxation processes that occur.

T_1 *relaxation*, also called longitudinal or spin–lattice relaxation, is the process of the return of protons to their original alignment with the static external magnetic field. Spin–lattice refers to the interaction of spins or protons with their surroundings. The T_1 relaxation time can be defined as the time required for the signal to decrease to 37% of its original value by longitudinal relaxation.

T_2 *relaxation*, also known as transverse or spin–spin relaxation, involves the loss of synchrony of precession among the protons. When the radio wave is switched off, the protons start to interact with their neighbors, giving up energy in random collisions. The bulk magnetization strength is decreased as the magnetic moments tend to cancel each other. The T_2 relaxation time could also be defined as the time required for the MR signal to decrease to 37% of its original value by transverse relaxation.

Figure 3.16 shows T_1 and T_2 relaxation curves. The two processes occur at the same time, while T_2 is always shorter than T_1. This means that the magnetic moments dephase faster than they return into alignment with the static main field. T_1 might be several hundred milliseconds, while T_2 is a few tens of milliseconds.

The decay of the MRI signal is characterized by exponential expressions. For the longitudinal relaxation:

$$S = S_0 \, e^{-t/T_1} \tag{3.30}$$

which means that the original signal, S_0, of the MRI decreases exponentially to S. The value of S_0 is influenced by factors such as the number of protons in the sample, length of time the radio wave was applied to the sample, sensitivity of the receiver coil, and overall sensitivity of the electronics. For transverse relaxation,

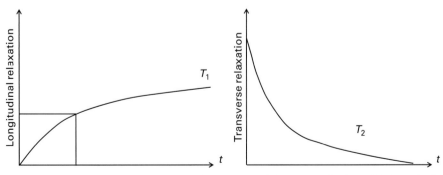

Figure 3.16 T_1, T_2 relaxation curves. T_1 shows return of protons to original state, aligning with the main field (i.e. the return to the original state is an exponential growth). T_2 shows loss of synchrony of the protons, and they lose some energy as they interact with each other.

$$S = S_0 \, e^{-t/T_2} \tag{3.31}$$

The overall effect of the two forms of relaxation can be obtained by combining the two equations:

$$S = S_0 \, e^{-t/T_1} \, e^{-t/T_2} \tag{3.32}$$

3.6.3 Pulse sequences

RF pulses must be applied so that coherent signals can be induced in receiver coils. The pulses are applied in specific sequences to produce signals that yield information about the sample. In every case, the RF pulse needs to tip the magnetization vector at some angle with respect to the static main field.

3.6.3.1 Free induction decay

This is the simplest pulse sequence, where the net magnetization vector is tipped by 90° (see Figure 3.17). The signal is induced in the coil immediately after applying the RF pulse. There are two major problems with this sequence:

- It is difficult to record the MR signal immediately after the 90° RF pulse is transmitted, because the transmitted signal is much stronger than that received at the coil. The large transmitted pulse produces ringing in the receiver coil which dissipates over several milliseconds, and during this time the coil is unable to receive any signal.
- T_2 relaxation is masked by another phenomenon, termed T_2^*, which is indistinguishable from the T_2 relaxation process, and is caused by magnetic field inhomogeneities across the sample that produce variations in the frequency of precession within the sample volume.

3.6.3.2 Spin echo

This sequence begins with an RF pulse that tips the net magnetization vector to 90°, so that the individual spins come into phase. The nuclei then start to dephase through the

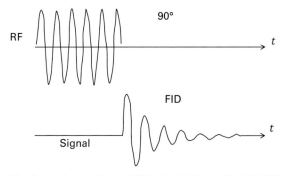

Figure 3.17 The free induction decay (FID) signal followed by 90° RF pulse.

effect of interaction of spins with each other (T_2 relaxation) and magnetic field inhomogeneities (T_2^* relaxation).

In order to remove the T_2^* effect, a 180° rephasing pulse is applied at time T after the initial RF pulse. This rephasing pulse flips all the spins. Thus, it takes spins that are precessing rapidly, and flips them over so that their phase is now behind the spins with lower precession rate. Flipping the slower spins sets them ahead of the mean precession rate. After a certain time, the faster spins catch up with the average spins, and the slower spins are caught by the average spins, so that all spins are in phase. When this happens, the spins are said to have "rephased." If dephasing has progressed for a time T between the initial RF pulse and the 180° pulse, then a time T is required after application of the rephasing pulse for the spins to rephase. The time after the initial RF pulse that the moment of exact rephasing occurs is referred to as T_E (time to echo) and is equal to $2T$. The entire sequence is repeated at a time T_R (repetition time) after the first 90° pulse. The repetition time T_R is at least 10 times T_E. Figure 3.18 illustrates the spin-echo pulse sequence.

3.6.3.3 Inversion recovery

This sequence starts with an initial 180° RF pulse that inverts spins. At a time T_I (inversion time) after the initial 180° pulse, a 90° pulse is applied. After this the inversion recovery sequence is the same as for spin echo. At a time T after the 90° pulse, a 180° rephasing pulse is given which produces a rephased signal at a time $T_E = 2T$ after the 90° pulse. As in all pulse sequences, the time between one complete pulse sequence and the next is defined as T_R.

The 180° pulse used at the beginning of inversion recovery allows more time for longitudinal relaxation of spins between pulse sequences than the smaller (e.g. 90°) pulses used in spin echo. Figure 3.19 shows the inversion recovery pulse sequence.

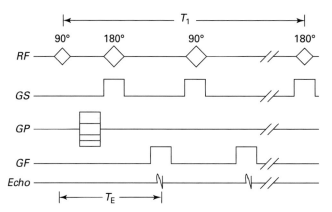

Figure 3.18 The spin-echo pulse sequence. A 90° RF pulse is applied, followed by a 180° rephasing pulse. GS, GP, and GF are the slice select, phase encoding, and frequency encoding gradients (to be discussed in detail later in this chapter). "Echo" is the signal received from the slice being imaged.

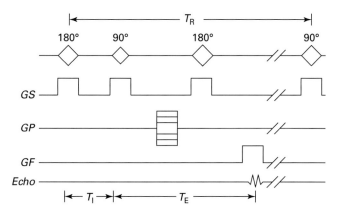

Figure 3.19   The inversion recovery pulse sequence. A 180° RF pulse is followed by a 90° pulse.

3.6.4 Spatial encoding

In order to form an image or to determine the origin of spectral information, the MR signals must be related to their points of origin within a sample. This is known as spatial encoding [3.1].

3.6.4.1 Sensitive point method

If the magnetic field is made to vary gradually across the patient, the frequency of precession and hence the resonance frequency of protons will also vary. So if the magnetic field is stronger at the patient's head and decreases gradually towards the feet, and an RF pulse is transmitted, then the pulse will resonate with protons somewhere along the patient. Selection of the gradient and the pulse frequency will result in resonance with protons in a selected transverse slice of the patient. The slice thickness is determined by the bandwidth of the RF pulse.

The procedure can be repeated in the other two orthogonal planes by using gradients to define sagittal and coronal planes. The intersection of the three planes defines a "sensitive point" for data acquisition. The procedure is repeated for each voxel. One main limitation with the sensitive-point technique is that excessive time is required to obtain enough information to construct an image. This technique only uses frequency encoding to establish a unique resonance frequency for each voxel in the patient. But signals may also be encoded according to their phase, and they may also be encoded by frequency a second time by using the Fourier transform.

3.6.4.2 Two-dimensional Fourier transform method

The most commonly used method of spatial encoding in commercial MRI systems is the two-dimensional Fourier transform (2DFT).

The *first step* is the activation of a slice-select gradient while a narrow-bandwidth RF pulse is sent. Only protons at the resonance frequency are nutated to a specific angle by the RF pulse; all other protons are unaffected. This gradient is usually applied in the

Z-direction. The other two axes are encoded by frequency and phase of the RF signals returning from the tissue.

The *second step* in the scheme is to apply a phase-encoding gradient in a direction perpendicular to the slice-encoding gradient. This gradient is turned off before any RF pulses are applied. When the gradient is turned on, it divides the slices into columns with different precessional frequencies, and when it is off, the protons return to the precessional frequency set by the main magnet; hence no difference in frequency exists from one column to the next. However, protons in the columns that earlier experienced a higher frequency of precession will have rotated further during the time that the phase-encoding gradient was on. Thus, when the gradient is turned off, the magnetization is locked in, with protons in different columns precessing at different phases of rotation. So the difference between columns is encoded by the phase of rotation [3.1].

The *third step* is to apply the frequency-encoding gradient at the time the RF signal is received from the patient. The effect of this gradient is to divide the slice into rows. While the RF receiver is turned on, protons in different rows precess at different frequencies, and the rows are encoded according to their frequency of rotation. Because the frequency-encoding gradient is turned on only during signal reception or "readout," it is often referred to as a "read gradient."

The *fourth step* of 2DFT is to apply the Fourier transform, which permits a complex data set to be acquired in a single set of measurements over a short period of time. The Fourier transform determines the contributions that were made by different pixels by transforming the MR signal acquired as a function of time to its mathematical representation as a function of frequency.

The *fifth step* is to repeat steps 1 to 4 a number of times and average the result. This averaging reduces the contribution of noise to the final data. The *sixth step* is to change the magnitude of the phase-encoding gradient and then repeat steps 2 to 5. The number of times that this step is carried out determines the number of columns into which the slice will be divided. In the seventh and *final step* of the 2DFT method, the second Fourier transform operates on the complex signal obtained after all of the phase-encoding steps have been completed.

The 2DFT method reduces the time significantly compared with the sensitive-point technique. The acquisition time, T_{aq}, required to obtain an image using this method is given by:

$$T_{aq} = N_a N_p T_R \qquad (3.33)$$

where N_a is the number of the signal averages, N_p is the number of phase-encoding steps, and T_R is the pulse repetition time (that is, the time the imager must wait to complete the selected pulse sequence).

3.6.5 Tissue contrast in MRI

There are many differences among human tissues in their relaxation times (T_1, T_2) and proton density $N(H)$. What is required is to maximize the contrast (difference in signal) between two materials in an MR image.

3.6.5.1 Spin echo

The strength intensity, S_{SE}, of the MR signal during a spin-echo pulse sequence is given by:

$$S_{SE} = N(H)\left(1 - 2e^{-(T_R - T_E/2)/T_1} + e^{-T_R/T_1}\right)e^{-T_E/T_2} \quad (3.34)$$

where $N(H)$ is the number of spins, T_1 is the longitudinal relaxation time constant, T_2 is the transverse relaxation time constant, T_E is the time to echo, and T_R is the pulse sequence repetition time.

T_1 and T_R appear together in an "exponential growth" term. Spin density, $N(H)$, appears as a scaling factor. If the spin density is doubled, the signal strength is doubled. If the only difference between two materials is in T_1, then the material having the shorter T_1 would produce a stronger signal at intermediate values of T_R. Generally, longer T_R values and shorter T_E values are always preferred for spin-echo imaging. Table 3.2 shows rules of thumb for contrast in spin-echo imaging [3.1].

3.6.5.2 Inversion recovery

The strength intensity of the MR signal during an inversion recovery pulse sequence is given by:

$$S_{IR} = N(H)\left(1 - 2e^{-T_I/T_1} + 2e^{-(T_R - T_E/2)/T_1} - e^{-T_R/T_1}\right)e^{-T_E/T_2} \quad (3.35)$$

where T_I is the inversion time (time between the initial 180° pulse and the next 90° pulse). The difference between this equation and the equation above is the complicated exponential growth term. T_1 weighting is influenced by both T_R and T_I.

3.6.6 Components of an MRI system

Main magnet: In MRI, the main magnet supplies the static main field. There is a wide range of field strengths from millitesla up to 10 tesla (used for research purposes). The higher the magnetic field strength, the better the signal; but T_1 also increases, which affects the selection of parameters for the pulse sequence. This in turn affects noise and patient motion. Higher field strengths also cause increased RF heating, difficulty in keeping magnetic field homogeneity, and chemical shift artifacts. Chemical shift artifacts occur because higher field strengths shift the resonance frequencies of fat and water molecules. This leads to the conclusion that lower field strengths might be better for imaging purposes.

Table 3.2 Rules for contrast in spin-echo imaging

T_R	T_E	Weighting	Factors for stronger signal
Short (~avg. T_1)	Short	T_1	Shorter T_1
Long (>4 T_1)	Short	$N(H)$	Greater $N(H)$
Long	Moderate (~ avg. T_2)	T_2	Longer T_2

There are two types of magnets: electromagnets and permanent magnets.

- *Electromagnets*: By twisting a conducting wire into the form of a coil, an electromagnet is formed. Two types of electromagnets are used in MR systems: resistive and superconductive. Any wire that carries an electric current is surrounded by a magnetic field, but a portion of this current is dissipated in the wire as heat because the conducting wire resists the flow of electrons. Thus resistive-type magnets must be water-cooled. For higher field strengths, conducting wires with zero resistance (superconducting wires) are needed. To maintain superconductivity, conductors must be kept near liquid helium temperature (−269 °C). This temperature is close to absolute zero (0 K, or −273 °C). Liquid helium is circulated around the superconducting wire in an insulating chamber called a dewar. A second insulating chamber, containing liquid nitrogen at −196 °C, is used to help maintain the helium in its liquid state. Superconducting magnets used in clinical MRI provide field strengths up to 2 tesla.
- *Permanent magnets*: These are made of ferromagnetic materials that have field strengths of up to 0.3 tesla.

Gradient coils: These provide the gradients needed for the spatial encoding of the MR signal. The generated magnetic field is much lower than the magnetic field of the main system magnet (Figure 3.20).

Radio-frequency coils: These coils send and receive the radio pulses. When pulses are transmitted into the patient, the coil is the source and the patient is the receiver. When the MR signal is read out, the patient is the source and the coil is the receiver. Accurate positioning of the patient within the sending coil is required to ensure that the region of interest is being imaged. The same coil may send and receive radio pulses.

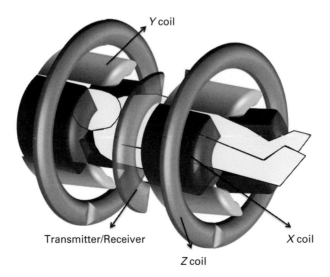

Figure 3.20 Magnetic field gradients in the x, y, and z directions.

The surface coil is practical for many parts of the human body. This is a loop of conducting material that is placed adjacent to the body part being imaged. One of the fundamentals of the surface coils is that the sensitivity of the coil decreases beyond a distance equal to the coil diameter, so coil positioning is an issue for performance.

Electronic components: A signal generator is used to produce the transmitted radio wave, where its magnitude is amplified with an RF amplifier. The receiver electronics include a mixer that combines the received signal with a reference signal at or near the Larmor frequency. The effect of mixing the signals is to subtract out the Larmor frequency, leaving only the small shifts in frequency that are used for spatially encoding the MR signal.

3.7 Summary

Medical imaging modalities and their associated technologies have revolutionized human lives by aiding our understanding of human health and disease. The diagnostic and therapeutic applications of medical imaging have revealed many secrets of the complexities of the human body. Early detection of cancer through diagnostic procedures (e.g., X-ray, CT, and MRI) has significantly increased the chances of survival for many patients worldwide. Medical imaging can be considered both as a science and as a tool to investigate human anatomy and to better understand its physiology and biochemistry. By reviewing basic equations of image formation in common imaging modalities, we hope that this chapter has served as a refresher of the basic physics involved in biomedical imaging.

3.8 Exercises

3.1 Describe the functions of the components in a basic X-ray tube.
3.2 Describe the mechanical features of the four generations of CT scanners.
3.3 Describe the *parallel-beam* back-projection reconstruction technique.
3.4 Create a model, using a phantom, resembling real-case X-ray attenuation among multiple layers with homogenous and inhomogeneous material.
3.5 Create a phantom to relate X-ray projections to 3D reconstructions from CT.
3.6 Explain the motion effects in MRI reconstruction. Construct a phantom to quantify the effects of linear motion on the quality of the reconstructed image.
3.7 Describe the collimator types used in nuclear medicine. Why is the converging collimator superior in some cases?
3.8 Why does refraction cause loss of resolution in ultrasound images?
3.9 What is the meaning of the piezoelectric effect?
3.10 List some artifacts that are present in ultrasound images.
3.11 Estimate the frequency shift for a 5 MHz ultrasound source moving toward a stationary detector in water at a speed of 15 cm/s. Is the frequency shifted to a higher or lower value?
3.12 List some medical applications of Doppler ultrasound.

References

[3.1] W. R. Hendee and E. R. Ritenour, *Medical Imaging Physics*. Hoboken, NJ: Wiley (2002).
[3.2] M. Ter-Pogossian, *The Physical Aspects of Diagnostic Radiology*. New York: Harper & Row (1967).
[3.3] W. R. Hendee, *Physical Principles of Computed Tomography*. Boston: Little Brown & Co. (1983).
[3.4] A. C. Kak and M. Slaney, *Principles of Computerized Tomographic Imaging*. New York: IEEE Press. (1987).
[3.5] R. K. Cacak, Measuring patient dose from computed tomography scanners. In Seeram, E. (ed.), *Computed Tomography*. Philadelphia: W.B. Saunders (2001) 199–208.
[3.6] H. Anger, Scintillation camera. *Rev. Sci. Instrum.* **29** (1958) 27.
[3.7] T. Budinger, Physical attributes of single-photon tomography. *J. Nucl. Med.* **21** (1980) 579–592.
[3.8] R. van Heertum, Current advances in hepatic SPECT imaging. In *Clinical SPECT Symposium*. Washington DC: American College of Nuclear Physicians (1986) 58–64.
[3.9] L. Friman and B. Soderberg, Spleen–liver ratio in RES scintigraphy: A comparison between posterior registration and emission computed tomography. *Acta Radiol.* **28** (1987) 439–441.
[3.10] B. Khan, P. Ell, P. Jarritti *et al.*, Radionuclide section scanning of the lungs in pulmonary embolism. *Br. J. Radiol.* **54** (1981) 586–591.
[3.11] K. F. Graff, Ultrasonics: Historical aspects. *Ultrasonics Symposium*. Phoenix: IEEE Conference Publications (1977) 1–10.
[3.12] W. McDicken, *Diagnostic Ultrasonics*. New York: John Wiley & Sons (1976).
[3.13] J. Reid and D. Baker, Physics and electronics of the ultrasonic Doppler method. In Bock. J. and Ossoining, K. (eds.), *Ultrasonographia Medica,* Vol. 1. *Proc. First World Congress on Ultrasonics in Medicine and SIDUO III*. Vienna Academy of Medicine (1971) 109.
[3.14] L. A. Shepp and B. F. Logan, The Fourier reconstruction of a head section. *IEEE Trans. Nucl. Sci.* **21** (1974) 21–43.

Appendix 3.1 Parallel beam filtered back-projection algorithm

CT construction of a single slice using the parallel beam filtered back-projection approach is illustrated in Figure A3.1. The MATLAB Code 3.1 below was used to implement the algorithm. It computes the parallel beam 2D projections of an object that is specified as a set of geometric shapes using the Radon transform.

Samples of filtered and unfiltered image reconstruction are shown in Figure A3.2. Code 3.2 shows a sample implementation of reconstruction from projections.

Mathematics of filtered back-projection technique for CT reconstruction

For better understanding of this important technique in CT reconstruction, mathematical details are presented.

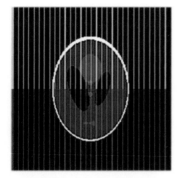
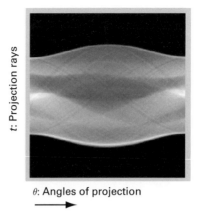

Rays enter in dark gray
and exit in light gray

t: Projection rays

θ: Angles of projection

Figure 3.A.1 Generated projections of a phantom brain using the Radon transform.

Code 3.1 Generate projections

function projections = generate_projections(IMG,THETA)

%% This MATLAB function takes an image matrix and vector of angles and then
%% finds the 1D projection (Radon transform) at each of the angles. It returns
%% a matrix whose columns are the projections at each angle.
%%

% pad the image with zeros so we don't lose anything when we rotate.
[iLength, iWidth] = size(IMG);
iDiag = sqrt(iLength^2 + iWidth^2);

%adding zeros as if to widen and lengthen the dimensions of the image so as
%not to lose info when rotation occurs. The addition is equal to the
%original image i.e. expanding the spatial support

LengthPad = ceil(iDiag -iLength) + 2;
WidthPad = ceil(iDiag -iWidth) + 2;

padIMG = zeros(iLength+LengthPad, iWidth+WidthPad);
padIMG(ceil(LengthPad/2):(ceil(LengthPad/2)+iLength-1), ...
    ceil(WidthPad/2):(ceil(WidthPad/2)+iWidth-1)) = IMG;

% loop over the number of angles, rotate 90-theta (because we can easily sum
% if we look at stuff from the top), and then add up. Don't perform any
% interpolation on the rotation.

% for movie generation
n = length(THETA);

projections = zeros(size(padIMG,2), n);
for i = 1:n
    tmpimg = imrotate(padIMG, THETA(i), 'bilinear', 'crop');
    projections(:,i) = (sum(tmpimg))';
end

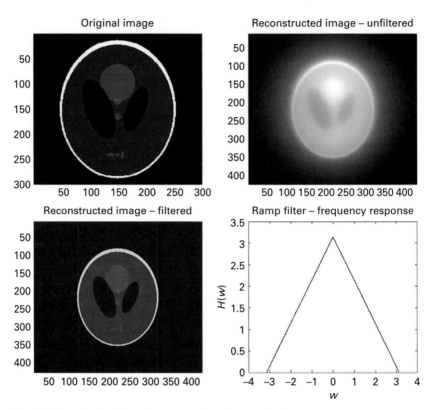

Figure 3.A.2 Sample filtered and unfiltered reconstructions from projections.

In order to obtain the projections $g_\theta(R)$, Figure A3.3, the Radon transform is used, which has the following formula

$$g_\theta(R) = \int_0^{2\pi} \int_0^\infty f(r,\phi)\delta\left(r\cos(\theta-\phi)-R\right)rdr\,d\phi, \qquad (3.A.1)$$

where $R = x\cos\theta + y\sin\theta$ (from Figure 3.6).

In back-projection, the measurements obtained are projected back along the same line. For a single projection at an angle θ

$$b_\theta(x,y) = \int_{R=-\infty}^\infty g_\theta(R)\delta(x\cos\theta + y\sin\theta - R)dR \qquad (3.A.2)$$

is the back-projected density for angle θ.

Adding up projections at all angles,

$$f_b(x,y) = \int_0^\pi b_\theta(x,y) = \int_0^\pi d\theta \int_{-\infty}^\infty g_\theta(R)\delta(x\cos\theta + y\sin\theta - R)dR.$$

$$= \int_0^\pi d\theta \int_{-\infty}^\infty g_\theta(R)\delta\left(r\cos(\theta-\phi)-R\right)dR.$$

Code 3.2 Reconstruction from projections

```
function [reconstructed_image,filter_response,w] = ...
            reconstruct_from_projection(projections,THETA,filter_type)

%% This is a MATLAB function that takes filtered back projections
%% PR is a matrix whose columns are the projections at each angle.
%% THETA is a row vector of the angles of the respective projections.

% figure out how big our image is going to be.
n = size(projections,1);
sideSize = n;

% filter the projections
[filtered_projections,filter_response,w] = filter_projections(projections,filter_type);

% convert THETA to radians
thetas = (pi/180)*THETA;

% set up the image
m = length(thetas);
reconstructed_image = zeros(sideSize,sideSize);

% find the middle index of the projections
midindex = (n+1)/2;

% set up x and y matrices
x = 1:sideSize;
y = 1:sideSize;
[X,Y] = meshgrid(x,y);
xproj = X -(sideSize+1)/2;
yproj = Y -(sideSize+1)/2;

% loop over each projection
for i = 1:m
   disp(['On angle', num2str(THETA(i))]);

   % figure out which projections to add to which spots
   filtIndex = round(midindex + xproj*cos(thetas(i)) +...
                     yproj*sin(thetas(i)));

   % if we are "in bounds" then add the point
   cur_reconstruction = zeros(sideSize,sideSize);
   spota = find((filtIndex > 0) & (filtIndex <= n));
   newfiltIndex = filtIndex(spota);
   cur_reconstruction(spota) = filtered_projections(newfiltIndex(:),i);

   reconstructed_image = reconstructed_image + cur_reconstruction;
end
reconstructed_image = reconstructed_image./m;
```

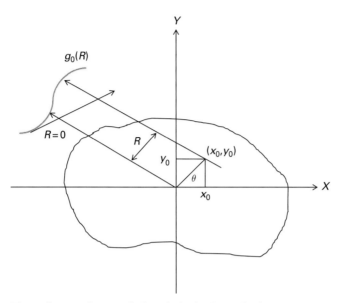

Figure 3.A.3 The Radon transform applied to obtain the CT projections.

The result is often called the laminogram reconstruction, which usually causes artifacts and distortions owing to the impulse response that causes blurring. In order to correct for the blurring, filtered back-projection is implemented, and the following steps are followed:

(a) A 1D Fourier transform is applied to the result, to obtain $\mathcal{F}\{g_\theta(R)\}$.
(b) Each projection is filtered by weighting $\mathcal{F}\{g_\theta(R)\}$ by a factor ρ.
(c) An inverse 1D Fourier transform is applied on the result of (b), to obtain $a_\theta(R) = \mathcal{F}^{-1}\{\mathcal{F}\{g_\theta(R)\} \times |\rho|\}$.
(d) Laminogram reconstruction is performed: $\int_0^\pi d\theta \int_{-\infty}^{\infty} a_\theta(R)\delta(x\cos\theta + y\sin\theta - R) \, dR$.

In general, filtered back-projection is fast, as it does not include 2D Fourier transforms.

Part II
Stochastic models

4 Random variables

4.1 Introduction

Statistical experiments are conducted in order to infer information about various processes and thus to guide decision making. The effectiveness of a certain drug on a particular disease, surgical procedures, therapy techniques, or demographic effects on disease are a few examples of statistical inference based on a statistical experiment.

A statistical experiment may be described in terms of a population, a phenomenon to be investigated, and a scaling procedure to quantify the spread of the phenomena in a population. Traditionally, a statistical experiment E is described in terms of a trilogy:

- the sample space Ω, which is the set of all possible elementary outcomes (the 'alphabet' of the experiment);
- the field σ_F, which is the set of all measurable events;
- probability measure P, which is a positive scalar function measuring the occurrence of the events; i.e. it assigns probabilities to events on σ_F.

That is, $E = \{\Omega, \sigma_F, P\}$. [4.1]

The form and level of complexity of each of these components depend on the specifics of the experiment. The power of statistical theory is in its ability to describe experiments of varying levels of complexity. This chapter will discuss the basic elements that describe statistical experiments. In particular, we shall focus on the concepts of random variables and random process. In the following chapter we discuss their generalizations to random fields.

Navigating through the extensive literature of statistics is not easy; indeed, it is a difficult task given space limitations as well as the purpose of the book. We must therefore say upfront that there is no unique approach to selecting what subjects to cover and what is an appropriate level of rigor. However, our experience dictates that understanding the foundations of statistical theory is essential for many approaches to image analysis. This chapter is a tour of some of the common terminologies and basics of statistical modeling that are essential to appreciate the material covered in the book. The chapter aims to make the statistical literature accessible, so that readers can learn more beyond what is covered here.

4.2 Statistical experiments

We follow the tradition of describing a statistical experiment in terms of $E = \{\Omega, \sigma_F, P\}$.

4.2.1 Sample space Ω

The sample space Ω enumerates the elementary outcomes of an experiment, and by construct, various combinations of them as well. For example, if $a_1, a_2, \ldots, a_N \in \Omega$ for some $N \in \mathbb{N}$ are the elementary outcomes of E (i.e. its single-valued possibilities), one might think that combinations of these outcomes should be included in Ω. However, some combinations may never happen. Hence, it is the tradition to list only the elementary outcomes (elements of the alphabet) in Ω, and the events (all possible combinations of the elementary outcomes, or the 'dictionary' of the experiment) are given a special entity, denoted by a *field* or *algebra* σ_F.

4.2.2 Field (algebra) σ_F

As the events need to be scaled or measured, an enumeration procedure is needed to generate the dictionary of events. Those that will not happen will be given zero weight or measure. Therefore, desirable characteristics of σ_F will be such that it will be *closed* under all countable (may be infinite in number) inclusions of elementary events, such as *unions*. Specifically, we define σ_F for events $A_1, A_2, \ldots, A_N \in \Omega$ and $N \in R$ such that:

(a) The empty set (or null event) $\emptyset$ and the sample space (sure event) Ω must be in σ_F.
(b) $A_1, A_2, \ldots, A_N \in \Omega$ implies that $\cup_{i=0}^{\infty} A_i \in \sigma_F$ for all $A_1, A_2, \ldots, A_N \in \Omega$.
(c) If $A_i \in \sigma_F$ then $\overline{A_i} \in \sigma_F$, where $\overline{A_i}$ is the complement of A_i.

The above requirements are all natural results of the field σ_F being an inclusive space that spans (includes) all measurable events.

4.2.3 Probability measure P

The probability measure P is a function that assigns weights to the events in σ. It is the tradition to have a positive scale normalized to the unit interval. Events may be related (dependent) or unrelated (independent) to each other. Events also may be joint (share some elementary outcomes) or disjoint (share no elementary outcomes) in their constructs. Therefore, the probability measure P must satisfy the following requirements (axioms):[4.2]

(a) $P(A_i) \geq 0$ for all events $A_1, A_2, \ldots, A_N \in \Omega$ and $N \in \mathbb{N}$.
(b) The empty set (or null event) $\emptyset$ has zero weight and the sample space (sure event) Ω has a weight of 1; that is, $P(\emptyset) = 0$ and $P(\Omega) = 1$.
(c) If $A_1, A_2, \ldots, A_N \in \Omega$ then $P(\cup_{i=1}^{N} A_i) = \Sigma_{i=1}^{N} P(A_i)$ if the events $A_1, A_2, \ldots, A_N \in \Omega$ are **mutually** disjoint, i.e. mutually exclusive.

As a consequence of axioms (b) and (c), if $\overline{A_i}$ is the complement of A_i, then $P(\overline{A_i}) = 1 - P(A_i)$.

4.2 Statistical experiments

Example 4.1 Consider a histology experiment conducted on cells from a tissue specimen taken during a procedure to determine the existence of cancer. In this experiment tissue is treated and viewed under a microscope, with viewed cells being cancerous (C) or noncancerous (NC). As biopsies are performed after reasonable suspicion to justify doing them, the weights of the C and NC events differ with procedure. The radiologist orders the pathology to confirm diagnosis that cannot be made with certainty. A pathologist may err. Hence, there are levels of pathological tests as well. A possible statistical experiment may be described as follows:
$\Omega = \{C, NC\}$, $\sigma = \{\emptyset, \Omega, C, NC\}$, $P(C) = \gamma$ and $P(NC) = 1 - \gamma$.

Example 4.2 Consider the same experiment as in Example 4.1, in which the agent used to prepare the tissue produced inconclusive results when viewing the cells under the microscope. The histologist chart showed unspecified cells (US) under these circumstances. That is, the sample space became: $\Omega = \{C, NC, US\}$. As these events are independent, the sigma algebra would be simply the collection of five possibilities: $\sigma = \{\emptyset, \Omega, C, NC, US\}$, and the probability measure will be such that $P(C) = \gamma$, $P(NC) = \beta$ and $P(US) = 1 - (\gamma + \beta)$.

Example 4.3 Consider the experiment of recording the life span of cells in a specimen under the effect of an agent. Suppose that the viewing domain of the microscope allows individual cells to be viewed and tracked, and that it is possible to tag each cell as it moves within the specimen until its death. A counting experiment is expected to be a tedious one, especially if the cells move a lot, but a histogram may be constructed indicating the number of cells that die with time.

Events containing similar elementary outcomes are called *joint*, while those with no common elementary outcomes are classed as *disjoint* Probability measures on disjoint events are *additive*. Events with no bearing on each other are called *independent*. Probability measures on independent events are *multiplicative*. As cause and effect is a natural rule of physics, it is also logical to ask the likelihood of related events with respect to each other. *Conditional probability* addresses this issue, providing the value of the probability of an event given that another event took place as the ratio of their joint probability normalized by the probability of the second event. We formally define these concepts as follows.

DEFINITION 4.1 *Two events A_1 and A_2 in the same sample space Ω are said to be disjoint if their intersection is empty; i.e., $A_1 \cap A_2 = \emptyset \in \Omega$.* ∎

DEFINITION 4.2 *Two events A_1 and A_2, not necessarily in the same sample space Ω, are said to be independent if their joint probability measure is multiplicative; i.e., $P(A_1 \cap A_2) = P(A_1) P(A_2)$.* ∎

DEFINITION 4.3 *The conditional probability measure of event A_1 given the occurrence of event A_2, where A_1 and A_2 are not necessarily in the same sample space Ω, is denoted by $P(A_1 | A_2)$ and is defined by: $P(A_1|A_2) = \dfrac{P(A_1 \cap A_2)}{P(A_2)}$ provided that $P(A_2) \neq 0$.* ∎

The expression for the conditional probability in Definition 4.3 is usually called Bayes' Theorem. As a direct corollary of the above definitions, independent events do not affect the value of the conditional probability measure. Likewise, disjoint events have a zero-valued joint probability measure and, consequently, a zero-valued conditional probability measure.

Example 4.4 Consider events $A_1, A_2 \in \Omega$ where A_1 is a subset of A_2; that is, $A_1 \subset A_2$. It follows that the conditional probability $P(A_1|A_2) = \dfrac{P(A_1)}{P(A_2)} \leq P(A_1)$ and that the joint probability measure $P(A_1 \cup A_2) = P(A_2)$.

A stimulus may affect a set of events even though they are disjoint. In this case, conditional probabilities enable the overall effect of that stimulus to be measured. For example, suppose that an experiment produces three disjoint events $A_1, A_2, A_3 \in \Omega$ such that $A_i \cap A_j = \Phi$; $i, j \in [1, 3]$. We can measure the effect of a stimulus (i.e., another event) B on the set of events by noting that $B = \bigcup_{i=1}^{3} (B \cap A_i)$, and since the intersections are disjoint as well, then the probability measure $P(B)$ is additive with respect to the components $P(B \cap A_i)$; i.e., $P(B) = \sum_{i=1}^{3} P(B \cap A_i)$, which can be written in terms of conditional expectations as: $P(B) = \sum_{i=1}^{3} P(B|A_i)P(A_i)$. This can be generalized to a larger number of events in what is known as the *total probability theorem*, which is stated below.

THEOREM 4.1 *Consider a set of events $A_1, A_2, \ldots, A_N \in \Omega$ and $N \in R$. Suppose the events are mutually disjoint, i.e., they span the sample space Ω. Consider an event $B \subset \Omega$. We can show that $P(B) = \sum_{i=1}^{N} P(B|A_i)P(A_i)$.*

The proof of the total probability theorem follows from the fact that the probability measure of disjoint events is analytically additive.[4.2]

In general, listing the events in Ω and σ_F will be a difficult if not impossible task with real-world problems. Likewise, obtaining the corresponding functional form for the probability measure P will be hard to accomplish. A logical task for statisticians has been to search for automatic procedures to generate events and their probability measure for particular experiments. The general approach that has evolved to accomplish this uses the concept of random functions, commonly referred to as *random variables*. This type of function maps events in the sample space and the sigma algebra, which may be quite abstract, into another representation in the Cartesian domain. In this domain, it is possible to assign a scale (measure or weight) using the common tools of calculus. We examine this concept next, as a prelude to describing multivariable experiments and complicated stochastic phenomena.

4.3 Random variables

4.3.1 Basic concepts

A random variable $X(\omega)$ is a function that maps from the sigma algebra σ_F into the real line R such that the event $\{\omega \in \Omega : X(\omega) \leq a\} \in \sigma_F$. As illustrated in Figure 4.1, the random variable maps events in σ_F into other forms of events (sets) defined on the real line; these sets are called *Borel* sets, and their "mass" corresponds to the probability of the events that the random variable goes between. For compact representation, we insist that the inverse mapping of the Borel sets should be events in σ_F; i.e., the set $\{X^{-1}(a) : a \in B \subset R\} \in \sigma_F$ for all Borel sets $B \subset R$. [4.3]

To avoid potential confusion over the difference between the sample space and the sigma algebra vis-à-vis the random variable, we use, as stated before, the alphabet of the experiment to represent Ω and its dictionary to represent σ_F. Recall that the sample space is formed of elementary outcomes. Measurable events form the sigma-algebra, based on measurability conditions. Random variables map events (in the sample space or the sigma-algebra) onto Borel sets. Hence, $X(\omega)$ is technically a mapping from σ_F into R. Of course, it is understood that events in σ_F are formed of elementary outcomes, i.e., must subsequently be contained in Ω. Like any function, $X(\omega)$ has a domain, which will be σ_F, and a range, which is the real line R. Hence, a shorthand for this relationship would be as follows: $X(\omega): \sigma_F \to R$.

Domains and ranges may be continuous or discrete. We will consider cases both where the mapping is between continuous entities, in which $X(\omega)$ will be denoted as a *continuous random variable*, and where the mapping is between discrete entities, in which $X(\omega)$ will be denoted as a *discrete random variable*. As the mapping is between events, the weights (measures) of the two ends of the mapping must be the same. That is, in the illustration shown in Figure 4.1, we must have $P(A) = P(B)$.

We shall provide a few illustrative examples to demonstrate the power of the random variable concept in describing a statistical experiment.

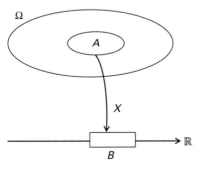

Figure 4.1 Illustration of the random variable as a mapping function from the sample space of the sigma algebra into Borel sets on the real line.

Random variables

Example 4.5 Consider the experiment in Example 4.1 above. Suppose we have a function $X(\omega)$ which takes an arbitrary value of 1 for C and -1 for NC. It is evident that we can establish events $\{\omega \in \Omega : X(\omega) \leq a\} \in \sigma_F$. In particular, we have the following possibilities:

$$\{\omega \in \Omega : X(\omega) \leq a\} = \begin{cases} \varnothing & \text{if } a < -1 \\ \Omega & \text{if } a > 1 \\ C & \text{if } a = 1 \\ NC & \text{if } a = -1. \end{cases}$$

The above example illustrates a discrete-valued random variable, which has a finite range and domain. Figure 4.2 illustrates this mapping.

Example 4.6 Suppose a statistical experiment has sample space $\Omega = \{\omega_i = i, i \in [1,8]\}$ consisting of eight elementary outcomes. Consider a function $X(\omega_i) = 5i$. We may illustrate that $X(\omega_i)$ is a discrete-valued random variable in Ω by examining whether $\{\omega \in \Omega : X(\omega) \leq a \in R\}$ is an event. It is evident that:

$$\{\omega \in \Omega : X(\omega) \leq a\} = \begin{cases} \varnothing & \text{if } a < 1 \\ \Omega & \text{if } a > 40 \\ \{i \in [1,8]\} \in \Omega & \text{if } a = 5i \end{cases}$$

Hence, $X(\omega_i) = 5i$ is a random variable.

The above illustrates the value of the random variable concept as an event generator. Equally important is to see whether the random variable will also enable measurability of the generated events. In other words, can we evaluate $P\big(\{\omega \in \Omega : X(\omega) \leq a\}\big)$? The ability to evaluate this quantity achieves the measurability requirements for the events in σ_F, and thus completely describes the statistical experiment. Indeed, the

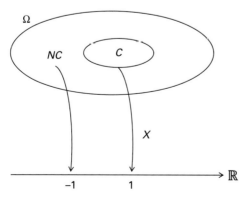

Figure 4.2 Illustration of the domain and range of a discrete-valued random variable.

quantity $P(\{\omega \in \Omega : X(\omega) \leq a\})$ has a special name in mathematical statistics: it is known as the cumulative probability distribution function (CDF). From its definition, the event shrinks as $a \to -\infty$ and expands as $a \to \infty$; therefore, the CDF is non-decreasing. Indeed, it is also monotonic (continuous from right); that is: $\lim_{\partial \to 0} P(\{\omega \in \Omega : X(\omega) \leq a + \partial\}) = P(\{\omega \in \Omega : X(\omega) \leq a\})$. As the CDF is a fundamental concept in the theory of statistics, we need to examine it in more detail. We will, for ease of notation, denote the CDF as $P(X \leq x)$ and will give it the special symbol $F_X(x)$. To make the notations consistent, we shall define the CDF formally as follows:

DEFINITION 4.4 *Given a random variable $X(\omega)$ defined for a statistical experiment $E = \{\Omega, \sigma_F, P\}$, the cumulative probability distribution (CDF) of $X(\omega)$ is a function on the real line which measures the event $\{\omega \in \Omega : X(\omega) \leq x\}$. We denote this function as $F_X(x) = P(\{\omega \in \Omega : X(\omega) \leq x \in B \subset R\}) = P(X \leq x)$, for every Borel set $B \subset R$.* ∎

The CDF, like any function, may be studied from the theory of calculus. Thus the concept of the random variable transforms the description of statistical experiments and statistical theory from an apparent guessing game into a well-founded mathematical theory. The monotonic nature and hence continuity of $F_X(x)$ is evident from the definition. We can easily infer the following properties of the CDF function $F_X(x)$:

(i) $0 \leq F_X(x) \leq 1$
(ii) $F_X(x)$ is differentiable over R.

DEFINITION 4.5 *The probability density function (PDF) $f_X(x)$ of a random variable X is the derivative of the CDF function; i.e., $f_X(x) = \dfrac{d F_X(x)}{dx}$.* ∎

We shall see later that both $f_X(x)$ and $F_X(x)$ enable various studies related to the experiment under consideration.

The differentiability of the CDF is a functional property due to its continuity, and does not imply that the random variable itself (the function that maps events to Borel sets on the real line) is continuous or discrete. The distinction between continuous and discrete random variables is in the form of the Borel sets that are generated from the mapping. A discrete random variable means that its domain may take only finite but discrete values, i.e., the Borel sets are discrete; whereas a continuous random variable has a continuous domain, i.e., the Borel sets are continuous. As a consequence of these characteristics, we may be able to define the probability of a point event for discrete random variables; i.e. $P(\{\omega_i \in \Omega : X(\omega_i) = x_i \in B \subset R\}) = P(X = x_i) \underset{=}{\text{def}} p_i$. Point events for continuous random variables are empty sets; i.e., their measures will be zero. The implications for these characteristics and differentiability of $F_X(x)$ are such that the following distinctions will be made between discrete and continuous random variables:

$$F_X(x) = \begin{cases} P(X \leq x) = \int_{-\infty}^{x} f_X(\alpha)\, d\alpha & \text{for continuous random variables} \\ P(X \leq x) = \sum_{i=-\infty}^{i=\infty} p_i u(x - x_i) & \text{for discrete random variables,} \end{cases}$$

where $p_i \underset{=}{\text{def}} P(X = x_i)$ and $u(x)$ is the unit step function. \hfill (4.1)

For the integer-valued case, the set $i \in R: X \leq x$ will be integer-valued and the upper limit of the summation in Eq. (4.1) will be easy to determine. If we use the generalized function representation, we may express the PDF for the discrete random variables in terms of the Dirac delta function, i.e., $\delta(x) = \dfrac{du(x)}{dx}$; hence,

$$f_x(x) = \sum_{i=-\infty}^{i=\infty} p_i \delta(x - x_i). \tag{4.2}$$

Therefore, a unified expression for the CDF may be written for both continuous and discrete random variables in terms of an integral functional only; i.e., $P(X \leq x) = \int_{-\infty}^{x} f_X(\alpha) \, d\alpha$. In practice, however, a clear distinction will be implicit in terms of the definition of the experiment and the values that events may take. Indeed, in principle, we may define a random variable to describe events that have both continuous and discrete domains. Below, we provide illustrative examples for the CDF and PDF for various random variables.

Example 4.7 Consider a random variable with the CDF shown in Figure 4.3 which has the following functional form:

$$F_X(x) = \begin{cases} 0 & \text{if } x < -1 \\ \dfrac{1}{3}(x+1) & \text{if } -1 \leq x < 0 \\ \dfrac{1}{3}(x+1) & \text{if } 0 \leq x < 1 \\ 1 & \text{if } 1 \leq x < \infty \end{cases}$$

∎

We note that the CDF in this example is not differentiable at $x = -1, 0, 1$. The problem, however, is at $x = 0$ where the CDF has a jump (discontinuity) of size $\dfrac{1}{3}$. We can address the behavior of the CDF at the jump by noting that: $P(X = 0) = P(X \leq 0) - P(X < 0) = \dfrac{2}{3} - \lim_{\varepsilon \to 0} P(X \leq 0 - \varepsilon) = \dfrac{2}{3} - \dfrac{1}{3} = \dfrac{1}{3}$.

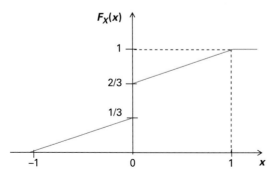

Figure 4.3   The CDF of a mixed random variable.

Hence, functional analysis enables us to address the various characteristics that the CDF may have.

4.3.2 Properties of the CDF and the PDF of a random variable

As the CDF is a probability measure for the event $\{\omega \in \Omega : X(\omega) \leq a\} \in \tilde{\sigma}$ then the positivity and upper bound of the CDF are evident. Likewise, as the name implies, the CDF is non-decreasing and monotonic, hence the continuity from the right is evident. We can infer the properties of the CDF for disjoint events as well as independent events using the basic definitions. We also note that the following identities follow straight from the definition of the CDF:

$$F_X(-\infty) = 0; \tag{4.3a}$$

$$F_X(\infty) = 1; \tag{4.3b}$$

$$F_X(x_1) \leq F_X(x_2) \text{ if } x_1 \leq x_2; \tag{4.3c}$$

$$\text{if } F_X(x_0) = 0, \text{ then } F_X(x) = 0 \text{ for all } x \leq x_0; \tag{4.3d}$$

The PDF, being a derivative of the CDF, is positive and summable. We can write the PDF for a discrete random variable as:

$$f_X(x) = \frac{F_X(x + \Delta x) - F_X(x)}{\Delta x} \tag{4.4}$$

The most important virtue of the CDF is its ability to provide a computational mechanism (or algorithm) to evaluate the probability measure through summation (discrete random variables) or integration (continuous random variables). Some examples will illustrate these concepts.

Example 4.8 Consider a statistical experiment defined within the boundaries illustrated in Figure 4.1. Suppose the mass function of the Borel sets is such that they have an exponential form:

$$m_B(\gamma) = f_X(x) = 0.5 \, e^{-0.25 \, x} u(x), \text{ for } \{\gamma \in B : m_B(\gamma) = 0.5 \, e^{-0.25 \, \gamma} u(\gamma)\} \in R.$$

We can evaluate the probability measure of the event $\{\omega \in \Omega : X(\omega) \leq a\} \in \sigma_F$ by the mass of its equivalent Borel set $\{\gamma \in B : m_B(\gamma) = 0.5 \, e^{-0.25 \, \gamma} u(\gamma)\} \in R$. In particular, we can evaluate the probability of such events as:

$$P\{\omega \in \Omega : a \leq X(\omega) \leq b\} \in \sigma_F = \int_a^b f_X(x) dx = 2(e^{-0.25 \, a} - e^{-0.25 \, b}).$$

Over the long history of statistics, various functional forms for $f_X(x)$ have been obtained for specific practical experiments. Some of the most common PDFs are listed in

Table 4.1 Common PDF functional forms.

Name	Continuous PDF	Discrete PDF
Uniform	$f_X(x) = \dfrac{1}{A-B}\left(u(x-B) - u(x-A)\right)$	$p_i = \dfrac{1}{N}; x \in \{x_i, i \in [A,B], N = B - A\}$
Exponential	$f_X(x) = A e^{-\beta x}\left(u(x-a) - u(x-b)\right),$ $a \leq b \in R$	$f_X(x) = A e^{-\beta x}\left(u(x-a) - u(x-b)\right),$ $a \leq b \in R$; discrete-valued
Gaussian	$f_X(x) = \dfrac{1}{\sqrt{2\pi\sigma^2}} e^{-\frac{(x-\mu)^2}{2\sigma^2}}, \; x \in R$	N/A
Cauchy	$f_X(x) = \dfrac{a/\pi}{a^2 + x^2}, x \in R$	N/A
Laplace	$f_X(x) = \dfrac{a}{2} e^{-a|x|}, \; x \in R$	N/A
Rayleigh	$f_X(x) = \dfrac{x}{a^2} e^{-\frac{x^2}{2\sigma^2}}, \; x \in R$	N/A
Maxwell	$f_X(x) = \dfrac{\sqrt{2}}{\sqrt{\pi}\, a^3} x^2 e^{-\frac{x^2}{2\sigma^2}} u(x)$	N/A
Gamma	$f_X(x) = \dfrac{\theta^{c+1} x^c e^{-\theta x}}{\Gamma(c+1)} u(x)$	N/A
Beta	$f_X(x) = \dfrac{\Gamma(\alpha_1 + \alpha_2) x^{(\alpha_1 - 1)} (1-x)^{(\alpha_2 - 1)}}{\Gamma(\alpha_1)\Gamma(\alpha_2)},$ $x \in (0,1)$ $f_X(x) = \dfrac{x^{(\alpha_1 - 1)} (1-x)^{(\alpha_2 - 1)}}{\beta(\alpha_1, \alpha_2)},$ $x \in (0,1)$	N/A
Binomial	N/A	$P(X = k) = p_k = \binom{n}{k} \theta^k (1-\theta)^{n-k},$ n: independent trails θ: probability of success in each trail
Poisson	N/A	$P(X = k) = p_k = \dfrac{\theta^k e^{-\theta}}{k!}, k$ $\in [0, \infty); \theta$ is frequency of occurrence of the event

Table 4.1. The parameters in the CDF forms in Table 4.1 represent the modes as well as resolution measures of the functions and will be addressed later on. It is important to remember the context of the definitions of the CDF and the PDF, and the brilliance of the statisticians, physicists and mathematicians who, over the years, have developed these tools that enable proper description and characterization of statistical experiments.

4.3.3 The conditional distribution

The CDF and the PDF may be defined for conditional events. For example, we may study the behavior of an event A defined such that $A = \{\omega \in \Omega : X(\omega) \leq x \in B \subset R\} \underset{\text{def}}{=} \{X \leq x\}, x \in R$ with respect to another event B which may or may not be defined on the same sample space. We can consider the conditional CDF as a measure of event $\{X \leq x|B\}$ in the same way we defined the conditional probability before:

$$F_{X|B}(x|B) \underset{\text{def}}{=} P(X \leq x|B) = \frac{P(X \leq x, B)}{P(B)} \qquad (4.5)$$

We point out that $\{X \leq x, B\}$ means that $\{\omega \in \Omega : X(\omega) \leq x \in R, B\}$, and the event may or may not be a subset of the same sample space Ω. It is straightforward to prove that the conditional CDF possesses all the properties of the CDF as discussed before. In particular, it is straightforward to justify the following properties: $F_{X|B}(\infty|B) = 1$, $F_{X|B}(-\infty|B) = 0$, and $P(x_1 \leq X \leq x_2) = F_{X|B}(x_2|B) - F_{X|B}(x_1|B)$ for $x_1 \leq x_2$ and $x_1, x_2 \in R$.

Indeed, the total probability theorem that we studied before may be expressed as follows: consider a partition $\mathsf{P} = \{B_1, B_2, \ldots, B_N\}$ on a sample space Ω with known a priori measures $P(B_i)$ for $i \in [1, N]$. Any event $A = \{\omega \in \Omega : X(\omega) \leq x \in B \subset R\}$ may be defined in terms of the partition P such that $A = \cup_{i=1}^{N} AB_i$, and the CDF for random variable X will be defined as follows:

$$F_X(x) \underset{\text{def}}{=} P(X \leq x) = P(A) = P\left(\bigcup_{i=1}^{N} AB_i\right) = \sum_{i=1}^{N} P(AB_i) \qquad (4.6)$$

$$= \sum_{i=1}^{N} P(A|B_i) P(B_i) = \sum_{i=1}^{N} F_{X|B_i}(x|B_i) P(B_i).$$

In the same way that we studied the probability density function (PDF) before, we can also define the conditional PDF; that is, for continuous random variables we have:

$$f_{X|B}(x|B) = \frac{d F_{X|B}(x|B)}{dx}. \qquad (4.7)$$

Example 4.9 Consider the two events $A_1 = \{\omega \in \Omega : X(\omega) \leq x \in R\}$ and $A_2 = \{\omega \in \Omega : X(\omega) \leq a \in R\}$. We can show that:

$$F_{X|A_2}(x|A_2) \underset{\text{def}}{=} \frac{P(X(\omega) \leq x, X(\omega) \leq a)}{P(X(\omega) \leq a)} = \begin{cases} 1 & \text{if } x \geq a \\ \frac{P(X(\omega) \leq x)}{P(X(\omega) \leq a)} = \frac{F_X(x)}{F_X(a)} & \text{if } x < a. \end{cases}$$

By derivatives, we obtain the conditional PDF

$$f_{X|A_2}(x|A_2) \underset{\text{def}}{=} \frac{d F_{X|A_2}(x|A_2)}{dx} = \begin{cases} 0 & \text{if } x \geq a \\ \frac{f_X(x)}{F_X(a)} & \text{if } x < a. \end{cases}$$

Example 4.10 Consider the events $A_1 = \{\omega \in \Omega : X(\omega) \leq x \in R\}$ and $A_2 = \{\omega \in \Omega : b < X(\omega) \leq a \in R, \, a > b\}$. We can show that:

$$F_{X|A_2}(x|A_2) \stackrel{\text{def}}{=} \frac{P(X(\omega) \leq x, b < X(\omega) \leq a)}{P(b < X(\omega) \leq a)} = \begin{cases} 0 & \text{if } x \leq b \\ 1 & \text{if } x \geq a \\ \frac{P(b \leq X(\omega) < x)}{P(X(\omega) \leq a)} = \frac{F_X(x) - F_X(b)}{F_X(a) - F_X(b)} & \text{if } b \leq x < a. \end{cases}$$

The conditional PDF will be:

$$f_{X|A_2}(x|A_2) \stackrel{\text{def}}{=} \frac{d F_{X|A_2}(x|A_2)}{dx} = \begin{cases} \frac{f_X(x)}{F_X(a) - F_X(b)} & \text{if } b \leq x < a \\ 0 & \text{otherwise.} \end{cases}$$

The conditional distribution is an important mechanism to measure the effects of a stimulus on a certain behavior, or the degree of dependency of events on each other. Later, we will generalize the concept of random variables to describe experiments that can create an indexed set of random variables, where the index is defined on the set of real numbers or on a graph; we will exploit the dependency of the random variables to perform clustering of classes to produce a meaningful description, and we will study various control mechanisms of experiments that can only be studied over a long period of observations.

4.3.4 Statistical expectation

The CDF and the PDF in Table 4.1 are described in terms of parameters that quantify the basic behavior of these functions, such as their mean value and the dispersion (variance) around that mean value. Over the years, statisticians have developed metrics that can be computed from the CDF or the PDF which provide important clues about the behavior of a statistical experiment. In fact, some of these metrics may provide an approximation or upper bounds of the probabilities of a certain event without actual calculation of the CDF and the PDF; thus a prediction may be possible for the behavior of events based on numerical calculations. Among these metrics is the statistical expectation which will be formally defined below.

DEFINITION 4.6 *Given a random variable X with PDF $f_X(x)$, its expected value $E(X)$ is defined by*

$$\mu = E(X) \stackrel{\text{def}}{=} \begin{cases} \int_{-\infty}^{\infty} x f_X(\alpha) \, dx & \text{for continuous random variables} \\ \sum_{i=-\infty}^{i=\infty} x_i p_i & \text{for discrete random variables} \end{cases} \quad \blacksquare \quad (4.8)$$

The expectation as defined above for a single random variable is a numerical indication of how symmetric the PDF is around the origin. Owing to the positivity constraints of the PDF, a zero expected value denotes symmetry, while a positive value indicates that the

PDF is biased towards the positive (right-hand side) of the origin, and a negative value indicates that the PDF is tilted to the left of the origin. Hence, in reality the quantity $E(X)$ provides the mean value of the PDF or its locus of "symmetry" on the x-axis. Therefore, $E(X)$ is the mean value or the average of the random variable X. We can define mathematically other forms of expectations, which include functions of random variables. For example, we may define the expected value of a function $g(X)$ as follows.

DEFINITION 4.7 *Given a random variable X with PDF $f_X(x)$, suppose we define a mapping $Y = g(X) : X \rightarrow \sigma_F$; i.e., the domain and range of $g(X)$ is similar to X. Then the expected value of $g(X)$ is defined by*

$$E\big(g(X)\big) = \begin{cases} \int_{-\infty}^{\infty} g(x) f_X(\alpha) \, dx & \text{for continuous random variables} \\ \sum_{i=-\infty}^{i=\infty} g(x_i) p_i & \text{for discrete random variables} \end{cases} \blacksquare \quad (4.9)$$

In this case, the mean is a special case of $g(X) = X$. The expectation of $g(X)$ measures the average of the function. As we shall see, *a function of a random variable is a measurable function*, and is therefore also a random variable. Hence, we may calculate $E(g(X))$ as above, using the PDF of a random variable X, or first calculate the PDF of $Y = g(X)$ and then calculate $E(Y)$ as follows:

$$E\big(g(X)\big) = E(Y) = \begin{cases} \int_{-\infty}^{\infty} y f_Y(\alpha) \, dy & \text{for continuous random variables} \\ \sum_{i=-\infty}^{i=\infty} y_i P(Y = y_i) & \text{for discrete random variables.} \end{cases}$$

$$(4.10)$$

The above result is fascinating, even though we have not formally derived it, and it has enormous practical implications in statistical analysis. This is due to the fact that calculating the PDF is not a simple matter, even for simple transformations. We focus on a few definitions which are special cases of $g(X)$ and provide some specific clues to the PDF of X.

DEFINITION 4.8 *Given a random variable X with PDF $f_x(x)$, the variance of X is defined as:*

$$\sigma^2 = E(X - \mu)^2 \underset{\text{def}}{=} \begin{cases} \int_{-\infty}^{\infty} (X - \mu)^2 f_X(\alpha) \, dx & \text{for continuous random variables} \\ \sum_{i=-\infty}^{i=\infty} (x_i - \mu)^2 p_i & \text{for discrete random variables.} \end{cases} \blacksquare$$

$$(4.11)$$

(Note that σ here is not the same as σ_F.) The variance measures the dispersion (width or concentration) of the PDF around the mean value. It serves to estimate the domain of the values that the random variable X may take. In fact, through the *Chebyshev inequality*, we can estimate the upper bound of the probability of a *normalized* event.

Fact The *Chebyshev inequality*.[4.1] Consider a random variable X with PDF having a mean value μ and variance σ^2. Define the normalized event $\{\omega \in \Omega : X(\omega) - \mu\} \in \sigma_F$. We can show that:

$$P(|X - \mu| \geq \varepsilon) \leq \frac{\sigma^2}{\varepsilon^2} \qquad (4.12)$$

The proof of the *Chebyshev inequality* follows directly from the definitions and the positivity of the density function. Its importance is in providing a measure for the concentration of the values of the random variable around its mean.

DEFINITION 4.9 *Given a random variable X with PDF $f_X(x)$, the kth moment of X around the origin is defined as:*

$$m_k = E(X)^k \stackrel{\text{def}}{=} \begin{cases} \int_{-\infty}^{\infty} x^k f_X(\alpha)\, dx & \text{for continuous random variables} \\ \sum_{i=-\infty}^{i=\infty} x_i^k p_i & \text{for discrete random variables.} \end{cases} \qquad (4.13)$$

The kth central moment $E(X - \mu)^k$ is obtained in a similar fashion by the proper substitution in the above equation. We now provide some examples to illustrate how the expectation values may be calculated for some of the PDFs in Table 4.1.

Example 4.11 Evaluate the mean and the variance of the Poisson distribution. This distribution is that of a counting random variable which estimates the instances of occurrences of a particular event, within a certain period, given the frequency of occurrence of any outcome or event.

$$E(X = k) = \sum_{k=0}^{\infty} k \frac{\theta^k e^{-\theta}}{k!} = \sum_{k=0}^{\infty} \frac{\theta^k e^{-\theta}}{(k-1)!}$$

$$= \theta \sum_{k=0}^{\infty} \frac{\theta^{k-1} e^{-\theta}}{(k-1)!} = \theta \sum_{m=-1}^{\infty} \frac{\theta^m e^{-\theta}}{(m)!} = \theta \left(\frac{\theta^{-1} e^{-\theta}}{(-1)!} + \sum_{m=0}^{\infty} \frac{\theta^m e^{-\theta}}{(m)!} \right) = \theta$$

Similarly,

$$E(X^2 = k^2) = \sum_{k=0}^{\infty} k^2 \frac{\theta^k e^{-\theta}}{k!} = \sum_{k=0}^{\infty} k \frac{\theta^k e^{-\theta}}{(k-1)!} = \left(\sum_{m=-1}^{\infty} (m+1) \frac{\theta^{m+1} e^{-\theta}}{(m)!} \right)$$

$$= \left(\sum_{m=0}^{\infty} (m+1) \frac{\theta^{m+1} e^{-\theta}}{(m)!} \right) = \theta \left(\sum_{m=0}^{\infty} (m+1) \frac{\theta^m e^{-\theta}}{(m)!} \right) = \theta(1 + \theta)$$

On the other hand, we note that $\text{var}(X) = E(X^2) - \mu^2$. Hence, it is immediately obvious that $\text{var}(X) = \theta$ for the Poisson distribution.

Example 4.12 Evaluate the mean and variance of the Cauchy distribution.

$$f_X(x) = \frac{a/\pi}{a^2 + x^2}, x \in R$$

The mean value is zero since $f_X(x)$ is an even symmetric function. The difficulty arrives with the variance, since the 2nd order expectation is infinite. Hence, the variance is undefined, but the parameter a measures the relationship between the maximum height and the span (width) of the PDF.

Knowledge of the PDF (or the CDF) enables the expectations to be computed. It is natural to ask whether knowledge of the expectations enables the determination of the functional form of the PDF. Unfortunately, it is not possible to infer the PDF from the expectations (moments), except in the case of the Gaussian PDF which is explicitly defined in terms of its mean and variance. But statisticians have studied mechanisms to generate the moments systematically through the so-called *moment generating function*, which is defined below.

DEFINITION 4.10 *Given a random variable X with PDF $f_X(x)$, the moment generating function $M(s)$ of X is defined as $M(s) = E(e^{sX})$.* ∎

The moments may be generated from $M(s)$ as follows.

$$E(X) = \lim_{s \to 0} \frac{dM(s)}{ds}; \quad E(X^2) = \lim_{s \to 0} \frac{d^2M(s)}{ds^2}.$$

In general, we can easily show that:

$$E(X^n) = \lim_{s \to 0} \frac{d^n M(s)}{ds^n}. \tag{4.14}$$

Example 4.13 Evaluate the moment generating function for the standard uniform PDF defined over the interval $x \in [0,b]$, $b \in R$.

$$M(s) = E(e^{sX}) = \frac{1}{b}\int_0^b e^{sx}dx = \frac{e^{bs} - 1}{bs}$$

It is evident that the mean value $b/2$, for example, may be obtained from the first derivative of $M(s)$ and taking the limit as s approaches zero (note the need for using l'Hôpital's rule).

One form of expectation function that mimics the moment generating function, yet offers the possibility of analyzing, and indeed constructing, the PDF of a random variable is known as the *characteristic function* and is defined as follows.

DEFINITION 4.11 *Given a random variable X with PDF $f_X(x)$, the characteristic function $\varphi_X(\mu)$ of X is defined as $\varphi_X(\mu) = E(e^{j2\pi\mu X})$, where the variable μ has dimensions of hertz (cycles/sec).*

$$\varphi_X(\mu) \underset{\text{def}}{=} \begin{cases} \displaystyle\int_{-\infty}^{\infty} e^{j2\pi\mu x} f_X(x)\, dx & \text{for continuous random variables} \\ \displaystyle\sum_{i=-\infty}^{i=\infty} e^{j2\pi\mu x_i} p_i & \text{for discrete random variables.} \end{cases} \quad \blacksquare \quad (4.15)$$

We note that $\varphi_X(\mu)$ is the conjugate of the Fourier transform, which is a unique mapping of the function $f_X(x)$. Thus a direct link is established between the PDF and the characteristic function, which is very useful in a number of applications.

Example 4.14 Evaluate the characteristic function for the standard uniform PDF defined over the interval $x \in [-b,b], b \in R$.

$$\varphi_X(\mu) = \frac{1}{2b}\int_{-b}^{b} e^{j2\pi\mu x}\, dx = \frac{e^{j2\pi\mu b} - e^{-j2\pi\mu b}}{2j(2\pi\mu)b} = \frac{\sin 2\pi\mu b}{2\pi\mu b} \underset{\text{def}}{=} \pi\,\text{sinc}(2\pi\mu b).$$

4.3.5 Functions of a random variable

Let us now consider how to apply calculus to functions of random variables in order to characterize a statistical experiment. The key issue is the measurability of functions of random variables; i.e., whether the mapping is actually constrained by the original domain (and range) of the original random variable. A random variable $X(\omega)$ is a mapping from the sigma algebra σ_F into the real line R such that the event $\{\omega \in \Omega : X(\omega) \leq a\} \in \sigma_F$, and we also insisted that the inverse mapping is an event, i.e., $\{X^{-1}(\alpha) : \alpha \in B \subset R\} \in \sigma_F$. Now let us define a function $Z(\omega) = g(X(\omega))$. It is evident from previous discussion that the transformation will generate events on R that must be Borel sets. Likewise, the inverse mapping will generate events that must be in Ω and σ_F, by construction. Hence, the measurability of $Z(\omega) = g(X(\omega))$ is evident and inherent. Figure 4.4 illustrates this concept, where the mappings of $X(\omega)$ and $Z(\omega)$ onto the real line produce Borel sets B_1 and B_2, which may be remapped back to the event $A \in \Omega$; i.e., $\{X^{-1}(\alpha) : \alpha \in B_1 \subset R\} = \{Z^{-1}(\beta) : \beta \in B_2 \subset R\} = A \in \sigma_F \subset \Omega$.

THEOREM 4.2 (see [4.3]): *If $X(\omega)$ is a random variable and $g(.)$ is a Borel function, then $Z(\omega) = g(X(\omega))$ is a random variable measurable by $X(\omega)$; i.e., the σ_F algebra generated by $Z(\omega)$ is a subset of the σ algebra generated by $X(\omega)$.*

As we have done before with random variables, we characterize $Z(\omega) = g(X(\omega))$ by its CDF or by its PDF. Depending on the functional form of $g(.)$, we may obtain the CFD $F_Z(z) \underset{\text{def}}{=} P(Z \leq z)$ in terms of $F_X(x) \underset{\text{def}}{=} P(X \leq x)$. Table 4.2 lists a few examples of the CDFs and PDFs of functions of random variables.[4.1]

4.3 Random variables

Table 4.2 The CDF and PDF of functions of random variables for various functional forms.

$Z(\omega) = g(X(\omega))$	CDF $F_Z(z)$	PDF $f_Z(z)$
$aX + b$; a and b are real constants	$F_X\left(\dfrac{z-b}{a}\right)$	$\dfrac{1}{\|a\|} f_X\left(\dfrac{z-b}{a}\right)$
X^2	$F_X(\sqrt{z}) - F_X(-\sqrt{z}) + P(X = -\sqrt{z})$	$\dfrac{1}{2\sqrt{z}}\left(f_X(\sqrt{z}) - f_X(-\sqrt{z})\right)$
Monotone increasing	$F_X\left(g^{-1}(z)\right)$	$f_X\left(g^{-1}(z)\right)\dfrac{d}{dz}\left(g^{-1}(z)\right)$
Monotone decreasing	$1 - F_X\left(g^{-1}(z)\right)$	$-f_X\left(g^{-1}(z)\right)\dfrac{d}{dz}\left(g^{-1}(z)\right)$
Continuous and $Z - g(X) = 0$ has countable number of real roots $x_1, x_2, \ldots, x_n, \ldots$	Integrate $f_Z(z)$	$\sum_k \dfrac{f_X(x_k)}{\|g'(x_k)\|}$
e^X	$F_X(\ln z); z > 0.$	$\dfrac{1}{z} f_X(\ln z)$
$\sqrt{X}$	$F_X(z^2)$	$2z f_X(z^2); z > 0.$

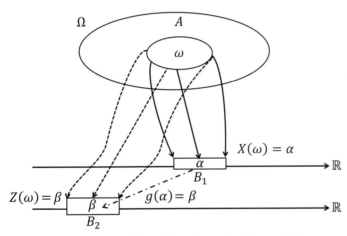

Figure 4.4 Illustration of the measurability of functions of random variables.

Derivations of the entries in Table 4.2 are straightforward and follow from the definitions of the CDF. The CDF should be obtained first, and then the derivative operator applied to obtain the PDF.

Functions of random variables form an important concept in mathematical statistics that enables statistical inference about one random variable (or, in general, a random process as will be studied later) in terms of another. Indeed, simulations of random variables from different distributions may be obtained from simulation of a random variable from the so-called standard uniform: i.e., $f_X(x) = 1$ for $x \in [0, 1]$. Such a form has been well studied, and various random number generators exist to generate samples from it. We will study simulations of random variables after briefly covering the case of random experiments that may be described by two random variables; this is a step towards generalization to a sequence of unstructured random variables, which will be followed by random variables that are defined on a graph or have a particular meaningful index. As our intention is to study random processes and random fields that have been useful for biomedical image analysis, we will not dwell on the details of random variables and statistical inferences beyond the basic background needed for our subsequent coverage.

4.4 Two random variables

Events in random experiments may take various forms, and may be better understood in terms of higher-dimensional mapping instead of one-dimensional. In this case, the measurability of the events on Ω or σ_F would be in terms of the mass of events (Borel sets) on multidimensional spaces. Consider two random variables $X_1(\omega)$ and $X_2(\omega)$. The events $\{\omega \in \Omega : X_1(\omega) \leq \alpha\} \in \sigma_F$ and $\{\omega \in \Omega : X_2(\omega) \leq \beta\} \in \sigma_F$ may be paired with respect to the two parameters α and β such that a new event $\{\omega \in \Omega : Z(\omega) = (X_1(\omega) \leq \alpha, X_2(\omega) \leq \beta) \leq \gamma = (\alpha, \beta)\} \in \sigma_F$ may be defined on the space $R_1 \times R_2$ as shown in Figure 4.5. We may express the random variable $Z(\omega)$ with respect to $X_1(\omega)$ and $X_2(\omega)$ as $Z(\omega) = (X_1(\omega), X_2(\omega))$, or in a vector, i.e. $Z(\omega) = \begin{pmatrix} X_1(\omega) \\ X_2(\omega) \end{pmatrix}$. We will be interested mainly in random variables defined on the same sample space; hence for simplicity we will write $Z = (X_1, X_2)$ and $Z = \begin{pmatrix} X_1 \\ X_2 \end{pmatrix}$.

In direct analogy to the case of single random variables, we may determine the probability mass distribution on the Borel sets defined on the plane $R_1 \times R_2$, by the

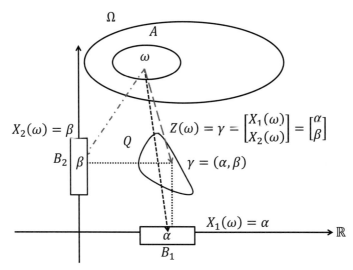

Figure 4.5 Illustration of the concept of two-dimensional random vectors for two random variables on the same sample space. For measurability, the sets $\mathbf{B}_1$, $\mathbf{B}_2$ and $\mathbf{Q}$ are Borel sets.

assignment $P_{X_1X_2} = P\left(Z^{-1}(Q)\right)$; hence, when dealing with a pair of random variables X_1 and X_2, we have three induced probability measures: $P_{X_1}(.)$, $P_{X_2}(.)$, and $P_{X_1X_2}(.)$. The mass distribution on R_1 represented by $P_{X_1}(.)$ consists of the unit mass distributed along R_1. Similarly, $P_{X_2}(.)$ represents a unit mass distributed along R_2, and $P_{XY}(.)$ represents a unit mass distributed along $R_1 \times R_2$. The measures $P_{X_1}(.)$ and $P_{X_2}(.)$ are related to $P_{X_1X_2}(.)$ as follows, where $\mathbf{B}_1$ and $\mathbf{B}_2$ are the Borel sets resulting from the mappngmapping $X(a)$ onto R_1 and R_2:

$$P_{X_1X_2}(\mathbf{B}_1 \times \mathbf{B}_2) = P(Z \in \mathbf{B}_1 \times \mathbf{B}_2) = P(X_1 \in \mathbf{B}_1, X_2 \in \mathbf{B}_2)$$
$$= P\left(X_1^{-1}(\mathbf{B}_1), X_2^{-1}(\mathbf{B}_2)\right). \qquad (4.16)$$

Now if $\mathbf{B}_1 = R_1$; i.e., the entire real line, then $X_1^{-1}(\mathbf{B}_1) = \Omega$, so that $P_{X_1X_2}(\mathbf{B}_1 \times \mathbf{B}_2) = P_{X_2}(\mathbf{B}_2)$. Similarly, if $\mathbf{B}_2 = R_2$, i.e. the entire real line, then $X_2^{-1}(\mathbf{B}_2) = \Omega$, so that $P_{X_1X_2}(\mathbf{B}_1 \times \mathbf{B}_2) = P_{X_1}(\mathbf{B}_1)$. We formally define these quantities below.

DEFINITION 4.12 *The probability measure $P_{X_1X_2}(.)$ defined on the Borel sets in the plane $R_1 \times R_2$ is called the joint probability measure induced by the joint mapping $(\alpha,\beta) = Z(\omega) = [X_1 \in \mathbf{B}_1, X_2 \in \mathbf{B}_2](\omega)$. The probability mass distribution is called the joint distribution. The probability measures $P(., X_2 \in \mathbf{B}_2) = P_{X_1}(.)$ and $P(X_1 \in \mathbf{B}_1,.) = P_{X_2}(.)$ are called the marginal probability measures induced by random variables X_1 and X_2, respectively. The corresponding probability mass distributions are called the marginal probability distributions.* ∎

DEFINITION 4.13 *The joint probability distribution function, or the joint cumulative distribution function for random variables X_1 and X_2, denoted by $F_{X_1X_2}(x_1,x_2)$, is defined by $F_{X_1X_2}(x_1,x_2) = P(X_1 \leq x_1, X_2 \leq x_2)$ for all values $x_1, x_2 \in R_1 \times R_2$. The special cases $F_{X_1X_2}(x_1,\infty) = P(X_1 \leq x_1, X_2 \leq \infty) = F_{X_1}(x_1)$ and $F_{X_1X_2}(\infty,x_2) = P(X_1 \leq \infty, X_2 \leq x_2) = F_{X_2}(x_2)$ are called the marginal distribution functions for random variables X_1 and X_2, respectively.* ∎

We follow the same development for the single random variable case and define the probability density function for two random variables.

FACT (see [4.5]) If the joint probability measure $P_{X_1X_2}(.)$ induced by X_1 and X_2 is absolutely continuous, a function $f_{X_1X_2}(.)$ exists such that: $\iint_Q f_{X_1X_2}(x_1,x_2)dx_1dx_2 = P_{X_1X_2}(\mathbf{B}_1 \times \mathbf{B}_2) = P_{X_1X_2}(Q)$ is called the probability density function for X_1 and X_2. Conversely, given $F_{X_1X_2}(x_1,x_2)$ and $f_{X_1X_2}(x_1,x_2)$ that satisfy the previous properties, there exist two random variables X_1 and X_2 defined on some sample space Ω with joint probability distribution and density functions $F_{X_1X_2}(x_1,x_2)$ and $f_{X_1X_2}(x_1,x_2)$, respectively.

We may list the main properties of $f_{X_1X_2}(.)$ as we did for single random variables; specifically, we note that:

(i) $f_{X_1X_2}(.) \geq 0$, $x_1, x_2 \in R_1 \times R_2$

(ii) $\iint_{-\infty}^{\infty} f_{X_1X_2}(x_1,x_2)dx_1dx_2 = 1$

(iii) $\int_{-\infty}^{x_1}\int_{-\infty}^{x_2} f_{X_1X_2}(\alpha,\beta)d\alpha\, d\beta = F_{X_1X_2}(x_1,x_2)$

(iv) $f_{X_1X_2}(x_1,x_2) = \dfrac{\partial^2 F_{X_1X_2}(x_1,x_2)}{\partial x_1 \partial x_2}.$

Example 4.15 Consider two jointly continuous and positive random variables X_1 and X_2 with the following joint density function:

$$f_{X_1X_2}(x_1,x_2) = \begin{cases} 24\, x_1 x_2 & \text{for } x_1 + x_2 \leq 1 \\ 0 & \text{otherwise.} \end{cases}$$

Find $f_{X_1}(x_1)$, $f_{X_2}(x_2)$ and $F_{X_1X_2}(x_1,x_2)$.

Solution The required quantities may be obtained by integrating $f_{X_1X_2}(x_1,x_2)$ over the specific region (see Figure 4.6).

$$f_{X_1}(x_1) = \int_{-\infty}^{\infty} f_{X_1X_2}(x_1,x_2)dx_2 = \int_0^{1-x_1} 24 x_1 x_2 dx_2 = 12 x_2 (1-x_1)^2;\ 0 \leq x_1 < 1.$$

Also,

$$f_{X_2}(x_2) = \int_{-\infty}^{\infty} f_{X_1X_2}(x_1,x_2)dx_1 = \int_0^{1-x_2} 24 x_1 x_2 dx_1 = 12 x_2 (1-x_2)^2;\ 0 \leq x_2 < 1.$$

The cumulative distribution function will be computed from the basic definition:

$$F_{X_1X_2}(x_1,x_2) \underset{\text{def}}{=} P(X_1 \leq x_1, X_2 \leq x_2) = \int_{-\infty}^{x_1}\int_{-\infty}^{x_2} f_{X_1X_2}(\alpha,\beta)d\alpha\, d\beta = \int_0^{x_1}\int_0^{x_2} 24\alpha\beta\, d\alpha\, d\beta$$

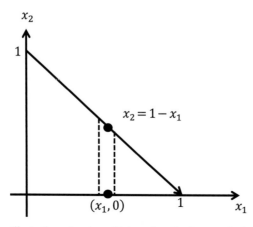

Figure 4.6 Illustration of region of integration for the marginal density $f_{X_1}(x_1)$.

given that $x_1 + x_2 \leq 1$, which leads to

$$F_{X_1 X_2}(x_1, x_2) = \begin{cases} 6 x_1^2 x_2^2 & x_1 + x_2 \leq 1 \\ 0; & \text{otherwise.} \end{cases}$$

We may address the important issue of dependence of random variables here. We maintain, from Definition 4.2 and Example 4.9, that events $\{\omega \in \Omega: X_1(\omega) \leq \alpha\}$ and $\{\omega \in \Omega: X_2(\omega) \leq \beta\}$ are independent if their joint probabilities distribute; that is

$$P\Big(\{\omega \in \Omega: X_1(\omega) \leq \alpha\} \{\omega \in \Omega: X_2(\omega) \leq \beta\}\Big)$$
$$= P\Big(\{\omega \in \Omega: X_1(\omega) \leq \alpha\}\Big) P\Big(\{\omega \in \Omega: X_2(\omega) \leq \beta\}\Big)$$
$$\stackrel{\text{def}}{=} P(X_1 \leq x_1) P(X_2 \leq x_2) = F_{X_1}(x_1) F_{X_2}(x_2)$$

Note that in the above example, $F_{X_1 X_2}(x_1, x_2)$ has a separable form, but the two random variables are not independent, owing to the restrictions $x_1 + x_2 \leq 1$. The independence concept will come in handy in various applications, including simulations of random variables.

4.4.1 Statistical expectation in two dimensions

Expectations in two dimensions follow in the same manner as for the one-dimensional case (see Definitions 4.5 and 4.6). In particular, the expected value of a function $g(X_1, X_2)$ of random variables X_1 and X_2 is defined as follows:

DEFINITION 4.14 *Given a pair of random variables (RV) X_1 and X_2, suppose we define a mapping* $Y = g(X_1, X_2) : \begin{pmatrix} X_1 \\ X_2 \end{pmatrix} \to \sigma_F$; *i.e., the domain and range of $g(X_1, X_2)$ is similar to* $\begin{pmatrix} X_1 \\ X_2 \end{pmatrix}$. *Then the expected value of $g(X_1, X_2)$ is defined by*

$$E\Big(g(X)\Big) = \begin{cases} \displaystyle\iint_{-\infty}^{\infty} g(x_1, x_2) f_{X_1 X_2}(x_1, x_2) dx_1 dx_2 & \text{for continuous RV,} \\ \displaystyle\sum_{i=-\infty}^{i=\infty} \sum_{j=-\infty}^{j=\infty} g(x_{1i}, x_{2j}) p_{i,j} & \text{for discrete RV,} \end{cases} \quad (4.17)$$

where $f_{X_1 X_2}(x_1, x_2)$ is the probability density function for continuous random variables and $p_{i,j}$ is the probability mass function for discrete random variables.

DEFINITION 4.15 *Given a pair of random variables X_1 and X_2, the covariance function is defined as:*

$$Cov(X_1, X_2) = E\left(X_1 - \mu_1\right)(X_2 - \mu_2)$$

$$= \begin{cases} \displaystyle\iint_{-\infty}^{\infty} (x_1 - \mu_1)(x_2 - \mu_2) f_{X_1 X_2}(x_1, x_2) dx_1 dx_2 & \text{for continuous RV} \\ \displaystyle\sum_{i=-\infty}^{i=\infty} \sum_{j=-\infty}^{j=\infty} (x_{1i} - \mu_1)(x_{2j} - \mu_2) p_{i,j} & \text{for discrete RV,} \end{cases} \quad (4.18)$$

where μ_k, $k = 1, 2$ are the marginal means as defined in Definition 4.5. That is, for any random variable X_k, we have:

$$\mu_k = E(X_k) = \begin{cases} \displaystyle\int_{-\infty}^{\infty} x_k f_{X_k}(x_k) dx_k & \text{for continuous random variables} \\ \displaystyle\sum_{i=-\infty}^{i=\infty} x_{ki} p_{ki} & \text{for discrete random variables,} \end{cases}$$

where $f_{X_k}(x_k)$ is the probability density function for continuous random variable X_k and p_k is the probability mass function for discrete random variable X_k. ∎

A special case for Definition 4.14 that does not include the marginal means is called the *autocorrelation* R, i.e., $R = E(X_1, X_2)$.

We note that all the properties of the expectation operators in higher dimensions are similar to those in one dimension.

In two dimensions (or multi-dimensions, in general), the random variables may possess various degrees of "relatedness," which may span the entire scale from *fully related* to completely *unrelated* or independent. We define the relatedness in terms of *correlation coefficient* ρ; i.e.,

$\rho = \frac{Cov(X_i, X_j)}{\sigma_i \sigma_j}$, where σ_i is the standard deviation of random variable X_i.

If the covariance is zero, then the two random variables are said to be *uncorrelated*. If the two random variables are independent, then their covariance becomes zero, and therefore, by definition, the two random variables become uncorrelated. We note that the converse is not true, except in the case of Gaussian random variables, which will be considered later.

4.4.2 Functions of two random variables

It is natural to study the mappings (transformations) of two random variables as we did with single random variables. Here we consider the transformation $\boldsymbol{Y} = g(X_1, X_2)$, where $g(.)$ is a general function. We use the boldface letter $\boldsymbol{Y}$ to represent the functional form for $g(.)$, which may be a vector. A given realization (certain value or instant of $\boldsymbol{Y}$) will be represented by small boldface letter $\boldsymbol{y}$. The key issue is the measurability of $g(.,.)$, which may be understood in a similar fashion to the one-dimensional case; see Figure 4.4. It is straightforward to show that under normal conditions, $g(.,.)$ is measurable and, therefore, we may define a complete functional description for it in terms of the probability distribution function $P(\boldsymbol{Y} = g(X_1, X_2) \leq \boldsymbol{y})$. We consider a few cases below.

Example 4.16 Consider two jointly continuous random variables X_1, X_2 with probability density function $f_{X_1 X_2}(x_1, x_2)$. Define a summation function $Z = X_1 + X_2$. If Z is a measurable random variable, its CDF may be calculated as follows:

$$F_Z(z) \underset{\text{def}}{=} P(Z \leq z) = P(X_1 + X_2 \leq z) = \int_{-\infty}^{\infty} \int_{-\infty}^{z-x_1} f_{X_1 X_2}(x_1, x_2) dx_1 \, dx_2$$

and the density function $f_Z(Z)$ would be evaluated as follows:

$$f_Z(z) = \frac{d}{dz} \int_{-\infty}^{\infty} \int_{-\infty}^{z-x_1} f_{X_1 X_2}(x_1, x_2) dx_1 \, dx_2 = \int_{-\infty}^{\infty} \left(\frac{d}{dz} \int_{-\infty}^{z-x_1} f_{X_1 X_2}(x_1, x_2) \, dx_1 \right) dx_2.$$

The inner differentiation may be evaluated using Leibnitz' rule, i.e.,

$$\frac{d}{dz} \int_{a(z)}^{b(z)} g(y, z) dy = \frac{db(z)}{dz} g(b(z), z) - \frac{da(z)}{dz} g(a(z), z) + \int_{a(z)}^{b(z)} \frac{\partial}{\partial z} g(y, z) dy$$

Hence,

$$f_Z(z) = \int_{-\infty}^{\infty} f_{X_1 X_2}(z - x_2, x_2) dx_2 = \int_{-\infty}^{\infty} f_{X_1 X_2}(x_1, z - x_1) dx_1 \quad (4.19)$$

Special case If X_1, X_2 are independent, then the joint density becomes separable, and $f_Z(Z)$ will have the following form:

$$f_Z(z) = \int_{-\infty}^{\infty} f_{X_1}(z - x_2) f_{X_2}(x_2) dx_2 = \int_{-\infty}^{\infty} f_{X_1}(x_1) f_{X_2}(z - x_1) dx_1 \quad (4.20)$$

Equation (4.20) is the *convolution* integral. For this case, the CDF would be: $F_Z(z) = \int_{-\infty}^{\infty} F_{X_1}(z - x_2) f_{X_2}(x_2) dx_2 = \int_{-\infty}^{\infty} f_{X_1}(x_1) F_{X_2}(z - x_1) dx_1$. For illustration, let us consider the simple case where both X_1, X_2 are independent and have uniform distribution. Let $f_{X_1}(x) = 1$; $x \in [1, 2]$ and $f_{X_2}(x) = 0.25$; $x \in [0, 4]$. It is straightforward to show that

$$f_Z(z) = \begin{cases} 0 & z \leq 1 \\ 0.25(z - 1) & z \in (1, 2] \\ 0.25 & z \in (2, 5] \\ 0.25(6 - z) & z \in (5, 6] \\ 0 & z > 6. \end{cases}$$

Table 4.3 Some one-dimensional functions of two random variables, and the corresponding CDF and PDF.

$Z = g(X,Y)$	CDF $F_Z(z)$	PDF $f_Z(z)$
$Z = X_1 + X_2$	$\int_{-\infty}^{\infty}\int_{-\infty}^{z-x_1} f_{X_1X_2}(x_1,x_2)dx_1\,dx_2$	$\int_{-\infty}^{\infty} f_{X_1X_2}(x_1, z-x_1)dx_1$
$Z = \max(X_1, X_2)$	$\int_{-\infty}^{z}\int_{-\infty}^{z} f_{X_1X_2}(x_1,x_2)dx_1\,dx_2 = F_{X_1X_2}(z,z)$	$\dfrac{d}{dz}F_{X_1X_2}(z,z)$
$Z = \min(X_1, X_2)$	$F_{X_1}(z) + F_{X_2}(z) - F_{X_1X_2}(z,z)$	$f_{X_1}(z) + f_{X_2}(z) - \dfrac{d}{dz}F_{X_1X_2}(z,z)$
$Z = \dfrac{X_1}{X_2}$	$\int_{0}^{\infty}\int_{-\infty}^{x_2 z} f_{X_1X_2}(x_1,x_2)dx_1\,dx_2 + \int_{-\infty}^{0}\int_{\infty x_2 z}^{\infty} f_{X_1X_2}(x_1,x_2)dx_1\,dx_2$	$\int_{-\infty}^{\infty} \|x_2\| f_{X_1X_2}(x_2 z, x_2)dx_2$
$Z = \sqrt{X_1^2 + X_2^2}$	$\iint_{Q(z)} f_{X_1X_2}(x_1,x_2)dx_1\,dx_2;$ $Q(z): x_1^2 + x_2^2 \le z^2$	$\dfrac{d}{dz}F_Z(z)$
$Z = X_1 X_2$	$\int_{-\infty}^{0}\int_{z/x_1}^{\infty} f_{X_1X_2}(x_1,x_2)dx_1\,dx_2 + \int_{0}^{\infty}\int_{-\infty}^{\infty z/x_1} f_{X_1X_2}(x_1,x_2)dx_1\,dx_2$	$\int_{-\infty}^{\infty}\dfrac{1}{\|x_1\|}f_{X_1X_2}\left(x_1,\dfrac{z}{x_1}\right)dx_1$

Table 4.3 lists several examples of the distribution of functions of two random variables; all can be derived from the basic definitions. These functions map two random variables into a single random variable i.e. there is a reduction in dimensionality involved in the transformation. We will next consider the case where the functions of random variables are vectors.

4.4.3 Two functions of two random variables

As a step towards generalized representation of functions of random variables, let us consider vector representations of the random variables X_1 and X_2, i.e., $\boldsymbol{X} = \begin{pmatrix} X_1 \\ X_2 \end{pmatrix}$ and a functional form for that vector representation $\boldsymbol{Y} = \begin{pmatrix} Y_1 \\ Y_2 \end{pmatrix} = g(X_1, X_2) = g(\boldsymbol{X}) = \begin{pmatrix} g_1(X_1, X_2) \\ g_2(X_1, X_2) \end{pmatrix}$. This will be quite straightforward in the case where $g(.,.)$ is a linear mapping of X_1, X_2. In this case, we may write: $\boldsymbol{Y} = \begin{pmatrix} Y_1 \\ Y_2 \end{pmatrix} = A\boldsymbol{X} = \begin{bmatrix} a_{11} & a_{12} \\ a_{21} & a_{22} \end{bmatrix}\begin{pmatrix} X_1 \\ X_2 \end{pmatrix}$, for some constants $a_{ij}, i,j \in [1,2]$. If the transformation A is invertible, i.e., $H = A^{-1}$ exists, then $\boldsymbol{X} = H\boldsymbol{Y}$. The *Jacobian* of the transformation is defined as:

$$J = \begin{bmatrix} \dfrac{\partial h_1}{\partial y_1} & \dfrac{\partial h_1}{\partial y_2} \\ \dfrac{\partial h_2}{\partial y_1} & \dfrac{\partial h_2}{\partial y_2} \end{bmatrix}$$

Then the joint probability density function of Y_1 and Y_2 may be written in terms of the joint density $f_{X_1 X_2}(x_1, x_2)$ of random variables X_1, X_2 as follows:[4.5]
$f_Y(y) = f_X(Hy)|J|$, where $|.|$ stands for the determinant.

Example 4.17 Consider two jointly continuous random variables X_1, X_2 with probability density function $f_{X_1 X_2}(x_1, x_2)$. Consider the polar coordinates:

$$Y_1 = R = \sqrt{X_1^2 + X_2^2},$$

$$R \geq 0, \text{ and}$$

$$Y_2 = \theta = \tan^{-1}\left(\frac{X_2}{X_1}\right),$$

$$\theta \in (-\pi, \pi); \text{ i.e., } \begin{pmatrix} X_1 \\ X_2 \end{pmatrix} = \begin{pmatrix} r\cos\theta \\ r\sin\theta \end{pmatrix}.$$

We may define the Jacobian of the polar transformation as follows:

$$J = \begin{bmatrix} \dfrac{\partial h_1}{\partial y_1} & \dfrac{\partial h_1}{\partial y_2} \\ \dfrac{\partial h_2}{\partial y_1} & \dfrac{\partial h_2}{\partial y_2} \end{bmatrix} = \begin{bmatrix} \dfrac{\partial x_1}{\partial r} & \dfrac{\partial x_1}{\partial \theta} \\ \dfrac{\partial x_2}{\partial r} & \dfrac{\partial x_2}{\partial \theta} \end{bmatrix} = \begin{bmatrix} \cos\theta & -r\cos\theta \\ \sin\theta & r\cos\theta \end{bmatrix}; \text{ and } |J| = 1.$$

Hence,

$$f_{Y_1 Y_2}(y_1, y_2) = f_{R\theta}(r\theta) = r f_{X_1 X_2}(r\cos\theta, r\sin\theta).$$

4.5 Simulation of random variables

In this section we discuss how to simulate one- and two-dimensional random variables of general distributions, starting from a standard uniform distribution. This will form a link between distribution or density functions and deterministic functional forms, which represent instants or realizations of the random variables. Generating such instants may be used in a reverse fashion to estimate the density function using histograms. Simulation is an art and a well-studied subject in statistical design; stochastic systems are studied through simulations. Here we only scratch the surface to give the reader some feeling for the outputs of random experiments in the form of realizations of the random variables that map the sample space into Borel sets on the real line.

The fundamental step in the simulation is the simple observation that since the distribution function is monotone and non-decreasing, an inverse may be possible; hence mapping from uniform distribution to any other form is possible. We illustrate this as follows. Let X and Y be two random variables, not necessarily on the same sample space or with the same form of distribution. Suppose the two random variables are related to each through the monotonic transformation $Y = g(X)$. The distribution function of Y with respect to the distribution of X is as follows: $P(Y \leq y) = P\left(g(X) \leq y\right) = P(X \leq g^{-1}(y))$; hence, $F_Y(y) = F_X\left(g^{-1}(y)\right) = g^{-1}(y) = x$, if X is uniformly distributed. Hence, we may take $g(X) = F_Y(y)$. Therefore, if we generate a realization from X, a realization from Y is obtained by inverse mapping.

4.6 Summary

This chapter has introduced the basic concepts of statistical modeling which serve as building blocks for the material in the book. We have defined the concept of a random variable from an operational point of view and illustrated its significance in describing statistical experiments. The characteristics of a single random variable have been studied, including the probability distribution and density function, and the concept of statistical expectation. Extensions to functions of single random variables and joint distribution of two random variables were considered. The chapter concluded with the basics of simulation of one- and two-dimensional random variables.

4.7 Computer laboratory

A random variable of $U(0,1)$ can be easily converted to any other distribution such as the normal distribution. The methodology of generating random numbers has several forms. However, the algorithm most often used is the linear congruential generator (LCG), whose recursive formula is given by (A4.1), where Z_i is a sequence of integer values ranging from 0 to $m-1$, starting from a seed point Z_0:

$$Z_i = (a\, Z_{i-1} + c) \bmod m \tag{A4.1}$$

where m is the modulus, a is the multiplier, c is the increment, and all are non-negative values. In order to obtain numbers in the interval $[0, 1]$, the generated integer sequence should be divided by m to obtain $U_i = Z_i/m$. There are many variations of LCGs; the form used in this project is the multiplicative LCG where the addition of c is not needed, so the recursive formula of the generator can be given by

$$Z_i = a\, Z_{i-1} \bmod m. \tag{A4.2}$$

We may convert the generated uniform streams to follow a Gaussian distribution of zero mean and unit variance using the Box–Muller approach, described as follows.

If u_1 and u_2 are independent random variates (realization from random variable) from $U(0,1)$, then Z_1 and Z_2 are independent standard normal deviates (realization from $N(0,1)$) obtained as follows:

$$Z_1 = \sqrt{-2 \ln u_1} \cos 2\pi u_2 \qquad (A4.3a)$$

$$Z_2 = \sqrt{-2 \ln u_1} \sin 2\pi u_2 \qquad (A4.3b)$$

The approach is to run the random generator to get a very large number of samples of a uniform random variable, then extract the even-ordered terms to be u_1 and the odd-ordered terms to be u_2, in order to guarantee their independence. See, for example, Rubinstein [4.6].

Task 1 (a) Generate three streams (1D, 2D and 3D) of random numbers with 100,000 samples each; you can use the MATLAB function for random number generation.
(b) Visualize the generated samples. *Hint*: you can use a scatter plot.
(c) Compute the histograms of the three streams, and then normalize them to produce an estimate of the probability density function (PDF).
(d) Visualize the PDFs of the three streams. Are the samples uniformly distributed? Do the PDFs represent a standard uniform distribution? Comment.

Task 2 Use the streams generated in Task 1 to do the following,
(a) Convert the generated streams to a standard normal distribution.
(b) Visualize the data samples. Are they normally distributed with mean 0 and unit variance?
(c) Compute the normalized histogram (PDFs) of the data samples from (a) and visualize the distribution. Comment on it.

Task 3 Use the streams generated in Task 2 to do the following;
(a) Convert the 1D normal variate to a normal distribution with mean -2 and standard deviation 3.
(b) Convert the 2D normal variate to a normal distribution with mean vector
$$M = \begin{bmatrix} 1 \\ 2 \end{bmatrix} \text{ and covariance matrix } \Sigma = \begin{bmatrix} 4 & 4 \\ 4 & 9 \end{bmatrix}.$$
(c) Convert the 3D normal variate to a normal distribution with mean vector
$$M = \begin{bmatrix} 5 \\ -5 \\ 6 \end{bmatrix} \text{ and covariance matrix } \Sigma = \begin{bmatrix} 5 & 2 & -1 \\ 2 & 5 & 0 \\ -1 & 0 & 4 \end{bmatrix}.$$
(d) For (a), (b) and (c) estimate the mean and covariance matrix and compare the estimated values with the ground truth ones. Comment.

4.8 Exercises

4.1 Given a probability space (Ω, σ_F, P), let A,B,C be the events such that $P(AB|C) = 1$. Prove/disprove the following:
(a) $P(AB) = 1$
(b) $P(ABC) = C$
(c) $P(A|C) = 0$.

4.2 Given a sample space $\Omega = \{\omega_1, \omega_2, \omega_3, \omega_4\}$:
(a) Construct the smallest σ_F-algebra σ_1 that contains the two sets $A = \{\omega_1, \omega_2\}$ and $B = \{\omega_3, \omega_4\}$.
(b) Construct the smallest σ_F-algebra σ_2 that contains the two sets $A = \{\omega_1, \omega_4\}$ and $B = \{\omega_2, \omega_3\}$.
(c) What members of σ_1 are σ_2 measurable?

4.3 Let $\mu(.)$ be a nonnegative finitely additive set function on the field σ_F. Show that
$$\mu\left(\bigcup_{n=1}^{\infty} A_n\right) \geq \sum_{n=1}^{\infty} \mu(A_n)$$

4.4 Let $A_1, A_2, \ldots, A_n$ be arbitrary subsets of a set. Describe explicitly the smallest σ-field σ_F containing $A_1, A_2, \ldots, A_n$. How many sets are there in σ_F? That is, give an upper bound that is attainable.

4.5 Derive the entries in Table 4.2.

4.6 Derive the entries in Table 4.3.

References

[4.1] A. Papoulis, *Probability, Random Variables and Stochastic Processes*, 3rd Edition, New York: McGraw-Hill (1991).
[4.2] R. Ash, *Real Analysis and Probability*, New York: Academic Press (1972).
[4.3] P. E. Pfeiffer, *Concepts of Probability Theory*, 2nd Edition, New York: Dover (1978).
[4.4] W. Feller, *An Introduction to Probability Theory and its Applications*, Vol. **1**, New York: Wiley (1968).
[4.5] W. Davenport, *Random Processes*, New York: McGraw-Hill (1970).
[4.6] R. Rubinstein, *Simulation and the Monte Carlo Method*, New York: Wiley (1981).

5 Random processes

5.1 Definition and general concepts

Recall that a random variable $X(\omega): \Omega \to R$ is a function that maps events in Ω to the real line R. For example, as we indicated in Chapter 4, consider a probability space (Ω, σ_F, P) where $\Omega = \{\omega_1, \omega_2, \omega_3, \omega_4\}$, with $P(\omega_1) = 0.1$, $P(\omega_2) = 0.3$, $P(\omega_3) = 0.4$, $P(\omega_4) = 0.2$. The random variable $X(\omega)$ will map the elementary events into measurable counterparts on the real line with unit masses equal to the probabilities. These mappings are: $x_1 = X(\omega_1)$, $x_2 = X(\omega_2)$, $x_3 = X(\omega_3)$, and $x_4 = X(\omega_4)$.

We also considered a sequence of random variables, $\{X_1(\omega), X_2(\omega), \cdots X_N(\omega)\}$, which maps events from Ω into an N-dimensional space. We did not restrict the set N to any order or any structure. The sequence of random variables is simply a collection of random variables that may be described by a joint probability distribution $F_{X_1 X_2 \cdots X_N}(x_1 x_2 \cdots x_N)$ or a joint density function $f_{X_1 X_2 \cdots X_N}(x_1 x_2 \cdots x_N)$. The convergence of the sequence of random variables to a particular distribution can be studied in terms of a limiting process which determines the degree and type of convergence [5.1], [5.2]. The mapping of events associated with random variables has been restricted to be real values, which define measurable sets on the real line, known as *Borel* sets. The mass of the *Borel* set corresponds to the measure or the probability of the corresponding event on the sample space Ω or the σ_F-algebra.

We are interested in cases where the mapping is not a specific value, but a sequence of values (waveform). A *group*, or an indexed set, of random variables which maps events on the sample space Ω or the σ-algebra to other sequences in the real or the complex domain is called a *random process*. We shall formally define the random process after we have illustrated the physical meaning entailed.

Figure 5.2 illustrates a doubly indexed function $X(\omega,t)$ which generates a function (deterministic) for each elementary event $\omega \in \Omega$ for the same experiment in Figure 5.1. These functions $X(\omega_i,t)$, $i \in [1,4]$, $t \in R$ are called *realizations*, or *sample functions*, of the *random process* $X(\omega,t)$. The probability that $X(\omega_i,t)$ would result is $P(\omega_i)$. Suppose we sample the deterministic realizations $X(\omega_i,t)$, $i \in [1,4]$, $t \in R$ with respect to the parameter $t \in R$. The resulting samples define a random variable with realizations that have measures $P(\omega_i)$. For example, as shown in Figure 5.2, the samples at t_1 and t_2 define two distinct random variables. This is consistent with the definition of the random process. At instant t_1, the amplitude of the waveforms will be equal to

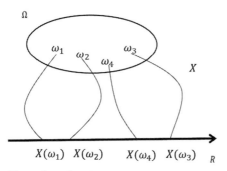

Figure 5.1 Illustration of random variable as mapping of events to the real line.

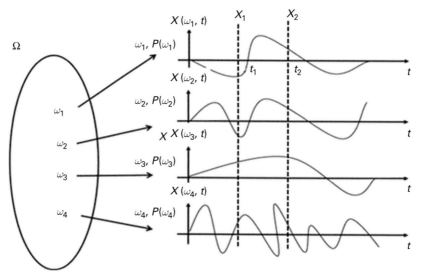

Figure 5.2 Illustration of a random process generating an ensemble of realizations of size four. Sampling the realizations of the random process $\mathbf{X}(\omega, \mathbf{t})$ with respect to the index $\mathbf{t}$ results in random variables.

$$x_1 = \text{amplitude}(X_1) = X(\omega, t_1) = \begin{cases} X(\omega_1, t_1) & \text{with probability } P(\omega_1) \\ X(\omega_2, t_1) & \text{with probability } P(\omega_2) \\ X(\omega_3, t_1) & \text{with probability } P(\omega_3) \\ X(\omega_4, t_1) & \text{with probability } P(\omega_4) \end{cases}$$

The amplitude (or the value of the sample function at a certain time instant) defines a random variable $X_1(\omega, t_1) = X(\omega, t_1) = X_1$.

Similarly, at $t = t_2$ the amplitude of the waveforms will be equal to

$$x_2 = \text{amplitude}(X_2) = X(\omega, t_2) = \begin{cases} X(\omega_1, t_2) & \text{with probability } P(\omega_1) \\ X(\omega_2, t_2) & \text{with probability } P(\omega_2) \\ X(\omega_3, t_2) & \text{with probability } P(\omega_3) \\ X(\omega_4, t_2) & \text{with probability } P(\omega_4) \end{cases}$$

which defines another random variable $X_2(\omega,t_2) = X(\omega,t_2) = X_2$. We may repeat the process and define other random variables on the indexing set $t \in R$. If we look at a particular realization $X(\omega_i, t)$ we get a *deterministic* function with the index $t \in R$ being the independent variable. This can be generalized when the sample space Ω contains an infinite number of points (or elementary events) or when the σ-algebra has a countable number of measurable events. In this case, the number of sample functions will be infinite. We are now in the position to formally define a random process.

DEFINITION 5.1 *A random process $X(\omega,t)$ is an indexed set of random variables where the index t belongs to some set $T \in R$.* ∎

5.1.1 Description of random processes

The index t may represent a time, position, angle, temperature, etc. The index set T may be finite or infinite; it may be one interval or a set of intervals in R; it may be numerable (e.g., integer-valued or rational values but countable) or denumerable (e.g., continuous values). We may describe a random process $X(\omega,t)$ by two general approaches: the first approach is in terms of a set of random variables $\{X(.,t), t \in T\}$ in which case, a random variable $X_i(.,t_i)$ is associated with "time" instants (or indexing parameters) t_i. The second approach is in terms of a set of realizations or function of the index t $\{X(\omega,.) \omega \in \Omega, t \in T \subset R.\}$. For each choice of the elementary outcome ω (or a combination of elementary outcomes), a time function $X(.,t); t \in T$ is chosen. Each such function is called a sample function or realization.

Figure 5.3 illustrates the two approaches to describing a random process. Of course, we are interested in a compact description, and the ensemble of realizations may not be practical when the possibilities are too large. We shall keep the two approaches for now as we impose certain structure on the events and the indexing function.

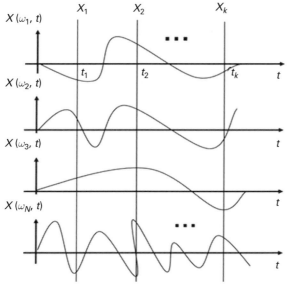

Figure 5.3 Illustration of a random process as an ensemble of realizations of size N or in terms of an indexed set of random variables of size k.

5.1.2 Classification of a random process

The random process $X(\omega,t)$ is a collection of N random variables. Based on the type of the random variables and the indexing set, the process can be classified in a number of ways. For example, we may use the form of the joint distribution of the sequence of the random variables comprising the random process. If the sequence is jointly Gaussian, we say the process is Gaussian. If the sequence has a joint Poisson distribution, we say the process is Poisson, and so on. We may then classify the process based on the invariance of the sequence to the sampling instants. We shall later study, in detail, a class of random processes known as *stationary random processes*, for which the joint distribution of the sequence of random variables does not change with a shift in the sample; i.e., $F_{X_1 X_2 \cdots X_N}(x_1 x_2 \cdots x_N) = F_{X'_1 X'_2 \cdots X'_N}(x'_1 x'_2 \cdots x'_N)$ where the sequences $X_1 X_2 \cdots X_N$ and $X'_1 X'_2 \cdots X'_N$ are separated by a shift Δ on the indexing set (e.g., time).

Classification of a random process may also be done with respect to the elementary outcomes and the indexing set. Here we can list four classifications for the random process based on whether the random variable $X(\omega)$ is discrete or continuous, and whether the index $t \in T \subset R$ is discrete or continuous. That is::

$X(\omega,t)$ will be a discrete random process with discrete parameters if both $X(\omega)$ and t are discrete.

Likewise $X(\omega,t)$ will be a continuous random process with continuous parameters if both $X(\omega)$ and t are continuous.

On the other hand, if $X(\omega)$ is continuous and t is discrete, the random process $X(\omega, t)$ is said to be continuous with discrete parameters.

The fourth class is for $X(\omega)$ is discrete and t continuous.

We illustrate these classifications by the following example.

Example 5.1 Discrete random process with discrete parameters. Toss a fair coin N times; $\Omega = \{h, t\}$ for one toss. Let

$$X_i \triangleq \begin{cases} 1 & \text{if a head occurs in toss } i \\ 0 & \text{if a tail occurs in toss } i \end{cases}$$

The number of sample functions (realizations) – 2^N. Let the index set $T = \{1, 2, 3, \ldots, N\}$. Therefore, an ensemble may be generated accordingly. For example, if $N = 3$, we have 8 realizations, and $T = \{1, 2, 3\}$; $\Omega = \{\omega_1, \omega_2 \cdots \omega_8\}$. The ensemble can be reconstructed as shown in Figure 5.4 below.

Example 5.2 Discrete random process with continuous parameters. Let $X(\omega,t) = A(\omega) \cos(2\pi ft + \theta(\omega))$, where f is a constant and $A(\omega)$ and $\theta(\omega)$ are random variables.

5.1 Definition and general concepts

	X_1	X_2	X_3
TTT	0	0	0
TTH	0	0	1
THT	0	1	0
THH	0	1	1
HTT	1	0	0
HTH	1	0	1
HHT	1	1	0
HHH	1	1	1

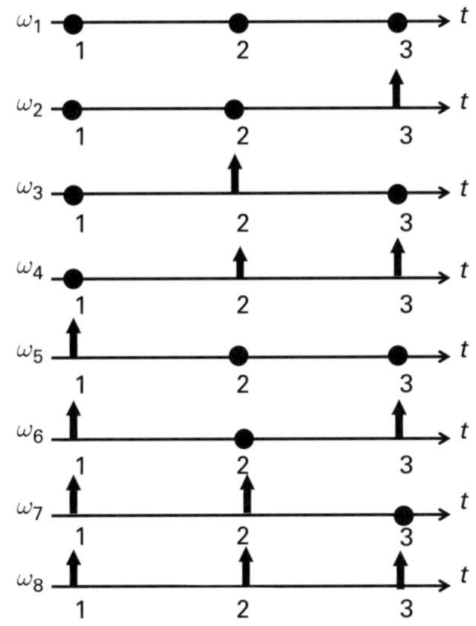

Figure 5.4 Construction of an ensemble from a simple statistical experiment involving tossing a fair coin three consecutive times. A total of eight waveforms (realization) may be obtained, each with equal probability.

Hence

$$Y(\omega, t) = \begin{cases} 1 & X(\omega, t) > 0 \\ 0 & X(\omega, t) = 0 \\ -1 & X(\omega, t) < 0 \end{cases}$$

Therefore, $Y(\omega, t)$ would take only discrete values for any $t \in T$. A typical sample function will be as in Figure 5.5. This resembles the output of a clipping circuit, which generates binary output from a sinusoidal input.

Example 5.3 Continuous random process with discrete parameters. Consider a sequence of independent and identically distributed (*iid*) random variables $X(t_i)$. If the density function $f_{X_i}(x_i) \equiv f_X(x)$ is continuous in x (e.g., Gaussian, Laplacian, Maxwell), and the set $T = \{t_1, t_2, t_3, \ldots\}$, i.e., discrete, then $X(\omega,t)$ will be a continuous random process with discrete parameters.

Example 5.4 Continuous random process with continuous parameters. Let $X(\omega,t) = A(\omega) \cos(2\pi f t + \theta(\omega))$, where f is a constant and $A(\omega)$ and $\theta(\omega)$ are continuous random variables,

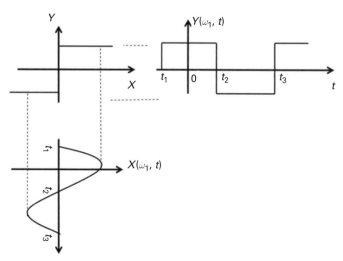

Figure 5.5 Construction of an ensemble from a clipping circuit with sinusoidal input.

$t \in T$ and T is continuous; e.g., let $A(\omega) = 3$, $(\omega) \sim U(0, 2\pi)$ $X(\omega,t) = 3\cos(2\pi ft + \theta(\omega))$ where U denotes a uniform density function. We can generate ensembles as follows:

$$\omega_1: \theta = 0 \quad X(\omega_1,t) = 3\cos(2\pi ft)$$
$$\omega_2: \theta = \pi/2 \quad X(\omega_2,t) = 3\cos(2\pi ft + \pi/2) = -3\sin(2\pi ft)$$
$$\omega_\infty: \theta = 2\pi \quad X(\omega_\infty,t) = 3\cos(2\pi ft + 2\pi) = 3\cos(2\pi ft).$$

Convention: We will be using $X(\omega,t) = X(t) = X_t = X$, but we will also use the full notation where necessary to avoid confusing a random process with a random variable.

5.1.3 Continuity of a random process

A deterministic function $X(t)$ is said to be *right* continuous if $\lim_{h \to 0, h>0} X(t_0 + h) = X(t_0)$, and *left* continuous if $\lim_{h \to 0, h>0} X(t_0 - h) = X(t_0)$. In a random function (random process), we have several kinds of continuity criteria.

DEFINITION 5.2 *A random process X_t is continuous in probability at t_0, if for all $\epsilon > 0$*

$$\lim_{t \to t_0} P(|X_t - X_{t_0}| > \epsilon) = 0. \blacksquare$$

DEFINITION 5.3 *A random process X_t is continuous in the mean square sense (m.s.s) if*

$$\lim_{t \to t_0} E(|X_t - X_{t_0}|^2) = 0. \blacksquare$$

DEFINITION 5.4 *A random process X_t is continuous with probability 1, if for all $\epsilon > 0$*

$$P(\lim_{t \to t_0} |X_t - X_{t_0}| > \epsilon) = 0. \blacksquare$$

5.1.4 The Kolmogorov consistency conditions

Let (Ω, σ_F, P) be a probability space, and let T be any index set. If $\{X_t; t \in T\}$ is a random process defined on Ω, then for any arbitrary finite subset of T, e.g. $t_1, t_2, \ldots, t_n$, the random variables $X(t_1), X(t_2), \ldots, X(t_n)$ will have the finite-dimensional distribution function

$$F_{X_n}(x_1, x_2, \ldots, x_n; t_1, t_2, \ldots, t_n) \triangleq P\Big(X(t_1) \leq x_1, X(t_2) \leq x_2 \ldots X(t_n) \leq x_n\Big). \quad (5.1)$$

Now, the collection of all finite-dimensional distribution function forms a *complete statistical description* of the random process provided that the following conditions hold:

$$K1: \lim_{X_n \to \infty} F_{X_n}(x_1, x_2, \ldots x_n; t_1, t_2, \ldots t_n) = F_{X_{n-1}}(x_1, x_2, \ldots x_n; t_1, t_2, \ldots, t_n), \quad (5.2)$$

for any subset $\{t_1, t_2, \ldots, t_n\} \in T$. That is, $F_{X_{n-1}}(.)$ can be obtained from $F_{X_n}(.)$ by integrating out the last variable.

$$K2: \lim_{X_n \to \infty} F_{X_n}(x_1, x_2, \ldots, x_i, \ldots, x_l, \ldots x_n; t_1, t_2 \ldots, t_i, \ldots, t_l, \ldots, t_n)$$
$$= F_{X_n}(x_1, x_2, \ldots, x_l, \ldots, x_i, \ldots x_n; t_1, t_2 \ldots, t_l, \ldots, t_i, \ldots, t_n) \quad (5.3)$$

for all pairs (x_i, t_i) and (x_l, t_l) and for all n. In other words, $F_{X_n}(.)$ is invariant to the same permutations applied on (x_i, t_i) (meaning the index of x and t remains the same). Conditions $K1$ and $K2$ are known as the Kolmogorov consistency conditions.

DEFINITION 5.5 *A vector random process (stochastic process)* $X(t)$ *consists of* n *random processes, each with parameter t belonging to the same parameter set T; that is,*

$$X(t) = \{X_1(t), X_2(t), X_3(t), \ldots, X_n(t) | t \in T\}. \blacksquare$$

DEFINITION 5.6 *A complex random process* $x(t)$ *is given by* $X(t) = X_1(t) + j X_2(t)$, *where* $X_1(t), X_2(t)$ *are real random processes and* $j = \sqrt{-1}$. $\blacksquare$

5.2 Distribution functions for a random process

5.2.1 Definitions

As we pointed out before, one way of describing and studying a random process is by using joint distribution for finite subfamilies of random variables in the process. This means that we can define distribution functions for a stochastic process in a similar fashion to sequences of random variables.

DEFINITION 5.7 *The first-order distribution function* $F_X(x, t)$ *for a random process* $X = X(\omega, t)$ *is a function defined by* $F(x, t) \triangleq P\Big(X(\omega, t) \leq x\Big)$, *for every* $x \in R$ *and every* $t \in T \subset R$. $\blacksquare$

Random processes

In general, the distribution function of a random process is a function of the indexing parameter t.

DEFINITION 5.8 *The second-order distribution function of the process $X(\omega,t)$ is the function defined by $F(x_1, x_2; t_1, t_2) \triangleq P(X(\omega, t_1) \le x_1, X(\omega, t_2) \le x_2)$, for every pair of x_1 and $x_2 \in R$, and every pair of numbers $t_1, t_2 \in T$.* ∎

A distribution function of any order n is defined similarly.

5.2.2 First- and second-order probability distribution functions

The *first-order* distribution function of any fixed $t \in T$ is the ordinary distribution function for the random variable $X = X(\omega, t)$ selected from the family that makes up the process; that is, $F(x,t) = F_X(x)$. The *second-order* distribution function is the ordinary joint distribution function for the pair of random variables $X_1 = X(\omega, t_1)$ and $X_2 = X(\omega, t_2)$ selected from the process; that is, $F(x_1, x_2; t_1, t_2) = F_{X_1 X_2}(x_1, x_2)$. We shall develop these distributions with the help of Example 5.5 below.

Example 5.5 The process $X(\omega,t)$ has four sample functions $\Omega = \{\omega_1, \omega_2, \omega_3, \omega_4\}$ shown in Figure 5.6 below. Let $P(\omega_k) = p_k$ with $\sum_{k=1}^{4} p_k = 1$. The first- and second-order distribution functions of the process will be evaluated from basic definitions as follows.

(i) *First order distribution function $F_{X_1}(x_1; t_1)$:*
  - For $t = t_1$: none of the sample functions lie below amplitude a; hence,
  $$F(a, t_1) \triangleq P(X(\omega, t_1) \le a) \equiv 0.$$
  Since only $X(\omega_1, t_1)$ is below b on the plot, this implies that $F(b, t_1) = P(X(w, t_1) \le b) \equiv P_1$.
  - For $t = t_2$: none of the sample functions lies below amplitude a. Hence,
  $$F(a, t_2) = P(X(w, t_2) \le a) \equiv 0.$$

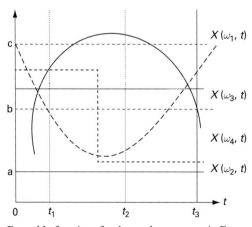

Figure 5.6   Ensemble functions for the random process in Example 5.5.

5.2 Distribution functions for a random process

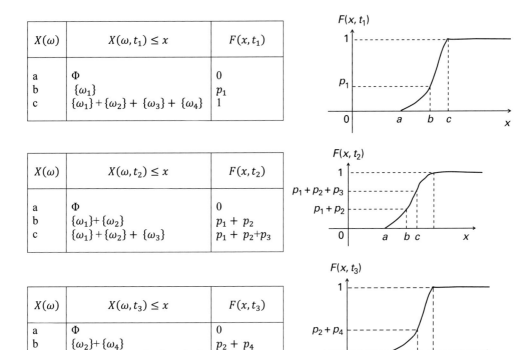

$X(\omega)$	$X(\omega, t_1) \leq x$	$F(x, t_1)$
a	Φ	0
b	$\{\omega_1\}$	P_1
c	$\{\omega_1\}+\{\omega_2\}+\{\omega_3\}+\{\omega_4\}$	1

$X(\omega)$	$X(\omega, t_2) \leq x$	$F(x, t_2)$
a	Φ	0
b	$\{\omega_1\}+\{\omega_2\}$	$P_1 + P_2$
c	$\{\omega_1\}+\{\omega_2\}+\{\omega_3\}$	$P_1 + P_2 + P_3$

$X(\omega)$	$X(\omega, t_3) \leq x$	$F(x, t_3)$
a	Φ	0
b	$\{\omega_2\}+\{\omega_4\}$	$P_2 + P_4$
c	$\{\omega_1\}+\{\omega_2\}+\{\omega_3\}+\{\omega_4\}$	1

Figure 5.7 First-order probability distribution functions for the random process in Example 5.5.

$X(\omega_1, t_2)$ and $X(\omega_2, t_2)$ lie below the value b. Hence; $F(b, t_2) \triangleq P\Big(X(\omega, t_2) \leq b\Big) = P_1 + P_2$.

$X(\omega_1, t_2)$, $X(\omega_2, t_2)$, and $X(\omega_3, t_2)$ lie below the value c. Hence, $F(c, t_2) = P\Big(X(\omega, t_2) \leq c\Big) = P_1 + P_2 + P_3$.

- For $t = t_3$: none of the sample functions is below a; hence, $F(a, t_3) = 0$; $X(\omega_2, t_3)$ and $X(\omega_4, t_3) \leq b$; hence, $F(b, t_3) = P_2 + P_4$. All sample functions are below c, so $F(c, t_3) = 1$.

We can summarize the results in the following table:
Similarly, we can obtain $F(x, t)$ for other values of the indexing parameter t, which defines another random variable with a different distribution function.

As an exercise, we may ask: is the process $X(\omega, t)$ first-order stationary? That is, does $F(x, t) = F(x, t + \Delta t)$?

(ii) *Second-order distribution function* $F_{X_1 X_2}(x_1, x_2; t_1, t_2)$: Using the values from the ensemble at t_1 and t_2, we can define various events and their measures, as shown in the following table.

x_1	x_2	$\{X(\omega,t_1) \leq x_1, X(\omega,t_2) \leq x_2\}$	$F(x_1,x_2; t_1,t_2)$
a	a	Φ	0
a	b	Φ	0
a	c	Φ	0
b	a	Φ	0
b	b	$\{\omega_1\}$	p_1
b	c	$\{\omega_1\}$	p_1
c	a	Φ	0
c	b	$\{\omega_1\} \cup \{\omega_2\}$	$p_1 + p_2$
c	c	$\{\omega_1\} \cup \{\omega_2\} \cup \{\omega_3\}$	$p_1 + p_2 + p_3$

Similarly, we can evaluate $F(x_2,x_3; t_2,t_3)$:

x_2	x_3	$\{X(\omega,t_2) \leq x_2, X(\omega,t_3) \leq x_3\}$	$F(x_2,x_3; t_2,t_3)$
a	a	Φ	0
a	b	Φ	0
a	c	Φ	0
b	a	Φ	0
b	b	$\{\omega_2\}$	p_2
b	c	$\{\omega_1\} \cup \{\omega_2\}$	$p_1 + p_2$
c	a	Φ	0
c	b	$\{\omega_2\}$	p_2
c	c	$\{\omega_1\} \cup \{\omega_2\} \cup \{\omega_3\}$	$p_1 + p_2 + p_3$

Similar evaluations can be used for other values of t_i and $t_j \in T$.

Comment: If the random process is defined, then the distribution functions of all finite orders are also defined (Kolmogorov [5.3]).

Example 5.6 Consider the following experiment of flipping a non-fair coin. The probability of a head is 1/3 and the probability of a tail is 2/3; i.e. $\Omega =$ {head, tail}, P(head) $= 1/3$ and p(tail) $= 2/3$. Let us define a random variable $X = X(\omega)$ such that:

$$X = \begin{cases} -1 & \text{if } \{\omega = \text{head}\} \\ 0 & \text{if } \{\omega = \text{tail}\}. \end{cases}$$

Hence, the distribution functions $F_X(x) = P(X \leq x) = \begin{cases} 0 & x \leq -1 \\ \dfrac{1}{3} & x < 0 \\ 1 & x \geq 0 \end{cases}$

Now, let us define a random process $X(\omega,t)$ such that:

$$X(\omega, t) = \begin{cases} \sin t & \text{if } \{\omega = \text{head}\} \\ 2t & \text{if } \{\omega = \text{tail}\} \end{cases}$$

5.2 Distribution functions for a random process

That is, the process has two sample functions $X(\omega_1, t) = \sin t$ and as shown in Figure 5.8.

We can determine the distribution function for $X(\omega, t)$ at any time t as follows (see Figure 5.9):

Exercise: (a) Is $X(\omega, t)$ first-order stationary? (b) Obtain the joint distribution function $t_1 = \pi/2$ and $t_2 = \pi$.

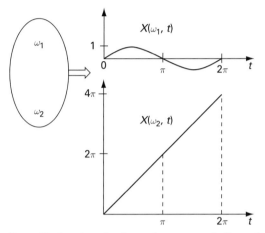

Figure 5.8 Ensemble functions for the random process in Example 5.6.

$X(\omega, \pi/4)$	$X(\omega, \pi/4) \le x$	$F(x, \pi/4)$
0	Φ	0
$1/\sqrt{2}$	$\{\omega_1\}$	1/3
$\pi/2$	$\{\omega_1\} + \{\omega_2\}$	1

$X(\omega, \pi/2)$	$X(\omega, \pi/2) \le x$	$F(x, \pi/2)$
0	Φ	0
1	$\{\omega_1\}$	1/3
π	$\{\omega_1\} + \{\omega_2\}$	1

$X(\omega, \pi)$	$X(\omega, \pi) \le x$	$F(x, \pi)$
0	$\{\omega_1\}$	1/3
2π	$\{\omega_1\} + \{\omega_2\}$	1
-1	Φ	0

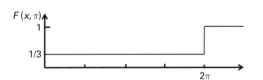

Figure 5.9 First-order probability distribution functions for the random process in Example 5.6.

5.3 Some properties of a random process

5.3.1 Stationarity

Since a random process is defined in terms of an indexed set of random variables, it is natural to ask about the effect of the indexing on the distribution function of the resulting sequence of random variables. The class of random processes in which shifting of the indexing parameter does not affect the joint distribution function of the sequence of random variables is quite special and possesses several interesting properties. This class is called stationary random processes.

DEFINITION 5.9 *The random process X is said to be stationary to order n if for any time deviation h, the following is true:*

$$F_n(x_1, x_2, \ldots, x_n\,;\, t_1, t_2, \ldots, t_n) = F_n(x_1', x_2', \ldots, x_n'\,;\, t_1 + h, t_2 + h, \ldots, t_n + h) \tag{5.4}$$

for all $t_1, t_2, \ldots, t_n \in T$ and all h such that $t_1 + h, t_2 + h, \ldots, t_n + h \in T$, where T is the index parameter set. ∎

It is evident that if the random process X is stationary to order n, then it is stationary to order $n - 1$, which follows from Kolmogorov consistency conditions.

5.3.2 The autocorrelation function

Correlation is a moment property that measures how random variables on the same statistical experiment are "*related*" to one another. Similarly, we may define correlations between random variables obtained by sampling of realizations of a random process $X(\omega, t)$.

DEFINITION 5.10 *The autocorrelation function, denoted by $R_{XX}(t,s)$ or $R_X(t,s)$ or $R(t,s)$, of a random process X is defined by the expectation: $R_X(t,s) = E\left(X(\omega, t)\,\overline{X(\omega, s)}\right)$.* ∎

Again, we may use shorthand forms for the random process $X(\omega, t)$ as: $X(t)$ or X_t, which will be clear from the context and will not be confused with random variables; hence, $R_X(t, s) = E\left(X(t)\,\overline{X(s)}\right)$. Suppose $X(t)$ is stationary to order 2 or more. Let $s = t + h$, and assume $x(\cdot)$ to be a *real-valued* random process; hence, $R_X(t,s) = E(X(t)\,X(t+h))$, which for a continuous parameter random process will be:

$$R_X(t, s) = \int\!\!\!\int_{-\infty}^{\infty} x_1 x_2\, f_{X_1 X_2}(x_1, x_2; t, t+h)\, dx_1 dx_2.$$
$$= \int\!\!\!\int_{-\infty}^{\infty} x_1 x_2\, f_{X_1 X_2}(x_1, x_2; 0, h)\, dx_1 dx_2 \tag{5.5}$$

By stationarity, $R_X(t,s)$ is a function of $h = |t - s|$, the time shift; hence, we may write: $R_X(t,s) = R(s,t) = R(t-s) = R(s-t) = R(|t-s|) = R(\tau); \quad \tau = |t-s|$. Consequently, for a process that is stationary to order 2 (at least) we have: $R_X(\tau) = E\left(X(t)X(t+\tau)\right) = R_X(-\tau)$; i.e., $R_X(\cdot)$ is symmetric.

DEFINITION 5.11 *A random process $X(t)$ is said to be stationary in the wide sense (w.s.s.) if:*

(a) $E(|X(t)|^2) < \infty$ for every $t \in T$, and
(b) $E(X(t)X(s)) = R(|t-s|)$ for every $t, s \in T$. ∎

It is evident that a process $X(t)$ that is stationary to order 2 and has finite second moment (i.e. $E(|X(t)|^2) < \infty$) is w.s.s. The converse is not true, in general. The proof is left as an exercise.

Example 5.7 Consider a sequence of random variables $\{X_n\}$ which are mutually independent, each with zero mean and variance σ_2. Show that the process $\{X_n\}$ is w.s.s. but not stationary to any order.
Proof:

(i) $E\left(|X(t)|^2\right) = \sigma^2 < \infty$

(ii) $E(X_k X_{k+n}) \triangleq R(n) = \begin{cases} \sigma^2 &, n = 0 \\ 0 &, n \neq 0 \end{cases}$

From (i) and (ii) it is obvious that $\{X_n\}$ is w.s.s. Now unless all X_n are identically distributed, $\{X_n\}$ will not be stationary even for order 1, because the distribution function will be in general a function of n.

Properties of $R(\tau)$: We can use the definitions to extract a number of properties of the autocorrelation function. Below are a few such properties; properties (i)–(iii) hold for real-valued random process.

(i) If the random variables are real, then the autocorrelation function is symmetric; that is, $R(\tau) = R(-\tau)$; hence, its Fourier transform will be also real and even.

We note that a *real* random process is symmetric, regardless of stationarity.

(ii) $R(0) = E\left(X(t)X(t+0)\right) = E\left(X^2(t)\right) \triangleq \sigma_X^2$, where σ_X^2 is the variance of the first-order probability distribution function of the process X.
(iii) $R(0) \geq \pm R(\tau)$. That is, the autocorrelation function has maximum value at the origin.

Proof:
We know that $E((X(t) \pm X(t+\tau))^2) \geq 0$; hence, $E(X^2(t)) \pm 2E(X(t)X(t+\tau)) + E(X^2(t+\tau)) = R(0) \pm 2R(\tau) + R(0) \geq 0$. Therefore, $R(0) \geq \pm R(\tau)$.

(iv) Consider a w.s.s. random process, and let $f(t)$ be any nonzero function, i.e. $f(t) > 0$ for all $t \in T$; then:

$$E\left(\left|\int_a^b X(t)f(t)dt\right|^2\right) = E\left(\int_a^b\int_a^b X(t)f(t)\overline{X}(s)\overline{f}(s)dtds\right)$$

$$= \int_a^b\int_a^b R(t-s)f(t)\overline{f}(s)dtds \geq 0.$$

Hence, $R(\tau)$ is nonnegative definite.

5.3.3 The autocovariance function

DEFINITION 5.12 Let $\eta_i \triangleq E(X(t_i))$; the autocovariance function $C(t_1,t_2)$ is defined as:

$$C(t_1,t_2) = E\left(X(t_1) - \eta_1\right)\left(\overline{X(t_2)} - \overline{\eta_2}\right)$$
$$= E\left(X(t_1)\overline{X(t_2)}\right) - \eta_1\overline{\eta_2} - \overline{\eta_2}\eta_1 + \eta_1\eta_2 \triangleq R(t_1,t_2) - \eta_1\overline{\eta_2}. \blacksquare$$

Example 5.8 Consider the ensemble from a real-valued random process $X(\omega,t)$ shown in Figure 5.10. For the particular choice of t_1 and t_2, we have $\mu_1 \triangleq E(X(t_1)) = 1$ and $\mu_2 \triangleq E(X(t_2)) = 0$. Let us define random variable $Y \triangleq (X(\omega,t_1) - \mu_1)(X(\omega,t_2) - \mu_2)$. Hence, $Y(\omega_1) = (2-1)(-\frac{8}{3}) = -\frac{8}{3}$, $Y(\omega_2) = (1-1)(3) = 0$, $Y(\omega_3) = (3-1)(4) = 8$, and $Y(\omega_4) = (-2-1)(2) = -6$. Therefore, $E(Y) \triangleq E(X(\omega,t_1) - \mu_1)(X(\omega,t_2) - \mu_2)$
$\triangleq C(t_1,t_2) = (-8/3)(1/2) + (0)(1/3) + 8(0) + (-6)1/6 = -7/3$.

5.3.4 The cross-correlation function

DEFINITION 5.13 *Consider two processes $X_1(t)$ and $X_2(t)$ defined on the same indexing parameter set T. The cross-correlation function $R_{X_1X_2}(t_1,t_2) = R_{12}(t_1,t_2)$ is defined as $R_{12}(t_1,t_2) = E\left(X_1(t_1)\overline{X_2(t_2)}\right)$.* $\blacksquare$

Let $R_{11}(\tau) \triangleq E(X_1(t)\overline{X_1}(t+\tau))$ and $R_{22}(\tau) \triangleq E(X_2(t)\overline{X_2}(t+\tau))$. The following properties can be easily shown to hold:

(i) $R_{12}(t_1,t_2) = R_{21}(t_2,t_1)$
(ii) $R_{11}(0) + R_{22}(0) \geq \pm 2R_{12}(\tau)$

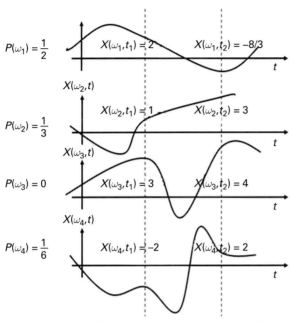

Figure 5.10 Sample functions of the random process in Example 5.8.

Proof:
$E(|X_1(t) \pm X_2(t+\tau)|^2) \geq 0$; hence by expansion we obtain:

$$E\left(X_1(t) \pm X_2(t+\tau)\right)\left(\overline{X_1(t)} \pm \overline{X_2(t+\tau)}\right) = E\left(X_1(t)\overline{X_1}(t)\right) \pm E\left(X_1(t)\overline{X_2}(t+\tau)\right) \pm$$

$$E\left(X_2(t+\tau)\overline{X_1}(t)\right) + E\left(X_2(t+\tau)\overline{X_2}(t+\tau)\right) \triangleq R_{11}(0) + R_{22}(0) \pm 2R_{12}(\tau) \geq 0.$$

Therefore, $R_{11}(0) + R_{22}(0) \geq \pm 2R_{12}(\tau)$.

DEFINITION 5.14 *The correlation coefficient:*

$$r_{12}(\tau) \triangleq \frac{R_{12}(\tau)}{\sqrt{(R_{11}(0) R_{22}(0))}} \cdot \blacksquare \qquad (5.6)$$

Let $X_1(t) = X$ and $X_2(t+\tau) = Y$. Since $|R_{12}(\tau)|^2 \leq R_{11}(0)R_{22}(0)$, $|r_{12}(\tau)| \leq 1$.

5.3.5 Time average

Consider a random process $X(t)$; $t \in (-\infty, \infty)$, the time average of $X(t)$ is defined as $\lim_{T\to\infty} \frac{1}{2T} \int_{-T}^{T} X(t)dt$, for a set $T \in R$. The time autocorrelation function is defined as

$$R(\tau) = \lim_{T \to \infty} \frac{1}{2T} \int_{-T}^{T} X(t)X(t+\tau)\, dt.$$ Note that both the time average and the time autocorrelation functions are random.

DEFINITION 5.15 *The time average (or time mean) of a function $f(\cdot)$ over the interval (a, b) is given by:*

$$A(f; a : b) \triangleq \frac{1}{b-a} \int_a^b f(t)\,dt, \quad b > a. \blacksquare \tag{5.7}$$

Some properties of $A\,(f(\cdot))$:

(i) $A(c) = c$, for any constant function $f(\cdot) = c$.
(ii) Linearity: $A(af(\cdot) + bg(\cdot)) = a\,A(f(\cdot)) + bA(g(\cdot))$
(iii) Positivity: If $f(\cdot) \geq 0$ then $A(f(\cdot)) \geq 0$.
(iv) $A(f(\cdot))$ exists if and only if $A\,(|f(\cdot)|) < \infty$.
(v) $|A\,(f(\cdot))| \leq A(|f(\cdot)|)$.
(vi) $|A\,((f(\cdot))g(\cdot)))|^2 \leq A(|f(\cdot)|^2)A(|g(\cdot)|^2)$ (Schwarz inequality).

DEFINITION 5.16 *Suppose $f(\cdot)$ and $g(\cdot)$ are real or complex-valued functions defined on the whole real line R. The time autocorrelation function $R_f(\cdot)$ for the function $f(\cdot)$ is given by*

$$R_f(\tau) \triangleq A\left(f(t)\overline{f(t+\tau)}\right) \equiv \frac{1}{b-a} \int_a^b f(t)\overline{f(t+\tau)}\, dt, \quad b > a. \tag{5.8}$$

The time cross-correlation function for $f(\cdot)$ and $g(\cdot)$ is given by

$$R_{fg}(\tau) \triangleq A\left(f(t)\overline{g(t+\tau)}\right) \equiv \frac{1}{b-a} \int_a^b f(t)\overline{g(t+\tau)}\, dt. \tag{5.9}$$

We note that if $a \to \infty$ and $b \to \infty$, then the definitions for $A(f(\cdot))$ and $R_f(\tau)$ are the same as before. $\blacksquare$

DEFINITION 5.17 *A sample function $X(\omega,.)$ from a stationary random process is said to be typical (in the wide sense) if and only if $A(X(\omega,\cdot)) = \mu_X$ and $R_X(\omega,\tau) = R_X(\tau)$, $\forall\ \tau$.* $\blacksquare$

DEFINITION 5.18 *A random process which has the property that any time average of one sample function $X(\omega,\cdot)$ is equal to the corresponding time average of any other sample function is called a regular random process.* $\blacksquare$

5.3 Some properties of a random process

Note that regularity implies that time-averaged properties are invariant to shifts over $\omega \in \Omega$. On the other hand, stationarity implies that the statistical properties are invariant to shifts over $t \in T$.

DEFINITION 5.19 *A random process is said to be* ergodic *if it is both regular and stationary.*∎

Ergodicity, when achieved, makes it possible to use time averages of sample functions of the random process as approximations to the corresponding ensemble averages (or expectations).

5.3.6 The power spectrum of a random process

Consider a function $g(\cdot)$ which is absolutely integrable; i.e., $\int_{-\infty}^{\infty} |g(t)|\, dt < \infty$. The Fourier transform of $g(.)$, $G(f)$ is: $G(f) = \int_{-\infty}^{\infty} g(t) e^{-j2\pi ft} dt$. The inverse Fourier transform is: $g(t) = \int_{-\infty}^{\infty} G(f) e^{j2\pi ft} df$. Now consider a w.s.s. random process $X(t)$ which is real-valued, with zero mean, and an autocorrelation function $R_X(\tau)$. Let us define a random variable

$$g_T(\lambda) \triangleq \int_{-T}^{T} X(t) e^{-j2\pi\lambda t} dt.$$

Let us also define the quantity $S_T(\lambda) = \dfrac{E\left(|g_T(\lambda)|^2\right)}{2T} \geq 0$. Hence,

$$S_T(\lambda) = \frac{1}{2T} E\left(g_T(\lambda) \cdot \overline{g_T}(\lambda)\right) = \frac{1}{2T} E \int_{-T}^{T} X(t) e^{-j2\pi\lambda t} \cdot \int_{-T}^{T} X(s) e^{j2\pi\lambda s} ds$$

$$= \frac{1}{2T} \iint_{-T}^{T} R_X(t-s) e^{-j2\pi\lambda(t-s)} dt\, ds \geq 0$$

Let us make the following change of variables: $t - s = u$, $v = s$; the Jacobian of the transformation is $\begin{pmatrix} u \\ v \end{pmatrix} = \begin{pmatrix} 1 & -1 \\ 0 & 1 \end{pmatrix} \begin{pmatrix} t \\ s \end{pmatrix}$; $\|j\| = 1$. This mapping is illustrated in Figure 5.11.

Hence,
$$S_T(\lambda) = \frac{1}{2T} \int_{-2T}^{0} R_X(u) e^{-j2\pi\lambda u} \int_{-(T+u)}^{T} dv\, du + \frac{1}{2T} \int_{0}^{2T} R_X(u) e^{-j2\pi\lambda u} \int_{-T}^{T-u} dv\, du$$

$$= \int_{-2T}^{0} \left(1 + \frac{u}{2T}\right) R_X(u) e^{-j2\pi\lambda u} du + \int_{0}^{2T} \left(1 - \frac{u}{2T}\right) R_X(u) e^{-j2\pi\lambda u} du$$

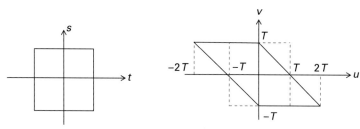

Figure 5.11 The transformation: $t - s = u$, $v = s$; $(t, s) \in [-T, T]$.

Therefore, we obtain $S_T(\lambda) = \int_{-2T}^{2T} \left(1 - \frac{|u|}{2T}\right) R_X(u) e^{-j2\pi\lambda u} du$. Now let us take the limit as $T \to \infty$ of the above quantity; that is,

$$\lim_{T \to \infty} S_T(\lambda) = \lim_{T \to \infty} \int_{-2T}^{2T} \left(1 - \frac{|u|}{2T}\right) R_X(u) e^{-j2\pi\lambda u} du \equiv \int_{-\infty}^{\infty} R_X(u) e^{-j2\pi\lambda u} du, \quad (5.10)$$

which will be finite if $\int_{-\infty}^{\infty} |R_X(u) e^{-j2\pi\lambda u}| du < \infty$, i.e. if the Fourier transform of $R_X(\tau)$ exists. We call this Fourier transform the power spectrum density function of the random process, which we formally define below.

DEFINITION 5.20 *The function $S(\lambda)$, which will be denoted by $S_X(f)$, is the Fourier transform of the autocorrelation function; i.e., $S_X(f) = \mathcal{F}(R_X(t))$.* ∎

Properties of the power spectral density function

(i) $R(\tau) = \int_{-\infty}^{\infty} S(f) e^{j2\pi f \tau} df$

(ii) $S(f) \geq 0$

(iii) $R(0) \triangleq E\left(X^2(t)\right) = \int_{-\infty}^{\infty} S(f) df$ (i.e., $R(0)$ = total power of the process).

(iv) If $X(t)$ is a real-valued random process, then $R_X(\tau)$ is real and even; hence, $S_X(f)$ will be also real and even; i.e., $S_X(f) = S_X(-f)$.

Power spectral density for nonstationary random process

We may still define the power spectral density function for a nonstationary random process, over a period T in the limit $S(f) = \lim_{T \to \infty} S_T(f)$, where $S_T(f)$ is the spectral density of the process over an interval T.

5.3.7 Cross-spectral density

Let $X_1(t)$ and $X_2(t)$ be two jointly w.s.s. processes; that is,

$$R_{12}(t_1, t_2) \triangleq E(X_1(t_1)\overline{X_2}(t_2)) \equiv R_{12}(|t_1 - t_2|) \triangleq R_{12}(\tau). \tag{5.11}$$

We define the cross-spectral density function

$$S_{12}(f) \triangleq \int_{-\infty}^{\infty} R_{12}(\tau)e^{-j2\pi f \tau}d\tau, \text{ and } R_{12}(\tau) \equiv \int_{-\infty}^{\infty} S_{12}(f)e^{j2\pi f \tau}df. \tag{5.12}$$

We note that $R_{12}(\tau) = R_{21}(-\tau)$, hence $S_{12}(f) = S_{21}(-f)$.

5.3.8 Power spectral density of discrete-parameter random process

Consider a zero-mean w.s.s. discrete-parameter random process $X(w,t_i) = \{X_i\}$. Hence, $E(X_i) = 0$, $E(X_iX_j) \triangleq R_X(i,j) \equiv R_X(i-j) \equiv R_X(j-i)$.

Let us define the quantity:

$$f_N(\lambda) \triangleq \sum_{k=-N}^{N} x_k e^{-j2\pi k\lambda} \quad \text{and} \quad S_N(\lambda) = \frac{1}{2N+1} E\left(f_N(\lambda)\overline{f_N}(\lambda)\right).$$

Hence,

$$S_N(\lambda) = \frac{1}{2N+1} \sum_{i=-N}^{N} \sum_{k=-N}^{N} R_x(i-k) e^{-j2\pi i\lambda} e^{j2\pi k\lambda}$$

$$= \sum_{m=-2N}^{0} \left(1 + \frac{m}{2N+1}\right) R_x(m) e^{-j2\pi m\lambda} + \sum_{m=1}^{2N} \left(1 - \frac{m}{2N+1}\right) R_x(m) e^{-j2\pi m\lambda}$$

$$= \sum_{m=-2N}^{2N} \left(1 - \frac{|m|}{2N+1}\right) R_x(m) e^{-j2\pi m\lambda}$$

Taking the limit as $N \to \infty$, we note that: $\lim_{N\to\infty} \sum_{m=-2N}^{2N} \frac{|m|}{2N+1} R_x(m) e^{-j2\pi m\lambda} \to 0$, provided

that $\sum_{m=-\infty}^{\infty} |m|R_x(m)| < \infty$. Hence,

$$\lim_{N\to\infty} S_N(\lambda) = \sum_{m=-\infty}^{\infty} R_X(m) e^{-j2\pi m\lambda} \triangleq S(\lambda) \tag{5.13}$$

which defines a power spectral density function for the discrete parameter w.s.s. random process. This is stated formally in the following definition.

DEFINITION 5.21 *The power spectrum density of a w.s.s. discrete-parameter random process is the function $S(\tilde{f})$ defined as:*

$$S(\tilde{f}) \triangleq \sum_{n=-\infty}^{\infty} R_X(n) e^{-j2\pi n \tilde{f}} \qquad (5.14)$$

i.e., the power spectrum equals the sequence Fourier transform of the sequence $R_X(n)$. ■

Notes:

(i) $S(\tilde{f}+1) = \sum_{n=-\infty}^{\infty} R_X(n) e^{-j2\pi n \tilde{f}} \cdot e^{-j2\pi n} = \sum_{m=-\infty}^{\infty} R_X(n) e^{-j2\pi n \tilde{f}} = S(\tilde{f})$;

i.e., $S(\tilde{f})$ is a periodic with period 1; hence, $R[n] = \int_{-1/2}^{1/2} S(\tilde{f}) e^{j2\pi m \tilde{f}} d\tilde{f}$ is the inverse sequence Fourier transform.

(ii) Although $R_X[n]$ is a discrete sequence, $S(\tilde{f})$ is a continuous function in the parameter $\tilde{f}$, which is called the discrete frequency and has units of *cycles*.

(iii) If the process $\{X_i\}$ is obtained by sampling the process $X(t)$ at a rate f samples/sec, then $\tilde{f} = f/f_s$, where f and f_s have units of cycles/sec, or Hz.

5.4 Linear systems with random inputs

The theory of systems is foundational for various branches of applied mathematics and has abundant applications in image analysis. We studied various properties of linear systems in Chapter 2. These properties apply for the case of a deterministic system with random input, as illustrated in Figure 5.12.

We review a few properties below for linear and time-invariant (LTI) systems.

Given an LTI system with system function (impulse response) $h(t)$, input $X(\omega,t)$, and output $Y(\omega,t)$ which are random processes defined on a common σ_F-algebra, we can easily prove that the following holds true (see [5.1]):

The system response:

$$Y(\omega, t) = \int_{-\infty}^{\infty} X(\omega, s) h(t-s) ds \qquad (5.15)$$

which is the well-known convolution integral.

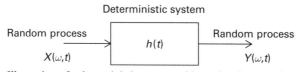

Figure 5.12 Illustration of a deterministic system with random input and output.

5.4 Linear systems with random inputs

The mean value:

$$E\big(Y(t)\big) = \int_{-\infty}^{\infty} E\big(X(s)\big) \cdot h(t-s)ds = \mu_X \int_{-\infty}^{\infty} h(t-s)ds \qquad (5.16)$$

where μ_X is the mean of the random process $X(t)$.

The autocorrelation function:

$$R_y(t, t+\tau) \triangleq E\big(Y(t)Y(t+\tau)\big) \equiv E\left(\int_{-\infty}^{\infty} X(s)h(t-s)ds \int_{-\infty}^{\infty} X(\gamma)h(t+\tau-\gamma)d\gamma\right)$$

$$= \iint_{-\infty}^{\infty} E\big(X(s)X(\gamma)\big) \cdot h(t-s)h(t+\tau-\gamma)dsd\gamma$$

$$\equiv \iint_{-\infty}^{\infty} R_x(s,\gamma)h(t-s)h(t+\tau-\gamma)dsd\gamma, \qquad (5.17)$$

which can be rewritten, using change of variables, as:

$$R_Y(t, t+\tau) = \iint_{-\infty}^{\infty} R_X(t-s, t+\tau-\gamma)h(s)h(\gamma)dsd\gamma$$

$$= \iint_{-\infty}^{\infty} R_X(t-s, t+\tau-\gamma)h(s)h(\gamma)dsd\gamma. \qquad (5.18)$$

Special case: $X(\omega,t)$ is a w.s.s. process:

$$R_X(t_1, t_2) = R_X(t_1 - t_2) = R_X(t_2 - t_1)$$
$$\Rightarrow R_X(t-s, t+\tau-\gamma) = R_X(\tau+s-\gamma)$$

Hence, $\displaystyle R_y(t, t+\tau) = \iint_{-\infty}^{\infty} R_x(\tau+s-\gamma)h(s)h(\gamma)dsd\gamma \equiv R_y(\tau) \qquad (5.19)$

Therefore, $Y(\omega, t)$ is also a w.s.s. process.

Power spectral density of the response of LTI systems

Consider the special case where the input $X(\omega,t)$ is a w.s.s. process. Taking the Fourier transform of the above equation, we obtain:

$$S_Y(f) = \int_{-\infty}^{\infty} R_Y(\tau)e^{-j2\pi f\tau}d\tau$$

$$= \int_{-\infty}^{\infty} \left(\iint_{-\infty}^{\infty} h(s)h(\gamma)R_X(\tau+s-\gamma)dsd\gamma\right)e^{-j2\pi f\tau}d\tau$$

Let $\beta = \tau + s - \gamma$; hence,

$$S_Y(f) = \iint_{-\infty}^{\infty} h(s)h(\gamma)R_X(\beta)e^{-j2\pi f(\beta-s+\gamma)}d\beta ds d\gamma \quad (5.20)$$
$$\equiv H(-f)H(f)S_X(f) \triangleq |H(f)|^2 S_X(f).$$

Example 5.9 Consider a LTI system with impulse response $h(t) = e^{-at}u(t), a > 0$. Suppose $X(\omega,t)$ is a white noise process with strength N_o. Evaluate the power spectral density of the response.

Solution: The Fourier transform of $h(t)$, $H(f) = \frac{1}{a+j2\pi f}$.

Let $R_X(\tau) = \frac{N_o}{2}\delta(\tau)$; hence $S_X(f) = \frac{N_o}{2}$, for all f.
It is easier to obtain $S_Y(f)$ first and then use the inverse Fourier transform to obtain $R_Y(\tau)$.

$$S_Y(f) \triangleq |H(f)|^2 S_X(f) \equiv \frac{N_o/2}{a^2 + (2\pi f)^2}.$$

$$R_Y(\tau) = F^{-1}\left(S_Y(f)\right) = \frac{N_o}{2}F^{-1}\left(\frac{1}{2a}\frac{2a}{a^2+(2\pi f)^2}\right) \equiv \frac{N_o}{4a}e^{-a|\tau|}.$$

5.5 Two-dimensional random processes

The statistical experiment may be defined such that, for each elementary outcome $\omega \in \Omega$, the realization $\{X(\omega, t)\ \omega \in \Omega, t \in T^N \subset R^N\}$ is an N- dimensional function of t. For the two-dimensional case, the process $X(\omega, t_1, t_2), (t_1, t_2) \in t^2 \subset R^2$ may be represented by an ensemble of two-dimensional functions of (t_1, t_2). All the properties which we developed above for the one-dimensional random process will apply. There are no topological restrictions on $t \in T^N \subset R^N$. Hence, the random process $\{X(\omega, t)\ \omega \in \Omega, t \in T^N \subset R^N\}$ may take various forms, and its realizations will be manifolds in $(N + 1)$-dimensional space (the extra dimension being the value of the process given a particular value of the vector).

For images, (t_1, t_2) is defined on a lattice, and the process $X(\omega, t_1, t_2), (t_1, t_2) \in T^2 \subset R^2$ defines what is known as a "random field." We will devote a separate chapter to random fields in which we study some basic forms of random processes that have shown great promise in image analysis over the past several decades.

5.6 Exercises

5.1 A random process $X(t)$ is w.s.s. and $X(0) = X(T)$; i.e, $E|X(0) - X(T)|^2 = 0$

(a) Show that $X(t)$ is a periodic process in the m.s.s.; i.e.,

$$E|X(t) - X(t+T)|^2 = 0$$

(b) Prove that the autocorrelation function is periodic with period T.

5.2 Consider the two random processes $X(t) = \cos(t+\theta)$ and $Y(t) = \cos(t-\theta)$, where θ is a random variable uniformly distributed on $(-\pi,\pi)$. Let $Z(t) = X(t) + Y(t)$.
(a) Show that $X(t)$ and $Y(t)$ are w.s.s.
(b) Compute $R_Z(t,s)$. Is $Z(t)$ w.s.s?

5.3 With $X(t)$ and $Y(t)$ as in Exercise 2, let $W(t) = \alpha X(t) + \beta Y(t)$, where α, β, and θ are mutually independent random variables, and α and β are identically distributed with

$$\alpha = \begin{cases} 1 & P(1) = 0.5 \\ -1 & P(-1) = 0.5 \end{cases}$$

(a) Compute $R_W(t,s)$ and show that $W(s)$ is w.s.s.
(b) Compute $R_{W^2}(t,s)$ and show that W^2 is not w.s.s.

5.4 In the following system, $X(t)$ is a zero-mean Gaussian random process, and each of the boxes represents a time-invariant linear filter with the transfer functions shown, e.g.,

$$H(f) = \int_{-\infty}^{\infty} h(t)e^{-j2\pi ft}dt, \quad j = \sqrt{-1}.$$

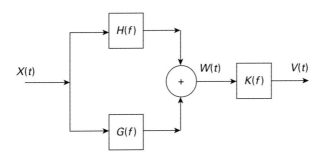

Compute $S_V(f)$ in terms of $R_X(\tau)$ (or $S_X(f)$), $H(f)$ (or $h(t)$), $G(f)$ (or $g(t)$), and $K(f)$ (or $k(t)$).

5.5 Determine which of the following functions are autocorrelation functions for some w.s.s. mean-square continuous random process and give reasons.
(i) $R(t) = t + e^{-|t|}$ (ii) $R(t) = \cos^2 t$
(iii) $R(t) = b$ for $|t| \leq a$, $R(t) = 0$ elsewhere
(iv) $R(t) = \exp(-t^2)$ (v) $R(t) = b|t-a|$, $t \in [0,a]$
(vi) $R(t) = e^{-|t|}\cos t$ (vii) $R(t) = \int_{-\infty}^{\infty} e^{-|t-\tau|}\cos\tau \, d\tau$

5.6 A random process is defined by: $X(t) = a\cos(2\pi Y + \theta)$, where Y and θ are independent random variables, θ is uniformly distributed over the interval $[0, 2\pi]$, and Y has a symmetric probability density $f_Y(y)$. Show that $X(t)$ is w.s.s. and find its spectral density function $S_X(f)$ in terms of $f_Y(y)$.

References

[5.1] A. Papoulis, *Probability, Random Variables and Stochastic Processes*, 3rd Edition. New York: McGraw-Hill (1991).
[5.2] P.E. Pfeiffer, *Concepts of Probability Theory*, 2nd Edition. New York: Dover (1978).
[5.3] A. Kolmogorov, *Grundbegriffe der Wahrscheinlichkeitsrechnung* (in German). Berlin: Julius Springer. Translation: A. Kolmogorov, *Foundations of the Theory of Probability*, 2nd Edition. New York: Chelsea (1956).

6   Basics of random fields

6.1   Introduction

This chapter describes the basics of random fields with focus on models that have been useful for image synthesis, filtering, segmentation, and registration. There is a vast literature on the subject. Besag [6.1], Geman and Geman [6.2], Derin and Elliott [6.3], and Dubes and Jain [6.4] are among the accessible literature in this area. Various books and monograms exist as well. Rue and Held [6.5], and Adler and Taylor [6.6] deal with some basics of random fields, and Blake et al. [6.7] contains examples of applied work on the random field in image analysis and computer vision. From an algorithmic point of view, Dubes and Jain [6.4] is excellent introductory reading.

In simple terms, a random field is a random process in which the index set is multi-dimensional. As random variables are the building blocks of random processes, they are also the basic ingredients of random fields. To introduce the subject of random fields, we provide examples of random experiments that produce outputs in one or more dimensions.

Figure 6.1 shows an ensemble of six waveforms, which may be obtained from electrodes measuring the brain-evoked potential (electroencephalogram or EEG signal). From a random experiment point of view, we may consider these six waveforms as realizations of a random process $X(\omega,t)$. Each signal may occur with a probability measure $P(\omega_i)$, $\omega_i \in \Omega$, $i \in [\ 1,6\ ]$, where Ω is the sample space. Then, as indicated in the previous chapter, sampling the ensemble at instances t_j will yield random variables $X_i = X(\omega,t_j)$; we note that the elementary outcome $\omega = \omega_i \in \Omega, i \in [\ 1,6\ ]$. The random process may be described by a collection of these random variables $\{X_1, X_2, \cdots X_N\}$. The probability distribution of $X(\omega,t)$ may be obtained from the limiting distribution of $\{X_1, X_2, \cdots X_N\}$ as $N \to \infty$. We have not imposed any structure on the index set. For stationary random processes, the Kolmogorov consistency condition relaxes the order of the index set (Chapter 5). Knowledge of the distribution function of the sequence of random variables enables calculation of the probability distribution of the random process as well as various characteristics of it, as studied in the previous chapter.

Now, let us consider the Landsat images in Figure 6.2, which were obtained by two different sensors (with different numbers of bands), during daylight, of the same area on August 26, 1984; September 11, 1984; November 14, 1984; January 17, 1985; March 22, 1985; April 23, 1985; July 28, 1985; August 13, 1985; January 04, 1986; and February 05, 1986 (obtained from the public domain US Geological Survey remote sensing archives; http://earthexplorer.usgs.gov/). If we co-register these images on the same coordinate system, then the pixels at a given location in all the

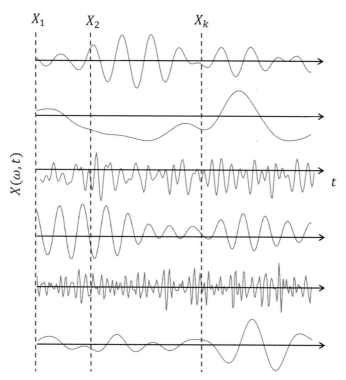

Figure 6.1 An ensemble of a random signal representing process $X(\omega,t)$.

realizations form a random variable that describes the changes of the environment being imaged over time. It is natural to assume that the pixel values would depend on their neighbors, since neighboring pixels would be most likely to belong to the same object or region. Given the characteristics of the imaging system (e.g., spatial resolution), the size of the neighborhoods of random variables may vary. The collection of random variables in the set of images form a special class of random processes known as random fields. The random field is described in terms of the random variables (global characteristics) and the neighborhoods (local characteristics). Hence, random fields defined on a lattice are different from one-dimensional (single parameter) random processes in one fundamental respect, in that the random variables at sites (pixel locations) are usually dependent on each other within a neighborhood, owing to the continuity of the domain of the regions. Therefore, the random fields are characterized by the particular distributions of the random variables and the neighborhood structure of their dependence. This dual dependence provides huge numbers of variations in ways to describe random fields.

The remote sensing example provides clues about the effect of the image acquisition (modality) of the particular sensor used. We may use multiple sensors to gain a better understanding of the region imaged. Likewise, one particular sensor may have a number of bands in order to provide better discrimination of the regions imaged. Hence, the random variables at each pixel may be vector quantities.

6.1 Introduction 133

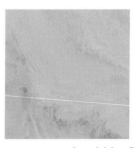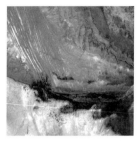

Acquisition Date: 26-AUG-84

Landsat Scene Identifier   LT51770421984255XXX04
Spacecraft Identifier   LANDSAT_5

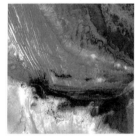

Acquisition Date: 11-SEP-84

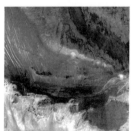

Acquisition Date: 14-NOV-84

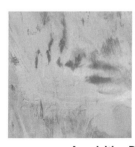

Acquisition Date: 17-JAN-85

Figure 6.2 An ensemble of realizations representing a random field $X(\omega,t)$. The index $t = [t_1\ t_2]$ is row and column location of the pixels in the realizations. The values of $X(.,t)$ may be a vector of measurements for different bands or fusion of sensor measurements.

134 Basics of random fields

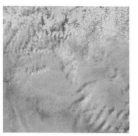 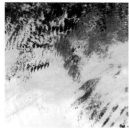

Acquisition Date: 22-MAR-85

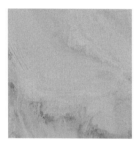 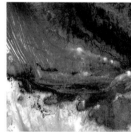

Acquisition Date: 23-APR-85

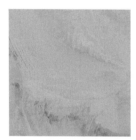 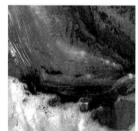

Acquisition Date: 28-JUL-85

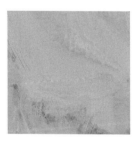 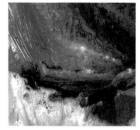

Acquisition Date: 13-AUG-85

Figure 6.2 (cont.)

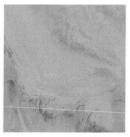 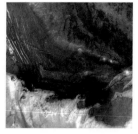

Acquisition Date: 04-JAN-86

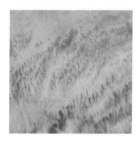 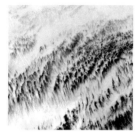

Acquisition Date: 05-FEB-86

Figure 6.2   (cont.)

Fusion of the information from various sensors may provide additional information. This is the case with biomedical imaging in particular, where ultrasound, X-rays, CT, MRI, PET, etc. each provide special details about the object being imaged. Fusion of CT and MRI, for example, of the human head provides enhanced information over either modality alone, since CT provides better imaging of the skull, while MRI provides better imaging of the soft tissues. In the example shown in Figure 6.3, we show 20 slices from CT and corresponding MRI slices for a patient who had a form of bone tumor near the hip area.

(a)   20 CT slices for this region of the hip
(b)   20 MRI slices for the same region of the hip as imaged with CT.

Techniques based on statistics and geometry can be employed to fuse multimodality images, in order to segment and reconstruct structures, for example. In the study involving CT and MRI in Figure 6.3, we were able to segment the tumor and track its volume. Figure 6.4 shows the tumor volume as treatment progressed. We note the importance of multimodality fusion, and the ability to segment tissues with low contrast, to discriminate tissues from tumor, and construct tumors with irregular shapes. CT may be obtained only once to set out a reference for bony structures, while multiple MRI scans can be obtained in order to quantify progress of treatments by co-registering the successive scans. These and many more are among the tools that can be acquired by using random field models in biomedical image analysis.

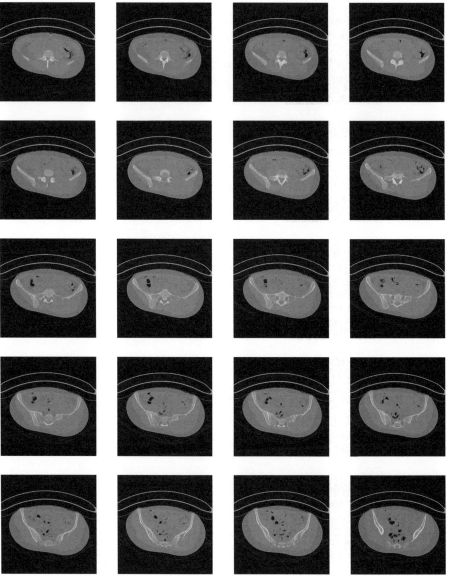

Figure 6.3 Multiple CT (this page) and MRI scans (next page) for an individual, showing progress of a tumor.

6.2 Graphical models

As we start our description of random fields, we summarize what we stated above: that a random field is a generalization of the stochastic process where the set of random variables is not only defined as a sequence, but also can be defined on a graph, tree, grid, etc. (see Figure 6.5).

6.2 Graphical models

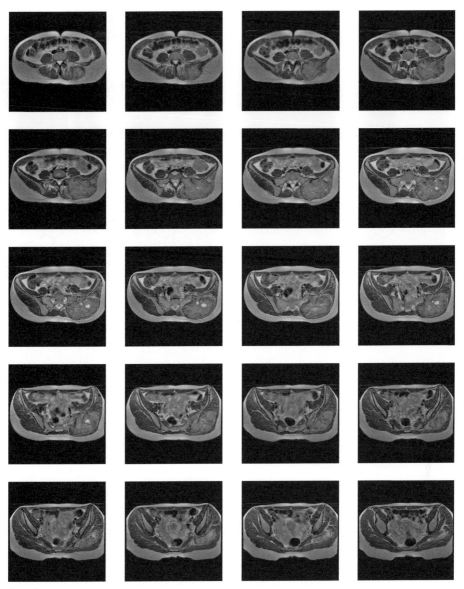

Figure 6.3 (cont.)

A Bayesian network is one of the graphical models that are used to visualize the structure of probabilistic models. A Bayesian network is an acyclic directed graph, which describes the probabilistic causality of events. Each vertex in the graph represents a variable of events, and each edge represents the probabilistic relationship between these events. Unlike the Bayesian network, a Markov random field is represented by an undirected graph, in which each edge captures the interdependency between two neighbors.

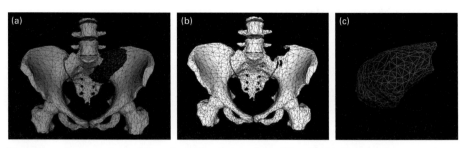

Figure 6.4 Extraction of a tumor in the hip region using fusion of the CT and MRI data. (a) Constructed volume with the tumor; (b) constructed volume minus the tumor; (c) the tumor volume.

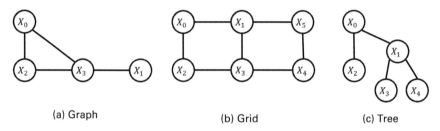

Figure 6.5 Illustration of graphical random field structures.

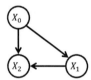

Figure 6.6 A simplified three-state graphical random field model.

Example 6.1 Consider a graphical model which consists of three events: X_0 represents whether a restaurant is open or not, X_1 whether I cook or not, and X_2 whether I eat or not. If the restaurant is open I will eat. Otherwise I will cook then eat. Figure 6.6 describes the relationship between these binary variables. The joint probability of all variables can be computed using the famous Bayes' rule:

$$P(X_2, X_1, X_0) = P(X_2|X_1, X_0)P(X_1, X_0) = P(X_2|X_1, X_0)P(X_1|X_0)P(X_0) \quad (6.1)$$

In order to compute this joint probability completely, we need to list the possible states and their transition probabilities, as shown below.

6.3 Markov system

The Markov system is described by a set of m states $\{s_1, s_2, \ldots, s_m\}$ and discrete time-steps $\{t_0, t_1, \ldots\}$, where in the tth time-step the system is in one of the available states $X_t \in \{s_1, s_2, \ldots, s_m\}$. Between each time-step, the next state is chosen randomly, where the current state determines the probability distribution for the next state. This can be written as follows:

$$P(X_{t+1} = s_i | X_t = s_j, \ldots, X_0 = s_k) = P(X_{t+1} = s_i | X_t = s_j) \quad (6.2)$$

Since the probability distribution of the next state depends only on the current state, the Bayesian network that describes the Markov system is a sequence.

The sequence of states that satisfies Eq. (6.2) is called a Markov chain. The process that generates this sequence is called a Markov process. The Markov chain is defined by its *transition probabilities*, the probability that a process at state S_j moves to a state S_j, in a single step. This transition probability is usually written in a matrix form A where a matrix element $a_{ji} \in A = P(X_{t+1} = s_i | X_t = s_j)$. Let us denote by $\pi_i(t)$ the probability that the chain is in state i at time t, and by $\pi(t)$ the vector of the state space probabilities at time t. Since the chain is started at a particular state, $\pi(0)$ is zero except at this particular state where it will be 1.

According to the Chapman–Kolomogrov theorem (e.g., [6.5]), the vectors of the state space probabilities at time t and time $t + 1$ are related to each other as follows: $\pi(t+1) = \pi(t) A$. Also, the vectors of the state space probabilities at time t and time 0 are related to each other as follows: $\pi(t) = \pi(0) A^t$. We illustrate these concepts in the example below.

Example 6.2 Consider a Markov system that describes the weather in a certain town. The states of the system are *Sunny*, *Cloudy*, and *Rainy*. Given the transition probabilities matrix

$$A = \begin{pmatrix} 0.5 & 0.35 & 0.15 \\ 0.15 & 0.6 & 0.25 \\ 0.4 & 0.1 & 0.5 \end{pmatrix}$$

if today is *Sunny* what is the expectation of the weather tomorrow and next week?

Solution Since the weather follows a Markov process, tomorrow's weather depends only on today's weather. Thus,

P(Sunny tomorrow | Sunny today) = 0.5
P(Cloudy tomorrow | Sunny today) = 0.35
P(Rainy tomorrow | Sunny today) = 0.15

Or, simply, if today is sunny then $\pi(0) = [1\ 0\ 0]$. Using the Chapman–Kolmogorov theorem, we get: $\pi(1) = \pi(0).A^1 = [\ 0.5\ 0.35\ 0.15\ ]$.

The expected weather next week (after 7 days) will be $\pi(7) = \pi(0).A^7$.

6.4 Hidden Markov model

The Markov model which describes the weather in Example 6.2 can be called an *observable* Markov model. This is because the output of the Markov process is the set of states; i.e., each state corresponds to an observable (physical) event. However, when the states are *unobservable* the system is called a hidden Markov model. Assume that we have two biased coins X_0 and X_1 with probabilities $P(H|X_0) = 0.6$ and $P(H|X_1) = 0.3$. One of the coins is selected randomly to be flipped, and a person observes only the output of the coin flips (i.e., does not know which coin is selected). Here, the states of the system are hidden, and the output {Head or Tail} (or $\{H,T\}$) is observed. The hidden Markov model (HMM) is defined by specifying the following items:

- The set of states $\{X_0, X_1,\ldots, X_n\}$; e.g. in the coin example $\{X_0, X_1\}$,
- The vector of the state space probabilities at time 0:$\pi(0)$,
- The transition probabilities matrix A
- The set of the output; e.g. in the coin example $\{H,T\}$,
- The output probabilities; e.g. in the coin example $P(H|X_0) = 0.6$ and $P(H|X_1) = 0.3$.

Example 6.3 Consider a hidden Markov model that describes the two biased flipped coins. Assume the transition probabilities matrix is

$$A = \begin{pmatrix} 0.75 & 0.25 \\ 0.35 & 0.65 \end{pmatrix}$$

If the current selected coin is X_0, i.e. $\pi(0) = [1\ 0]$, what is the probability that the observed output sequence $\{H,H,T,H\}$ is generated from the coin sequence $\{X_0,X_1,X_0,X_1\}$, $P(H,H,T,H,X_0,X_1,X_0,X_1)$?

Solution By Bayes' theorem, we can express the desired result as follows:

$$P(H,H,T,H,X_0,X_1,X_0,X_1) = P(H,H,T,H|X_0,X_1,X_0,X_1)P(X_0,X_1,X_0,X_1).$$

The quantities on the right are given by,

$$P(X_0,X_1,X_0,X_1) = P(X_0)P(X_1|X_0)P(X_0|X_1)P(X_1|X_0) = \pi_0(0) \times a_{01} \times a_{10} \times a_{01}$$
$$= 1 \times 0.25 \times 0.35 \times 0.25.$$

$$P(H,H,T,H|X_0,X_1,X_0,X_1) = P(H|X_0)P(H|X_1)P(T|X_0)P(H|X_1)$$
$$= 0.6 \times 0.3 \times 0.4 \times 0.3.$$

The HMM may describe three types of problems. First, given a model, what is the probability of a set of observed data? Second, given a model, what is the expected sequence of states that gives a certain set of observed data? Finally, given a set of observed data, how can we learn a good HMM to describe the data? Dynamic programming can be used to solve such problems.

6.5 Markov random field

The Markov random field (MRF) models have been widely used in image analysis, and there exists an enormous body of literature on the theory, algorithms and applications of MRF (e.g., [6.1]–[6.5]). Moreover, MRF models that have exponential priors belong to the class of Gibbs models. While a MRF is defined in terms of local properties, a Gibbs random field (GRF) describes the global properties of an image in terms of joint distribution of intensity for all pixels (e.g. [6.1]). This class of MRF with exponential priors, known as Markov–Gibbs random fields (MGRF), has been extensively used in image modeling (e.g., [6.4],[6.8],[6.9]).

As a generalization of the definitions of random variables in Chapter 4, a random field may be defined in terms of a triplet consisting of:

- a sample space,
- a class of Borel sets on the sample space, and
- a probability measure P whose domain is the class of Borel sets.

A random field model is a specification of the measure P for a particular class of random variables (e.g., random variables representing intensities at pixels in an image). Random fields defined on lattices (e.g., pixels in an image) can be identified as follows.

Denote by $S = \{1,2,\ldots,n\}$ a set of n sites (e.g., set of image pixels). Let $\mathcal{L} = \{1,2,\ldots,K\}$ denote the set of labels that are assigned to the sites, where K is the number of labels. Let the mapping $f: S \rightarrow \mathcal{L}$ denote a labeling $f = \{f_1, f_2, \ldots, f_n\}$ where $f_p \in \mathcal{L}$. The set of all labelings $\mathcal{L}^n$ is denoted by $\mathcal{F}$.

Let $F = \{F_1, F_2, \ldots, F_n\}$ be a set of random variables defined on S. Hence, we can define f as a configuration of the field F. The probability that a random variable F_p takes a value f_p can be written as $P(F_p = f_p)$. Then joint probability that describes the field F can be written as $P(F_1 = f_1, F_2 = f_2, \cdots, F_n = f_n)$. This simply can be rewritten as $P(F = f)$, which will be abbreviated as $P(f)$.

Example 6.4 Consider a simple image that consists of a row of four pixels. Each pixel can be assigned a label from one to three. In this case:

- $S = \{1,2,3,4\}$ is the set of sites;
- $L = \{1,2,3\}$ is the set of labels;
- $f = \{1,1,1\}, f = \{3,2,2\}$ and $f = \{2,2,1\}$ are examples of the labeling;
- The set of all labelings $\mathcal{F} \equiv \mathcal{L}^n = \{\ \{1,1,1\},\{1,1,2\},\{1,1,3\},\{1,2,1\},\cdots,$
$\{3,3,2\},\{3,3,3\}\ \}$;

- There are 81 different labelings, because the cardinality of $\mathcal{F}$ is 81 in this case; i.e., $|\mathcal{F}| = |\mathcal{L}^n| = 3^4 = 81$;
- The image can be represented by a random field F of four random variables $\boldsymbol{F} = \{F_1, F_2, F_3, F_4\}$.

The set of sites S can represent different graphical forms (e.g., tree, grid, graph, etc.); this helps to define a geometric neighborhood system N. N is mathematically defined by the set of all neighboring pairs $\{p, q\}$, where $\{p, q\} \in S$. In image modeling, S represents the set of image pixels. Since the image has a natural structure that is a 2D/3D array, this also helps to define a geometric neighborhood system N. Figure 6.7(a) illustrates an example for the neighbors of a pixel p on a grid up to 5th order. The most popular neighborhood system in 2D image analysis is the 1st-order neighbors, the four nearest neighbors sharing a side with the given pixel. The neighborhood of a pixel p, N_p, satisfies the following properties:

1. $p \in N_p$
2. If $p \in N_q$ then $q \in N_p$.

Example 6.5 Consider the 3×5 image shown in Figure 6.7(b). We can define the following neighborhoods based on the order of the symmetric MRF model:

- The 1st-order neighborhood of p is $N_p = \{a, b, c, d\}$,
- The 1st-order neighborhood of p is $N_c = \{p, f, z, g\}$.
  (Note: $p \in N_c$, since $c \in N_p$.)
- The 1st-order neighborhood of q is $N_q = \{x, y\}$.
- The 2nd-order neighborhood of p is $N_p = \{a, b, c, d, e, f, g, h\}$. ∎

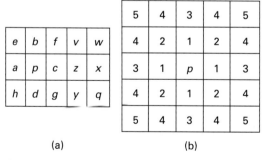

Figure 6.7 Illustration of the neighborhood systems on a 2D grid. (a) the first-order neighbors for p and q; (b) The neighbors up to the 5th order for a pixel p.

Geman and Geman [6.2] popularized the MRF models to engineers and computer scientists, as a powerful tool for image modeling. The MRF is viewed as associated to Gibbs random fields, as stated before. In this chapter, a variety of Markov–Gibbs random fields will be considered.

DEFINITION 6.1 (*Markov random field*) *A random field F, defined on S with respect to a neighborhood system N, is a discrete Markov random field if and only if the positivity, Markovianity, and homogeneity conditions are satisfied. This means that its probability density function* P(f) *satisfies the following properties:*

1. $P(f) > 0$ for all $f \in \mathcal{F}$ Positivity
2. $P(f_p | f_{s-p}) = P(f_p | f_{N_p})$ Markov property   (6.3)
3. $P(f_p | f_{N_p})$ is the same for all sites p Homogeneity

where $S-p$ denotes set difference (i.e., stands for all pixels in S except p), and $f_{N_p} = \{f_q | q \in N_p\}$ denotes all labels of pixels in N_p. ∎

The Markov property in the above definition states that a pixel is dependent directly only on its neighbors. This establishes a local model. A MRF is *homogenous* if $P(f_p|f_{N_p})$ is independent of the location of the site p in S. For a homogenous MRF, if $f_p = f_q$ and $f_{N_p} = f_{N_q}$ we can write $P(f_p|f_{N_p}) = P(f_q|f_{N_q})$ even if $p \neq q$.

Example 6.6 A random field that has $P(f_p|f_{N_p}) \propto \sum_{q \in N_p} |f_p - f_q|$ is a homogenous random field. However, a random field that has $P(f_p|f_{N_p}) \propto \sum_{q \in N_p} a_p |f_p - f_q|$, where a_p is a parameter whose value depends on the site p, is a non-homogenous random field. ∎

6.6 Gibbs model

In 1901, Gibbs used Boltzmann's distribution of energy states in molecules to express the probability of a whole system with many degrees of freedom being in a state with a certain energy [6.2].

DEFINITION 6.2 (*Gibbs random field*) *A random field F, which is defined on S with respect to a neighborhood system N, is a discrete Gibbs random field (GRF) if and only if the random variables in* **F** *obey a Gibbs distribution. A Gibbs distribution takes the following form:*

$$P(f) = Z^{-1} \exp(U(f)/T) \qquad (6.4)$$

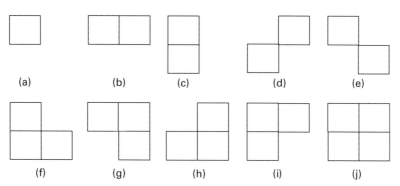

(a) (b) (c) (d) (e)

(f) (g) (h) (i) (j)

Figure 6.8 The clique types of the second-order neighborhood.

where Z is a normalizing constant called the partition function, T is a control parameter called temperature, and $U(f)$ is called the Gibbs energy [6.6], and is given by:

$$U(f) = \sum_{c \in C} V_c(f) \tag{6.5}$$

where $V_c(f)$ is known as the potential function (or the clique function), and C is the set of all cliques. ∎

Specifying the clique functions establishes a global model.

DEFINITION 6.3 *(Clique)* A clique is a set of pixels in which all pairs of pixels are mutual neighbors. ∎

Figure 6.8 illustrates the clique types for the 1st and 2nd-order neighborhood systems for a lattice. The single site, the horizontal and the vertical pair-site cliques are shown in Figure 6.8(a)–(c). This set of cliques belongs to the 1st-order neighboring system. In addition to this set shown in (a–c), diagonal pair-site cliques (Figure 6.8(d) and (e)), triple-site cliques (Figure 6.8(f)–(i)), and a quadruple-site clique (Figure 6.8(j)) are from the 2nd-order neighboring system.

Besag [6.1] studied the linkage between Gibbs and Markov models. He showed that a unique GRF exists for every MRF, and vice versa, as long as the GRF is defined in terms of cliques on a neighborhood system. A Gibbs random field describes the global properties of an image in terms of the joint distributions of labels for all pixels $P(f)$, whereas a Markov random field is defined in terms of local properties.

THEOREM 6.1 *(Hamersley–Clifford theorem [6.1])*: *A random field F is an MRF on S with respect to N if and only if F is a GRF on S with respect to N (i.e., its density can be factorized over the cliques on S with respect to N).*

In order to prove this theorem we need to prove that $P(f)$ satisfies Markov property if it is a Gibbs distribution. Below we summarize the main steps in the proof of this theorem (see [6.1]).

Proof Let $P(f)$ be a Gibbs distribution on S with respect to N. Conditional probability can be written as

$$P(f_p|f_{S-p}) = \frac{P(f_p, f_{S-p})}{P(f_{S-p})} = \frac{P(f)}{\sum_{\bar{f}_p \in L} P(\bar{f})}, \tag{6.6}$$

where $\bar{f} = \{f_1, f_2, \ldots, \bar{f}_p, f_{n-1}, f_n\}$ is any set of random variables which agrees with f at all sites except possibly p. Assume F is a GRF on S with respect to N then $P(f)$ is the Gibbs distribution, Eq. (6.4). Thus Eq. (6.6) can be rewritten as follows:

$$P(f_p|f_{S-p}) = \frac{\exp(-\sum_{c \in C} V_c(f)/T)}{\sum_{\bar{f}_p \in L} \exp(-\sum_{c \in C} V_c(\bar{f})/T)} \tag{6.7}$$

Let us divide C into two sets A and B, assuming that A consists of cliques containing p, and B consists of cliques that do not contain p. Then Eq. (6.7) can be written as:

$$P(f_p|f_{S-p}) = \frac{\left[\exp\left(\sum_{c \in A} V_c(f)/T\right)\right]\left[\exp\left(-\sum_{c \in B} V_c(f)/T\right)\right]}{\sum_{\bar{f}_p \in L}\left[\exp\left(-\sum_{c \in A} V_c(\bar{f})/T\right)\right]\left[\exp\left(-\sum_{c \in B} V_c(\bar{f})/T\right)\right]} \tag{6.8}$$

Since B does not consist of cliques containing p, we can say that $\exp\left(\sum_{c \in B}(\bar{f})/T\right) = \exp\left(\sum_{c \in B} V_c(f)/T\right)$. Thus this term can be outside the summation in the denominator. Finally, $P(f_p|f_{S-p})$ depends only on the potential of the cliques containing p, i.e. the neighborhood of p, and Eq. (6.5) can be rewritten as

$$P(f_p|f_{S-p}) = \frac{\exp(-\sum_{c \in A} V_c(f)/T)}{\sum_{\bar{f}_p \in L} \exp(-\sum_{c \in A} V_c(\bar{f})/T)} \cdot \frac{\exp(-\sum_{c \in B} V_c(f)/T)}{\exp(-\sum_{c \in B} V_c(f)/T)} \tag{6.9a}$$

$$= \frac{\exp(-\sum_{c \in A} V_c(f)/T)}{\sum_{\bar{f}_p \in L} \exp(-\sum_{c \in A} V_c(\bar{f})/T)} = \frac{P(f_p, f_{N_p})}{p(f_{N_p})} = P(f_p|f_{N_p}). \tag{6.9b}$$

This proves that a Gibbs random field is a Markov random field. ∎

6.7 Markov–Gibbs random field models

MGRF models have been successfully used in texture and general image analysis and synthesis (e.g. [6.3],[6.4],[6.9],[6.10]). The literature is rich with MGRF models, each of which tries to select the potential functions that are suitable for a specific system behavior. Here, we review some models and algorithms.

6.7.1 Auto-models

The Gibbs energy can be defined by specifying interactions between sites in the image. In most of the image processing and computer vision literature, the Gibbs energy has been defined in terms of the "single-site" clique and "two-site" cliques. This is called the pairwise interaction model. The single-site potentials are also called the external field. The single-site potential allows one to impose structure on a pattern from an outside source (e.g. the force of gravity acting on each pixel). The two-site potential influences the "attraction" or "repulsion" between neighboring pairs of pixels in the image. This potential parameter of the two-site clique is sometimes called a *bonding parameter* [6.9]. The different models corresponding to this form of the energy are typically called *auto-models*. Besag [6.1] formulated the energy function of these models as follows:

$$U(f) = \sum_{p \in S} V_p(f_p) + \sum_{\{p,q\} \in \mathcal{N}} V_{pq}(f_p, f_q) \tag{6.10}$$

where $V_p(.)$ is the potential function for single-pixel (single-site) cliques, and $V_{pq}(.,.)$ is the potential function for all cliques of size 2, with $V_{pq}(f_p, f_q) = V_{pq}(f_p, f_q)$ and $V_{pq}(f_p, f_p) = 0$.

The **auto-binomial model** is an example of a Gibbs model having an energy function of the form in Eq. (6.10), where

$$V_p(f_p) = \alpha f_p - \ln\left(\frac{K!}{f_p!(f_p - K)!}\right), \tag{6.11a}$$

$$V_{pq}(f_p, f_q) = \beta_q f_p f_q \tag{6.11b}$$

where α is called the potential parameter of the single-site clique. This parameter controls the influence of the external field. The potential parameter of the two-site clique is β_q, which influences the interaction between neighboring pairs. Note that the potential parameter α has no subscript. This means that it is constant for all the sites in the lattice. Thus this model is a homogenous MRF model. However, the potential parameter β_q of the two-site clique has a subscript q. This means that its value depends on the orientation (horizontal, vertical, diagonal, and anti-diagonal) of the neighbor q. This model is called an anisotropic model. On the other hand, in the isotropic models, $\beta_q = \beta$ is a constant that is independent of the orientation of the neighbors.

The **Derin–Elliott model** [6.3] can also be expressed in the framework of Eq. (6.10) as follows:

$$V_p(f_p) = \alpha f_p, \tag{6.12a}$$

$$V_{pq}(f_p, f_q) = \begin{cases} -\beta_q & f_p \neq f_q \\ \beta_q & f_p = f_q \end{cases} \tag{6.12b}$$

This model is a homogenous model, since α is constant for all the sites in the lattice. Also, it is an anisotropic model since β_q depends on the orientation of the neighbor q.

The **auto-normal model** is one of the popular continuous MRF models in image modeling. To take advantage of the mathematical properties of the Gaussian distribution, Besag [6.1] proposed the auto-normal model, which is a Gaussian Markov random field model. In such models, pixel p labels have jointly Gaussian distributions with means μ_p and variance σ^2, and correlations controlled by β_q. The auto-normal model is defined as

$$V_p(f_p) = \frac{(f_p - \mu_p)^2}{2\sigma^2}, \qquad (6.13\mathrm{a})$$

$$V_{pq}(f_p, f_q) = \beta_q \frac{(f_p - \mu_p)(f_q - \mu_q)}{2\sigma^2} \qquad (6.13\mathrm{b})$$

This model is a homogenous model since α is constant for all the sites in the lattice. Also, it is anisotropic, since β_q depends on the orientation of the neighbor q.

The **submodular model** was developed by Ali et al. [6.10], who studied asymmetric pairwise co-occurrences of the region labels. The model is chosen to guarantee more instances where the Gibbs energy function is submodular, so it can be globally minimized using a standard graph cuts approach in polynomial time. The Gibbs potential governing asymmetric pairwise co-occurrences of the region labels can be described as follows:

$$V_p(f_p) = 0, \qquad (6.14\mathrm{a})$$

$$V_{pq}(f_p, f_q) = \gamma \delta(f_p \neq f_p) \qquad (6.14\mathrm{b})$$

where the indicator function $\delta(A)$ equals 1 when the condition A is true and zero otherwise. To identify the homogeneous isotropic model that describes the labeling f, one needs to estimate only one potential value γ.

6.7.2 Aura-based GRF model

Elfadel and Picard [6.9] used the concept of an "aura set" from set theory to convert the nonlinear energy function of a homogeneous anisotropic GRF model to a linear sum of "aura" measures. For $A, B \subseteq S$ and neighborhood structure N_p, the aura of A with respect to B is defined by

$$O_B(A, N_p) = \bigcup_{p \in A} (N_p \cap B) \qquad (6.15)$$

Also, the aura of A w.r.t. B can be defined as the "dilation" of A with structure element N_p followed by intersection with B. The aura measure $m(A,B)$ is defined by

$$m(A, B) = \sum_{p \in A} |N_p \cap B| \geq |O_B(A, N_p)|. \qquad (6.16)$$

Figure 6.9 illustrates an example of an aura set. Elfadel and Picard [6.9] showed that the aura measures are the sum of co-occurrences as follows. The symmetric neighborhood

Figure 6.9 Example of an aura set. $\mathcal{A}$ is the set of zeros, $\mathcal{B}$ is the set of ones. Using the nearest four neighborhood system, the aura of $\mathcal{A}$ w.r.t. $\mathcal{B}$ is the set of ones in dark gray boxes. $m(\mathcal{A},\mathcal{B}) = 10$.

N_p is partitioned into M isotropic subneighborhoods and the lattice S is partitioned into label subsets $S_\ell = \{p \in S | f_p = \ell\}$, $\forall \ell \in \mathcal{L}$. Elfadel and Picard then proved that the aura measures are the sum of co-occurrences: $m(\ell_1, \ell_2) = \sum_{i=1}^{n} m^i(S_{\ell_1}, S_{\ell_2})$. Finally, they reformulated the anisotropic Gibbs energy function Eq. (6.4) (taking into account only the potential function for all cliques of size 2) using the aura measures as a linear cost function:

$$\sum_{\{p,q\} \in \mathcal{N}} V_{pq}(f_p, f_q) = \sum_{i=1}^{m} \sum_{\{\ell_1,\ell_2\} \in \mathcal{L}} V^i(\ell_1, \ell_2) m^i(\ell_1, \ell_2). \qquad (6.17)$$

Elfadel and Picard [6.9] used this linear formulation of the Gibbs energy in order to characterize various types of textures.

6.7.3 Other models

Gimel'farb [6.11] proposed a MGRF model that takes into account multiple pairwise pixel interactions. This model is used for images with textures that are spatially uniform. Such an image is classified by a histogram of its gray level differences. The author proposed an algorithm based on the maximum likelihood approach to estimate his model parameters. Compared with other models, the author claims that the parameters for his model are larger in number but simpler to estimate.

Zhu, Wu and Mumford [6.12] proposed the "filters, random fields, and maximum entropy" (FRAME) model. This model integrates filtering theory and MRF modeling using the maximum entropy principle. To model a set of texture images, they extract texture features by applying a set of filters to the observed images. The marginal distributions of the images are then estimated from the histograms of the filtered images. After that, they fit a distribution for this texture from the marginal distributions using maximum-entropy-based method. The authors claim that this model is more descriptive than conventional MRF models. However, it is computationally very expensive.

6.8 GRF-based image synthesis

The synthesis process consists in finding the configuration in "the set of all configurations" which maximizes the probability $P(f)$ (i.e., minimizes the Gibbs energy $U(f)$). The synthesis process is also called sampling. Sampling is the process of generating a realization of a random field, given a model whose parameters have been specified. Since the partition function Z is the sum of the Gibbs energy over all F, it is regarded as not computable. This complicates the sampling problem. Therefore, standard statistical procedures for sampling random variables such as rejection–acceptance and conditional probability decomposition (e.g. [6.13]) cannot be used in this case. Instead, image data is typically synthesized iteratively, using a Monte Carlo method such as the Metropolis exchange algorithm [6.14].

In this section, we discuss a set of iterative sampling algorithms. In all the experiments, we select the 2nd-order neighborhood system and the homogenous anisotropic pairwise interaction model, which is the Derin–Elliott model, Eq. (6.12). Therefore, the model parameters vector is $\theta = \{\alpha,\beta_1,\beta_2,\beta_3,\beta_4\}$, which corresponds to the set of cliques in Figure 6.8 (a–e).

6.8.1 Gibbs sampler algorithm

Geman and Geman [6.2] proposed a raster scan algorithm to sample GRF. This algorithm is called the Gibbs sampler. This algorithm requires K exponential functions to be computed in step (2) of Algorithm 1. Thus, its computation time is high. Figure 6.10 shows realizations of the Derin–Elliott model generated by Algorithm 1 with $N_{iter} = 50$. All images are binary images and have sizes 128×128.

Algorithm 1 Gibbs sampler

(See [6.1] and [6.4].)

1. Start with any random labeling f
2. For all $p \in P$ do:
    a. Compute probabilities P_l for $l \in L$ where $P_l = P(F_p = l | F_{N_p} = f_{N_p})$
    b. Set the label of site p to l with probability P_l
    c. End

Repeat step 2 for N_{iter}

6.8.2 Chen algorithm

Chen [6.15] proposed an algorithm for sampling a GRF. This algorithm eliminates the need for computing the partition function. This algorithm is similar to simulating annealing (e.g., [6.16]) except that no "cooling schedule" is required. Since the ratio of

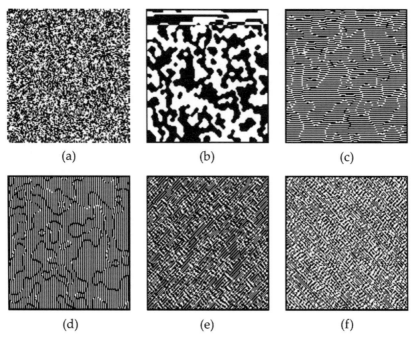

Figure 6.10 Gibbs sampler realization results. (a) The random input, (b) generated image with $\theta =$ {0.3,0.3,0.3,0.3,0.3}, (c) generated image with {0.0,1.0,1.0,1.0,1.0}, (d) generated image with {0.0,1.0,1.0,1.0,1.0}, (e) generated image with {0.0,1.0,1.0,5.01.0}, (f) generated image with {0.0,1.0,1.0,1.0,2.0}.

likelihoods in step 2b of Algorithm 2 does not depend on the partition function Z, it can be computed in practice by including only those cliques involving site p. Figure 6.11 shows realizations of the Derin–Elliott model generated by Algorithm 2 with $N_{iter} = 100$. All images are of size 64×64 and $\alpha = 0$. The results demonstrate that the change of model parameters affects the generated image.

Algorithm 2 Chen algorithm

(See [6.15] and [6.4])

1. Start with any random labeling f
2. For all $p \in P$ do:
   a. Choose $l \in L$ at random and let $\hat{f}_p = l$ and $\hat{f}_q = f_p$ for all $q \neq p$.
   b. Let $P = \min \left\{1, P(F = \hat{f}\,)/P(F = f)\right\}$
   c. Replace f by $\hat{f}$ with probability P
   d. End
3. Repeat step 2 for N_{iter}

6.8 GRF-based image synthesis

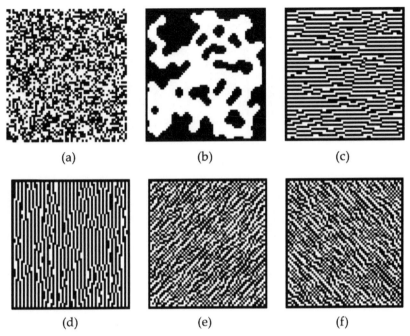

Figure 6.11 Chen algorithm realization results. (a) The random input, (b) generated image with θ = {0.0,0.3,0.3,0.3,0.3}, (c) generated image with {0.0,1.0,1.0,1.0,1.0}, (d) generated image with {0.0,1.0,1.0,1.0,1.0}, (e) generated image with {0.0,1.0,1.0,1.0,1.0}, (f) generated image with {0.0,1.0,1.0,1.0,1.0}.

6.8.3 Metropolis algorithm

Cross and Jain [6.17] described an exchange algorithm to generate textured images. This algorithm is based on the Metropolis algorithm (widely available; we will call this Algorithm 3) [6.14]. Unlike Chen's algorithm, the Metropolis algorithm computes the trial labeling by randomly selecting two sites with different colors and then interchanging their colors. This preserves the number of pixels at each label. Figure 6.12 shows realizations of the Derin–Elliott model generated by Algorithm 3 with $N_{\text{iter}} = 8$. All images are of size 64×64 and $\alpha = 0$. The results demonstrate that the change of model parameters affects the generated image.

In Algorithms 1 and 2, the number of raster scans N_{iter} of the image is critical. To generate a fine texture, the algorithm should be stopped at $50 < N_{\text{iter}} < 100$ (e.g. [6.4]).

Figure 6.13 shows the realizations of the Derin–Elliott model generated by Algorithm 1 at different iterations. All images are binary images and have sizes 128×128, and the model parameters vector $\theta = \{0.3, 0.3, 0.3, 0.3, 0.3\}$. Furthermore, in all sampling algorithms, the values of the model parameters are critical. As shown in Figure 6.12, and owing to these specific parameter values, the short-term correlations among neighboring pixels develop into long-term correlations. Hence, MRF exhibits a phase transition phenomenon (e.g., Pickard [6.18]).

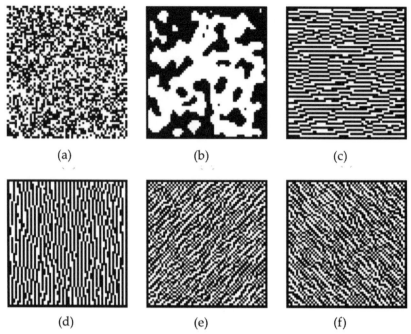

Figure 6.12 Metropolis algorithm realization results (a) the random input, (b) generated image with $\theta =$ {0.0,0.3,0.3,0.3,0.3}, (c) generated image with {0.0,1.0,1.0,1.0,1.0}, (d) generated image with {0.0,1.0,1.0,1.0,1.0}, (e) generated image with {0.0,1.0,1.0,1.0,1.0}, (f) generated image with {0.0,1.0,1.0,1.0,1.0}.

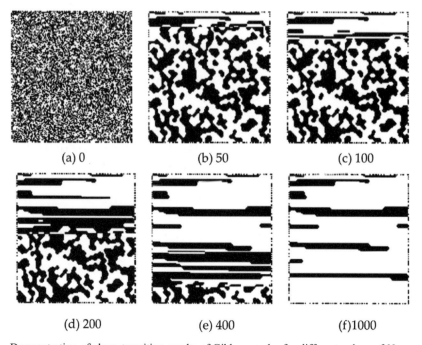

Figure 6.13 Demonstration of phase transition results of Gibbs sampler for different values of N_{iter}.

To avoid this phenomenon, the Metropolis algorithm preserves the number of pixels at each label constant using the exchange step as explained in Algorithm 3. However, the exchange process in this algorithm violates the positivity condition of MRF (Definition 6.1). Picard and Elfadel [6.8][6.9] provide more insights on the use of Gibbs–Markov models for texture synthesis.

6.9 GRF-based image analysis

Fitting a MRF model to an image requires that the parameters of the model be estimated from a sample of the image, and the degree of fit between a specific model and a given image must be assessed quantitatively. The literature is rich with works that propose different MGRF models suitable for a specific system behavior. Usually, these papers identify their model parameters using an optimization technique. This technique tries to maximize either the likelihood or the entropy of the proposed probability distributions.

Maximum likelihood estimation (MLE) is the most popular estimator used in estimating unknown parameters of a distribution (e.g., [6.11]). For the Gibbs probability distribution (GPD) with potential parameter θ, we have:

$$P(f;\theta) = Z^{-1}(\theta) \exp\left(-U(f;\theta)/T\right). \tag{6.18}$$

The log-likelihood function is defined by

$$\mathfrak{L}(f;\theta) = \log P(f;\theta) = -U(f;\theta)/T - \log\left(Z(\theta)\right) \tag{6.19}$$

$$\theta^* = \arg\max_{f \in \mathcal{F}} \left(-U(f;\theta)/T - \log\left(Z(\theta)\right)\right). \tag{6.20}$$

Equation 6.18 can be solved by the differentiation of the log-likelihood. However, the second term in Eq. 6.19, log(Z), is intractable. Thus, numerical techniques are usually used to find a solution for this problem.

In the maximum entropy principle (MEP), the observed statistics are represented as a set of constraints, and the MEP is used to estimate the model parameters. Many techniques (e.g., [6.12]) use MEP in texture modeling. MEP-based texture modeling techniques select statistics that characterize textures, and then infer the maximum entropy distribution subject to the constraint that the marginal probability of sufficient statistics with respect to the model should match the empirical probability of the same statistics in the training data.

In this section we discuss some popular methods used to estimate the parameters for MRF models.

6.9.1 Coding estimation

The coding method was proposed by Besag [6.1]. In this method, the image grid is partitioned into a number of disjoint sets of pixels, called coding patterns. The codings

Basics of random fields

1	2	1	2	1	2
2	1	2	1	2	1
1	2	1	2	1	2
2	1	2	1	2	1
1	2	1	2	1	2
2	1	2	1	2	1

(a)

1	2	1	2	1	2
3	4	3	4	3	4
1	2	1	2	1	2
3	4	3	4	3	4
1	2	1	2	1	2
3	4	3	4	3	4

(b)

Figure 6.14 Besag's scheme for coding sites. (a) First-order model and (b) second-order model.

are chosen such that the distribution of the pixel values within one coding pattern is independent of the pixel values of the other coding patterns. This simply means that a pixel and its neighbors cannot be members of the same coding pattern. The number of coding patterns is kept as low as possible to obtain the most efficient estimator. Thus we get two coding patterns for a 1st-order MRF (checkerboard) and four coding patterns for a 2nd-order MRF. These coding patterns are shown in Figure 6.14 (a) and (b), respectively. All pixels labeled j are used for the jth set of parameter estimates $j = 1, 2, 3, 4$. Using Bayes' formula and the MRF properties, we can conclude that the colors of sites in each coding are conditionally independent:

$$P(f_p, f_q | f_{N_p}, f_{N_q}) = P(f_p | f_{N_p}) P(f_q | f_{N_q}) \qquad (6.21)$$

The coding method estimates the vector parameters θ by finding the vector θ_j which maximizes the log-likelihood in coding j

$$\mathcal{L}_j(f; \theta_j) = \sum_{p \in S_j} \log \left(\frac{\exp(-U(f; \theta_j)/T)}{\sum_{\ell \in \mathcal{L}} \exp(-U(\ell; \theta_j)/T)} \right), \qquad (6.22)$$

where S_j is the set of pixels that have the code j. After optimizing $\mathfrak{L}_j(f;\theta)$, the estimated vector for the second-order model is defined as $\theta = \sum_j^4 \theta_j$.

6.9.2 Least square error method

The least square error (LSQR) method was proposed by Derin and Elliot [6.3], who reduced the problem to solving an over-determined linear system. They established different 3×3 label blocks of pixels. For a pixel p with label f_p and its neighborhood N_p of 8 pixels, the block is (f_p, f_{N_p}). Each different 3×3 block of labels establishes a block type. For two blocks around the pixels p and q, with $f_p \neq f_q$ and $f_{N_p} = f_{N_q} = f_{N_1}$, we can formulate the following:

$$U(f_p) - U(f_q) = \ln\left(\frac{P(f_q, f_{N_1})}{P(f_p, f_{N_1})}\right) \tag{6.23}$$

The ratio $P(f_q, f_{N_1})/P(f_p, f_{N_1})$ is estimated by counting the number of 3×3 blocks of type (f_q, f_{N_1}) and dividing by the number of blocks of type (f_p, f_{N_1}). A second-order binary MGRF has 256 such equations. In order to estimate the model parameters using least square methods, we need to solve this over-determined system of equations. Derin and Elliott [6.3], in their implementation, claimed accurate estimation by using the most frequently occurring block types. However, there is no consistent way to establish which are the most frequent block types.

6.9.3 Analytical method for parameter identification

The Gibbs potential governing asymmetric pairwise co-occurrences of the region labels described in Eq. (6.14a,b) has only one parameter γ. Then the GRF model of region maps is specified by the following Gibbs probability distribution:

$$P(\mathbf{f}) = \frac{1}{Z} \exp\left(\sum_{\{p,q\}\in N} V(\mathbf{f}_p; f_q)\right) = \frac{1}{Z} \exp\left(\gamma |T| F_{\text{neq}}(\mathbf{f})\right). \tag{6.24}$$

Here, $T = \{\{p,q\}: p,q \in S; \{p,q\} \in N\}$ is the family of the neighboring pixel pairs supporting the Gibbs potentials, $|T|$ is its cardinality, and $F_{\text{neq}}(\mathbf{f})$ denotes the relative frequency of the non-equal labels in the pixel pairs of that family:

$$F_{\text{neq}}(\mathbf{f}) = \frac{1}{|T|} \sum_{\{p,q\}\in N} \delta(f_p \neq f_q) \tag{6.25}$$

To completely identify this model, the potential value γ specifying the Gibbs potential has to be estimated. In doing so, the GRF model is identified using a reasonably close first approximation of the maximum likelihood estimation of γ. Using Eq. (6.24), the model log-likelihood can be written as follows:

Table 6.1 The proposed parameter estimation method for binary images of size 128 × 128

Actual γ	0.1	0.75	1.0	1.75
Proposed γ	0.12(0.009)	0.77(0.014)	1.04(0.013)	1.78(0.013)
CM	0.94(0.003)	1.02(0.0)	1.09(0.011)	1.79(0.066)
LSQR	0.11(0.016)	0.64(0.041)	0.85(0.054)	1.79(0.091)

$$L(\mathbf{f}|\gamma) = -\gamma \frac{|T|}{|S|} F_{neq}(\mathbf{f}) - \frac{1}{S} \log \sum_{\hat{\mathbf{f}} \in F} \exp\left(-\gamma |T| F_{neq}(\hat{\mathbf{f}})\right). \quad (6.26)$$

The model log-likelihood (6.26) can be approximated by truncating the Taylor's series expansion of $L(\mathbf{f}|\gamma)$ to the first three terms in the close vicinity of the zero potential, $\gamma = 0$:

$$L(\mathbf{f}|\gamma) \approx L(\mathbf{f}|0) + \gamma dL(\mathbf{f}|\gamma)/d\gamma + \frac{1}{2}\gamma^2 \frac{dL^2(\mathbf{f}|\gamma)}{d\gamma^2}. \quad (6.27)$$

In the vicinity of the origin $\gamma = 0$, the approximate log-likelihood (6.27) becomes (e.g., Ali et al. [6.10]):

$$L(\mathbf{f}|\gamma) \approx -|S|\log K + \gamma \frac{|T|}{|S|}\left(F_{neq}\left(\mathbf{f} - \frac{1}{K}\right)\right) - \frac{1}{2}\gamma^2 \frac{|T|}{|S|}\frac{K-1}{K^2}. \quad (6.28)$$

Let $\dfrac{dL(\mathbf{f}|\gamma)}{d\gamma} = 0$; hence, the MLE of γ would be:

$$\gamma* = \frac{K^2}{K-1}\left(\frac{K-1}{K} - F_{neq}(\mathbf{f})\right). \quad (6.29)$$

Example 6.7 Simulated texture images are generated using the Gibbs sampler Algorithm 2. Four different realizations of the binary GMRF model (6.24) are generated. Samples of these realizations for images of size 128 × 128 are shown in Figure 6.15. To obtain accurate statistics, 100 realizations are generated from each texture type (value of gamma). The analytical method, Eq. (6.26), is used to estimate the model parameter γ for these data sets. The means and the variances (written in parentheses) of the 100 realizations for each type are shown in Table 6.1.

For comparison purposes, the estimations of the coding method (CM) [6.1], and least square error method (LSQR) [6.10] are also illustrated. Notice that the analytical estimates of the GRF parameters outperform the classical methods (e.g., CM and LSQR). These statistical results highlight the robustness of the analytical estimation.

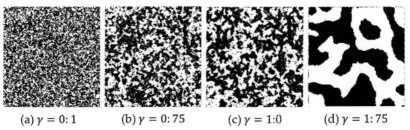

(a) $\gamma = 0:1$ (b) $\gamma = 0:75$ (c) $\gamma = 1:0$ (d) $\gamma = 1:75$

Figure 6.15 Samples of synthesized binary images of size 128×128.

The coding method [6.1] allows an easy formulation of the estimator for auto-binomial model. However, it is generally considered difficult to use reliably [6.3], and its performance varies widely for different data. In the LSQR method one must propose *ad hoc* alternatives to avoid zero probability. In the previous discussed methods and others proposed in the literature [6.1], the ranges where these methods work well are unknown. These regions of validity were investigated by Picard [6.8], as described below.

A given set of GRF parameters will synthesize a variety of texture patterns while its energy is being minimized as shown in Figure 6.15. The problem is which pattern should correctly be associated with the parameters. To answer this question, Picard [6.9] considered that the pattern is not in "equilibrium" unless its energy has decreased to some level where it has stopped changing. Figure 6.12 shows the realizations of the isotropic first-order Derin–Elliott model generated by Algorithm 3 at different iterations. The images are of size 64×64 and have 32 gray levels. The model parameters vector $\theta = \{0.0, 1.0, 1.0, 1.0, 1.0\}$. The synthesis is done at different temperature T values and different iterations i.

In Figure 6.16, when the parameter is estimated for samples at $N_{iter} = 100$, it will be accurate for the first two columns, but too low for the third column. Thus, Picard proposed that the first problem with the way estimation methods have been evaluated has to do with a lack of attention to the pattern's equilibrium. An estimate taken while the energy of a pattern is still decreasing should not be expected to fit the parameters which are synthesizing the pattern. This estimate needed to be adjusted upward.

To determine the region of validity of the parameter estimation methods, Picard [6.8] examined the Gibbs energy at different temperatures. For the GRF model that is used in experiments shown in Figure 6.16 and for a binary image, Figure 6.17 shows the average normalized energy over 40 000 iterations after equilibrium. From this figure we can see that two saturations occur, at high temperature $T > 100$ and cold temperature $T < 3$, so in these regions all values of model parameter map to the same energy. Thus, the parameters estimated in these regions are not unique.

The patterns corresponding to the energy at high-temperature binary noise and to the energy at low temperature are images with white on one half and black on the other. In the center, where the energy changes abruptly as in a true "phase transition," one finds patterns that appear to be generally closer to natural textures.

158   **Basics of random fields**

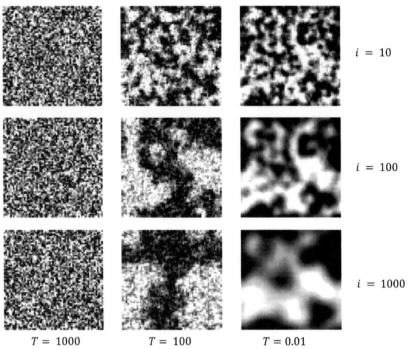

Figure 6.16   Equilibrium is reached after $N_{iter} = 10$ for $T = 1000$, $N_{iter} = 100$ for $T = 100$ and $N_{iter} = 1000$ for $T = 0.01$. (See Picard [6.8].)

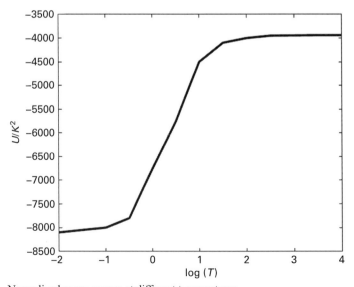

Figure 6.17   Normalized mean energy at different temperatures.

6.10 Summary

This chapter provides a short introduction to random fields. Techniques for segmentation and registration in subsequent chapters will show the importance of random fields in object modeling and characterization. There is a vast literature on theory, algorithms, and applications of random field modeling that illustrates the importance of this subject matter. Open-source implementation of a number of techniques associated with random fields is also available. In subsequent chapters we will study approaches for image segmentation, registration, and shape modeling using random field theory.

6.11 Exercises

6.1 For the four boxes shown in the figure, assume that within each box there are a large number of colored (red, green, and blue) balls. A robot chooses an initial box according to some random process. From this box, a ball is chosen at random, and its color is recorded as the observation. The ball is then replaced in the box from which it was selected. A new box is then selected according to the random selection process associated with that box, and the ball selection process is then repeated.
  (a) Plot the state diagram of this hidden Markov model (HMM).
  (b) State the parameters of this HMM.
  (c) Suppose the current selected box is Box 1. What is the probability that the robot will select from Box 3, three cycles of box selection from now, and ten cycles from now?
  (d) Suppose the current selected box is Box 3. What is the probability that the robot will select from Box 3, three cycles of box selection from now and ten cycles from now?
  (e) Comment on the results of (c) and (d).
  (f) Suppose the current selected box is Box 2. What is the probability that for the next six cycles the robot will select from "Box 4, Box 1, Box 3, Box 2, Box 4, Box 1"?
  (g) Suppose the current selected box is Box 4. What is the probability that the robot continues to select from Box 4 for *exactly n* cycles?
  (h) What is the expected value of n if the robot continues to select from Box 3 for *exactly n* cycles?
  (i) What is the probability of the following output sequence given the sequence in (f) {Red,Green,Red,Blue,Blue,Green,Red}?
  (j) Assuming the robot started from Box 1, compute P(Green, Blue, Red, Green, Box 1, Box 2, Box 3, Box 4).
  (k) Compute P(Red, Green,Blue).

| Box 1 | Box 2 | Box 3 | Box 4 |

6.2 Are the following statements true or false? Correct them where necessary:
  (a) The image which is synthesized using the Metropolis algorithm from a binary Gibbs random field with a temperature $T = 10^{-6}$ is almost a random noisy image.
  (b) Unlike the Chen algorithm for image synthesis, the Metropolis algorithm does not violate the positivity condition of MRF.
  (c) The coding method is a maximum likelihood estimator (MLE).
  (d) The interaction model with a potential function $V(f_p, f_q) \propto e^{\|-I_p - I_q^2\|} e^{\|-p-q^2\|}$ is a homogenous isotropic pairwise interaction model.
  (e) If pixels p and q are neighbors of a pixel r, then r must be a neighbor of both p and q.

6.3 Markov–Gibbs random field-based image synthesis and analysis:

0	1	0
1	0	1
0	1	0

I_1

−1	1	−1
1	−1	1
−1	1	−1

I_2

The 3 × 3 image I_1 given here is synthesized from the binary GRF:

$$p(f) = z^{-1} \exp\left(-\sum_{(p,q) \in \aleph} \beta_q f_p f_q\right)$$

  (a) Assume that the neighborhood system $\aleph$ is the first-order system and the interaction model is homogenous and isotropic. What are the signs of β_q?
  (b) Assume that the neighborhood system $\aleph$ is the second-order system and the interaction model is homogenous and anisotropic. What are the signs of β_q?
  (c) Repeat (a) using I_2.
  (d) Repeat (b) using I_2.
  (e) How do you select the signs of β_q such that for I_2 all the pixels in the same row have the same values?
  (f) How do you select the signs of β_q such that for I_2 all the pixels in the same column have the same values?
  (g) How do you select the signs of β_q such that for I_2 all the pixels in the image have the same values?

6.12 Computer laboratory

Task 1 Markov–Gibbs random field-based image synthesis

Assume that the Gibbs energy is identified by the second-order neighborhood system and the pairwise interaction model. The potential function is selected to be the Derin–Elliott model

$$V_p(f_p) = \alpha f_p,$$

$$V_{pq}(f_p, f_q) = \begin{cases} -\beta_q & f_p \neq f_q \\ \beta_q & f_p = f_q \end{cases}.$$

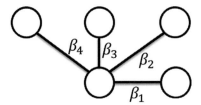

Using the Chen algorithm (Algorithm 2), do the following:
(a) Sample the binary Gibbs distribution which has the potential parameters
  i. $\alpha = 0$, $\beta_1 = -1.0$, and $\beta_2 = \beta_3 = \beta_4 = 1.0$
  ii. $\alpha = 0$, $\beta_2 = -1.0$, and $\beta_1 = \beta_3 = \beta_4 = 1.0$
  iii. $\alpha = 0$, $\beta_3 = -1.0$, and $\beta_2 = \beta_1 = \beta_4 = 1.0$
  iv. $\alpha = 0$, $\beta_4 = -1.0$, and $\beta_2 = \beta_3 = \beta_1 = 1.0$

(b) Sample the binary Gibbs distribution which has the potential parameters $\alpha = 0$, $\beta_q = 1/T$, where $T = 0.1$, $T = 0.001$, and $T = 1000$. Comment on the output realization.
(c) Sample the binary Gibbs distribution which has the potential parameters $\alpha = 0$, $\beta_q = 0.3$ with different numbers of iterations ($N_{iter} = 10$, 500, and 1000). Comment on the effect of the number of iterations on the final realization.
(d) Repeat (a–c) for a Gibbs distribution with 8 colors.
(e) Repeat (a–c) using the Metropolis algorithm and for a Gibbs distribution with 32 colors.

Task 2 Markov–Gibbs random field-based image analysis
(a) Using the coding method, estimate the parameters of the realizations which are generated in Task 1(a) and (c) (use sufficient N_{iter}). Sample the binary Gibbs distribution which has the estimated parameters.
(b) Repeat (a) using LSQR.

References

[6.1] J. E. Besag, Spatial interaction and the statistical analysis of lattice systems. *J. Roy. Stat. Soc. B* **36** (1974) 192–236.

[6.2] S. Geman and D. Geman, Stochastic relaxation, Gibbs distributions, and the Bayesian restoration of images. *IEEE Trans. Pattern Anal. Machine Intel.* **6** (1984) 721–741.

[6.3] H. Derin and H. Elliott, Modeling and segmentation of noisy and textured images using Gibbs random fields. *IEEE Trans. Pattern Anal. Machine Intel.* **9**(1) (1987) 39–55.

[6.4] R. C. Dubes and A. K. Jain, Random field models in image analysis. *J. Appl. Stat.* **16** (1989) 131–164.

[6.5] H. Rue and L. Held, *Gaussian Markov Random Fields: Theory and Applications*. Boca Raton, FL: Chapman and Hall/CRC (2005).

[6.6] R. J. Adler and J. Taylor, *Random Fields and Geometry*. Berlin: Springer (2007).

[6.7] A. Blake, P. Kohli and C. Rother, *Markov Random Fields for Vision and Image Processing*. Cambridge, MA: MIT Press (2011).

[6.8] R. W. Picard and I. M. Elfadel, Structure of aura and co-occurrence matrices for the Gibbs texture model. *J. Math. Imaging Vision* **2** (1992) 5–25.

[6.9] I. M. Elfadel and R. W. Picard, Gibbs random fields, co-occurrences, and texture modeling. *IEEE Trans. Pattern Anal. Machine Intel.* **16**(1) (1994) 24–37.

[6.10] A. M. Ali, A. A. Farag and G. Gimel'farb, Analytical method for MGRF model parameters estimation. In *Proc. 19th Int. Conf. Pattern Recognition (ICPR-08)* (2008) 1–4; DOI: 10.1109/ICPR.2008.4761339.

[6.11] G. L. Gimel'farb, Texture modeling with multiple pairwise pixel interactions. *IEEE Trans. Pattern Anal. Machine Intel.* **18**(11) (1996) 1110–1114.

[6.12] S. C. Zhu, Y. N. Wu, and D. Mumford, Filters, random fields and maximum entropy (frame): To a unified theory for texture modeling. *Int. J. Computer Vision* **27**(2) (1998) 107–126.

[6.13] W. J. Kennedy and J. E. Gentle, *Statistical Computing* (1980) Marcel Dekker.

[6.14] N. Metropolis, A. W. Rosenbluth, M. N. Rosenbluth, A. H. Teller and E. Teller, Equations of state calculations by fast computing machines. *J. Chem. Phys.* **21** (1953) 1087–1091.

[6.15] C. C. Chen, Markov random field models in image analysis. Unpublished PhD thesis, Michigan State University, East Lansing, 1988.

[6.16] P. J. M. van Laarhoven and E. H. L. Aarts, *Simulated Annealing: Theory and Application*. Reidel: Dordrecht (1987).

[6.17] G. R. Cross and A. K. Jain, Markov random field texture models. *IEEE Trans. Pattern Analysis Machine Intel.* **5** (1983) 25–39.

[6.18] D. K. Pickard, Inference for discrete Markov fields: the simplest nontrivial case. *J. Acoust. Soc. Am.* **82** (1987) 90–96.

7 Probability density estimation by linear models

Probability density estimation is a crucial step in stochastic system identification. In the random field models studied in Chapter 6 as well as the applications to follow in image analysis, probability density estimation is a fundamental component. The purpose of this chapter is to study approaches for density estimation that are local, i.e. may be identified using empirical measurements, which are assumed realizations of a random process or random field of a certain statistical experiment. Of interest to us are density models that have manageable numerical implementation and may be used at various levels of image analysis.

7.1 Introduction

Numerical methods for estimating the probability density function (PDF) of a random variable X (a random vector in general) are important in various signal and image analysis applications. Such estimates form the basis of optimal filtering, synthesis, and segmentation of an image or a signal. Indeed, PDF estimation is fundamental in Bayesian statistics and in a huge number of machine-learning applications [7.1].

Given a random sample $D = \{X_1, X_2, \cdots, X_N\}$ from a particular distribution with PDF $f(x)$ that is assumed to be continuous over a domain $[a, b] \subset \mathbb{R}$, the modes of $f_X(x)$ (i.e., the minima and maxima) are in the closed interval $[a, b]$. The estimate $\hat{f}(x)$ of the PDF can be obtained by a number of methods.

Density estimation has been heavily studied under two primary umbrellas: parametric and nonparametric methods. Nonparametric methods take the stance of letting the data represent themselves. These methods (an example being the Parzen window method [7.2]) achieve good estimation for any input distribution if enough data are observed. However, these methods have many parameters that need to be tuned [7.3]. One of the core methods on which nonparametric density estimation approaches are based is the k-nearest-neighbors (k-NN) method. These approaches calculate the probability of a sample by combining the memorized responses for the k nearest neighbors of this sample in the training data. In these estimators (e.g. the Parzen density estimator [7.2]), the amount of computation is directly related to the number of training samples. In order to reduce the computation, Fukunaga and Hayes [7.4] extracted a representative subset from the training data. This reduced subset was chosen such that the Parzen density estimation generated is very close to that generated with the full data set, in the sense of an entropy measure of similarity between the two estimates.

Silverman [7.5] proposed a kernel density estimator using the fast Fourier transform (FFT). A kernel density estimator is a weighted linear combination of shifted kernel functions, which possess certain characteristics such as positivity, integrability and compactness. Various kernels have been used, including the Gaussian, uniform, quadratic and triangular windows. Silverman estimated density using a univariate Parzen window on regular grids. This method exploits the properties of the FFT, where the FFT of the density estimate is the product of the FFTs of the kernel function and the data. However, this algorithm cannot be used in the general cases of density estimates. In order to reduce the number of kernel evaluations, Jeon and Landgrebe [7.6] proposed a simple branch-and-bound procedure that is applied to the Parzen density estimation. Girolami and He [7.7] proposed a Parzen window-based density estimator which employs condensed data samples. The advantage of nonparametric methods is their flexibility: they can fit almost any data well. However, they often have a high computational cost, and there is no opportunity to incorporate prior knowledge.

Parametric methods, on the other hand, are useful when the underlying distribution is known in advance or is simple enough to be modeled by a simple distribution function or a mixture of such functions. The parametric model is very compact (low memory and CPU usage) where only few parameters are required. Parameters of a mixture are typically estimated using expectation-maximization (EM) algorithms that converge to the maximum likelihood estimates of the mixture weights (prior probabilities of the mixture components) and parameters of each component [7.8]. After Laird et al. [7.9] extended the EM algorithm so that it could be used in estimating parameters from an incomplete data set, it became a popular approach in density estimation, and many versions of EM have been introduced elsewhere [7.8].

7.2 Nonparametric methods

A histogram is the simplest nonparametric density estimator. Given a random sample $D = \{X_1, X_2, \cdots, X_n\}$ from a particular distribution with PDF $f_x(x)$, a histogram can approximate any form of $f_x(x)$ as $n \to \infty$. For simplicity, from now on $f_x(x)$ will be written $f(x)$. It is well known that the probability $P(X \in \mathcal{R}) = \int_{\mathcal{R}} f_x(x)dx$, where $\mathcal{R}$ is a region with volume h^d in d dimensions of space $\mathbb{R}^d$. Assume that the volume h^d is very small, so this integral can be approximated by the product of the value of $f(x^*)$ with the volume of the region $\mathcal{R}: P(X \in \mathcal{R}) \approx f(x^*)h^d$. This integral can also be approximated by the ratio between the number of samples k falling within this region to the total number of samples n. Therefore, $f(x^*)$ can be approximated by:

$$\hat{f}(x) = \frac{k}{nh^d}. \qquad (7.1)$$

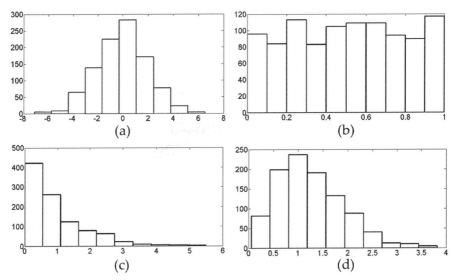

Figure 7.1 Illustration for histograms of different distributions. (a) Gaussian, (b) uniform, (c) exponential, and (d) Rayleigh.

Example 7.1 Consider a random sample $D = \{X_1, X_2, \cdots, X_{1000}\}$. Figure 7.1 shows histograms of the data for the following cases:

- D is drawn from a Gaussian distribution, with zero mean and variance four (Figure 7.1(a));
- D is drawn from a uniform distribution within interval $(0,1)$ (Figure 7.1(b));
- D is drawn from an exponential distribution with parameter 1 (Figure 7.1(c));
- D is drawn from a Rayleigh distribution with parameter 1 (Figure 7.1(d)).

Choosing the width h of the histogram bin is an important factor in obtaining an accurate estimate for $f(x)$. If h is small, in practice we have a finite number of training data, so as $h \to 0$, $\mathcal{R}$ will eventually contain no samples: $k = 0, f(x) = 0$, a useless result. On the other hand, if h is big, $\mathcal{R}$ will contain more samples, so $k/n \to P$; however, we then estimate only an average of $f(x)$, not $f(x)$ itself.

Example 7.2 Consider a random sample $D = \{X_1, X_2, \cdots, X_{1000}\}$. Figure 7.2 shows histograms of the data for the following cases:

- D is drawn from a Gaussian distribution with zero mean and variance 4 (Figure 7.2(a), with bin width $h \approx 2$);
- D is drawn from a Gaussian distribution with zero mean and variance 4 (Figure 7.2(a), with bin width $h \approx 4$);
- D is drawn from a Gaussian distribution with zero mean and variance 4 (Figure 7.2(b), with bin width $h \approx 6$).
- As shown above, the modes in the histogram can be enhanced or "buried" based on the selection of the bin. Hence, generalized nonparametric methods offer an advantage

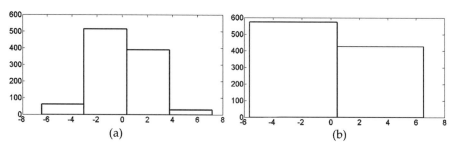

Figure 7.2 Illustration for a histogram of Gaussian distributions with bin of width (a) $h \approx 4$ and (b) $h \approx 6$.

over histogram-based estimation. These methods are adaptive to the data, and in general require no priors in the estimation process. However, they often have a high computational cost and involve large numbers of parameters that need to be estimated.

7.2.1 Kernel-based estimators

The kernel-based techniques are the most popular density estimation methods. The estimated $\hat{f}(x)$ for a d-dimensional data point x in space $\mathbb{R}^d$ is given by

$$\hat{f}(x) = \frac{1}{n}\sum_{i=1}^{n} |H|^{-0.5} K(|H|^{-0.5}(x - x_i)). \tag{7.2}$$

In this equation, H is a symmetric positive definite $d \times d$ bandwidth matrix, and the d-variate kernel $K(x)$ is a bounded function satisfying [7.15]

$$\int_{\mathbb{R}^d} K(x)\, dx = 1 \quad \lim_{\|x\|\to\infty} |x|^d K(x) = 0$$

$$\int_{\mathbb{R}^d} xK(x)\, dx = 0 \quad \int_{\mathbb{R}^d} xx^T K(x)\, dx = cI \tag{7.3}$$

where c is a constant and I is the identity matrix. The multivariate kernel can be generated from the product of d symmetric univariate kernels or by rotating a univariate kernel in $\mathbb{R}^d$. When the bandwidth matrix is chosen to be $H = h^2 I$, then the kernel density estimator in Eq. (7.2) will be:

$$\hat{f}(x) = \frac{1}{nh^d}\sum_{i=1}^{n} K\left(\frac{x - x_i}{h}\right). \tag{7.4}$$

In the case of one-dimensional data, $x \in \mathbb{R}$, the kernel estimator (7.4) has the following form:

$$\hat{f}(x) = \frac{1}{nh}\sum_{i=1}^{n} K\left(\frac{x - x_i}{h}\right). \tag{7.5}$$

where h is the "window" width. There are various kernels (windows) that have been studied in the literature, including the uniform and Gaussian PDFs [7.5]. In particular, the differentiability, integrability, and tail properties of the kernel-based estimator are well studied in the statistical literature [7.5]. In addition, the quality of the estimator has been examined in terms of statistical properties such as consistency and the effect of sample size.

7.2.2 Parzen window

In the Parzen window approach the width h is chosen, and then the number of samples k inside the window is calculated.

Example 7.3 Consider a one-dimensional random sample $D = \{1,2,1,1,2,3,3.5,3.5\}$, and find the density estimation

$$\hat{f}(2.5) = \frac{1}{\sqrt{2\pi} \times 8} \left(3e^{-\frac{1}{2}(2.5-1)^2} + 2e^{-\frac{1}{2}(2.5-2)^2} + e^{-\frac{1}{2}(2.5-3)^2} + 2e^{-\frac{1}{2}(2.5-3.5)^2} \right) = 0.2410$$

using the Parzen window approach. The relative frequencies of the values are illustrated in Figure 7.3.

Choose the window function to be unit step with width $h = 1$. Centering this window at 2.5, so simply using Eq. (7.1), the dataset $\{2,2,3\}$ will be inside this window. Therefore $k = 3$, and $\hat{f}(2.5) = \frac{k}{nh} = \frac{3}{8*1} = 0.375$.

Choose the window function to be a zero-mean unit variance Gaussian window, i.e. $h = 1$. Centering this window at 2.5, and therefore using Eq. (7.5), $\hat{f}(2.5) = \frac{1}{\sqrt{2\pi}*8} \left(3 * e^{-\frac{1}{2}(2.5-1)^2} + 2 * e^{-\frac{1}{2}(2.5-2)^2} + e^{-\frac{1}{2}(2.5-3)^2} + 2 * e^{-\frac{1}{2}(2.5-3.5)^2} \right)$.

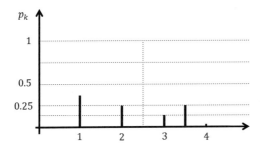

Figure 7.3 Relative frequencies of the values in the random sample in Example 7.3.

7.2.3 k-NN estimator

Unlike the Parzen window, in the k-NN approach the number of samples k is chosen first, and then the width h is adjusted.

Example 7.4 Consider a one-dimensional random sample $D = \{1,2,1,1,2,3,3.5,3.5\}$, and find the density estimation $\hat{f}(2.5)$ using k-NN with $k = 4$.

We need to select the window width such that the number of samples inside the window will be at least $k = 4$. A good choice for the width would be $h = 2$ with a unit step window function. Since the width of the function is 2, its height should be 0.5. Centering this window at 2.5, so simply using Eq. (7.1), the dataset $\{2,2,3,3.5,3.5\}$ will be inside this window. Therefore $k = 5$, and $\hat{f}(2.5) = \frac{k/2}{nh} = \frac{5/2}{8*1} = 0.3125$.

7.3 Parametric methods

As we said in the introduction to this chapter, these methods are useful when the underlying distribution is known or is simple enough to be modeled by a simple distribution function or a mixture of such functions. Figure 7.4 illustrates examples of these distributions:

$$\text{Gaussian} \quad \frac{1}{\sigma\sqrt{2\pi}}e^{-\frac{(x-\mu)^2}{2\sigma^2}}$$

$$\text{exponential} \quad \frac{1}{\sigma}e^{-\frac{x-\mu}{\sigma}}$$

$$\text{gamma} \quad \frac{(x-\mu)^{\gamma-1}}{\sigma^\gamma \Gamma(\gamma)}e^{-\frac{x-\mu}{\sigma}}$$

These distributions are controlled using different parameters. A location parameter, e.g. μ, shifts the PDF graph left or right on the horizontal axis. A scale parameter may stretch ($\sigma > 1$) or compress ($\sigma < 1$) the PDF graph. A shape parameter, e.g. γ, changes the PDF graph. The

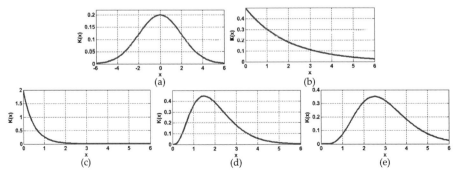

Figure 7.4 Examples of different well known distributions. (a) Gaussian ($\mu = 0, \sigma = 2$). (b) Exponential ($\mu = 0, \sigma = 2$). (c) Gamma ($\mu = 0, \sigma = 0.5, \gamma = 1$). (d) Gamma ($\mu = 0, \sigma = 0.5, \gamma = 4$). (e) Gamma ($\mu = 0, \sigma = 0.5, \gamma = 6$).

7.3.1 Maximum likelihood estimator (MLE)

Suppose a random sample $D = \{X_1, X_2, \cdots, X_n\}$ is drawn from a distribution $\varphi(\theta)$ with a vector of parameters $\theta = (\theta_1, \ldots, \theta_r)$. The goal is to estimate the vector θ. In this density estimation problem, we have data samples and know the distribution type, but the distribution parameters θ are unknown. The MLE method estimates θ by maximizing the log-likelihood of the data, $\log f(x_1, x_2, \cdots, x_n | \theta)$. The parameter θ is shown in the log-likelihood of the data to show the dependence of f on θ explicitly.

$$\begin{aligned}\theta_{MLE} &= \arg\max_\theta \, \log f(x_1, x_2, \cdots, x_n | \theta) \\ &= \arg\max_\theta \, \log \prod_{i=1}^n f(x_i|\theta) \\ &= \arg\max_\theta \sum_{i=1}^n \log f(x_i|\theta)\end{aligned} \qquad (7.6)$$

To solve Eq. (7.6): first we let $L(\theta) = \sum_{i=1}^n \log f(x_i|\theta)$, then we calculate

$$\frac{\partial L}{\partial \theta} = \left[\frac{\partial L}{\partial \theta_1}, \frac{\partial L}{\partial \theta_2}, \cdots, \frac{\partial L}{\partial \theta_r}\right]^T.$$ Finally, we find θ by letting $\frac{\partial L}{\partial \theta} = \mathbf{0}$.

Example 7.5 Assume that a box contains a large number of colored (red, green, and blue) balls. The numbers of the red, green, and blue balls are not equal. A robot chooses a ball, according to some random process, and the ball color is recorded as the observation. The ball is then replaced in the box. Given 100 observations from this experiment, $R = 45$ red balls, $G = 15$ green balls, and $B = 40$ blue balls, what is the MLE of the probability of choosing a green ball given the probability of choosing a red ball is 0.45?

- Since the numbers of the red, green, and blue balls are not equal, this means that the probabilities are also not equal.
- Assuming that the probability of choosing a green ball is μ, then the probability of choosing a blue ball is $1 - 0.45 - \mu = 0.55 - \mu$.
- From the observed data, we can see that there are 15 green balls chosen out of a total of 100 balls. Therefore we can expect that $\mu = 15/100$.
- Let us see what is the MLE:

$$L(\theta) = \sum_{i=1}^{100} \log f(x_i|\theta) = 45\log(0.45) + 15\log(\mu) + 40\log(0.55 - \mu)$$

$$\frac{\partial L}{\partial \theta} = \frac{\partial L}{\partial \mu} = \frac{15}{\mu} - \frac{40}{0.55 - \mu} = 0$$

$$\mu = \frac{15}{100}$$

Example 7.6 Consider a one-dimensional random sample $D = \{X_1, X_2, \cdots, X_n\}$, drawn independently and identically distributed (i.i.d.) from a 1D Gaussian distribution with mean μ and variance σ^2. Find the MLE of μ and σ.

According to the three steps explained in the previous section:

$$L(\theta) = \sum_{i=1}^{n} \log f(x_i|\theta) = \sum_{i=1}^{n} \log\left(\frac{1}{\sigma\sqrt{2\pi}} e^{-\frac{(x_i-\mu)^2}{2\sigma^2}}\right) = n\log\left(\frac{1}{\sigma\sqrt{2\pi}}\right) - \sum_{i=1}^{n}\frac{(x_i-\mu)^2}{2\sigma^2}$$

$$\frac{\partial L}{\partial \theta} = \left[\frac{\partial L}{\partial \mu}, \frac{\partial L}{\partial \sigma}\right]^T = \left[\sum_{i=1}^{n}\frac{x_i-\mu}{\sigma^2}, -\frac{n}{\sigma} + \sum_{i=1}^{n}\frac{(x_i-\mu)^2}{\sigma^3}\right] = [0, 0]$$

$$\mu_{\text{MLE}} = \frac{1}{n}\sum_{i=1}^{n} x_i \qquad \sigma^2_{\text{MLE}} = \frac{1}{n}\sum_{i=1}^{n}(x_i-\mu)^2$$

7.3.2 Biased versus unbiased estimator

An estimator of a parameter is unbiased if the expected value of the estimate is the same as the true value of the parameters. As an example, the estimator of Gaussian distribution mean μ_{MLE} shown in Example 7.5 is unbiased since

$$E[\mu_{\text{MLE}}] = E\left[\frac{1}{n}\sum_{i=1}^{n} x_i\right] = \frac{1}{n}\sum_{i=1}^{n} E[x_i] = \frac{1}{n} nE[x_i] = \mu \tag{7.7}$$

However, the estimation of Gaussian distribution variance σ^2_{MLE} shown in Example 7.5 is biased since

$$E[\sigma^2_{\text{MLE}}] = E\left[\frac{1}{n}\sum_{i=1}^{n}(x_i - \mu_{\text{MLE}})^2\right] = E\left[\frac{1}{n}\sum_{i=1}^{n}\left(x_i - \frac{1}{n}\sum_{j=1}^{n} x_j\right)^2\right]$$

$$= E\left[\frac{1}{n}\sum_{i=1}^{n}\left(x_i^2 - \frac{2}{n}\sum_{i=1}^{n} x_i x_j + \frac{1}{n^2}\left(\sum_{j=1}^{n} x_j\right)^2\right)\right] \tag{7.8}$$

$$= \left(1 - \frac{1}{n}\right)\sigma^2$$

This estimation can be modified such that it will be unbiased as follows:

$$\sigma^2_{\text{unbiased}} = \frac{1}{n-1}\sum_{i=1}^{n}(x_i - \mu_{\text{MLE}})^2 \tag{7.9}$$

We can see that as $n \to \infty$ there is no difference between the unbiased estimation Eq. (7.9) and the biased estimation Eq. (7.8).

7.3.3 The expectation-maximization (EM) approach

The EM algorithm is a general method of finding the maximum likelihood estimate of the parameters of an underlying distribution from a given data set when the data are incomplete or have missing values. To explain this, assume in Example 7.5 that the number of green balls G and the number of blue balls B are unknown. However, we know the sum of these numbers $G+B = 100 - 45 = 55$. In this case we cannot use the MLE approach, because, as shown in Example 7.5, MLE gives only two equations where we have three unknowns (μ, σ and G or B). We can solve this problem iteratively as follows:

- Estimate the expectation of the values G and B.
- Use these expected values to estimate the MLE of μ.
- Then update the expected values.
- Repeat these steps.

These steps are the main idea of the EM algorithm. Note that EM is an unsupervised method, but MLE is a supervised method.

Example 7.7 Assume that a box contains a large number of colored (red, green, and blue) balls. The numbers of red, green, and blue balls are not equal. A robot chooses a ball, according to some random process, and the ball color is recorded as the observation. The ball is then replaced in the box. After 100 observations from this experiment, the number of blue balls recorded is $B = 40$. What is the MLE of the probability of choosing a red ball?

Unlike Example 7.4, the number of green balls G and the number of red balls R are unknown. However, we know the sum of these numbers $G + R = 100 - 40 = 60$ (green and red balls). In this case we cannot use the MLE, because MLE gives only two equations and we have three unknowns (μ, σ, and number of green or red balls). We can solve this problem iteratively as follows:

- Start with initial $\mu = 0.1$
- Estimate the expectation of the values of G and R.

$$R = \frac{0.45}{0.45 + \mu}$$

$$G = \frac{\mu}{0.45 + \mu}$$

- Use these expected values to estimate the MLE of μ.

$$L(\theta) = \sum_{i=1}^{100} \log f(x_i|\theta) = R\log(0.45) + G\log(\mu) + 40\log(0.55 - \mu)$$

$$\frac{\partial L}{\partial \theta} = \frac{\partial L}{\partial \mu} = \frac{G}{\mu} - \frac{40}{0.55 - \mu} = 0$$

$$\mu = \frac{0.55 G}{40 + G}$$

- Update the expected values.
- Repeat these steps.
- After 10 iterations you will obtain the following: $G = 14.9760$, $R = 45.0240$, and $\mu = 0.1498$.

The EM algorithm can be summarized as follows:
- Given initial parameters θ^0
- Repeatedly
  - Re-estimate expected values of hidden variables C.
  - Then recalculate the MLE of θ using these expected values for the hidden variables C.

Assume a joint density function $f(x, C | \theta)$ for a complete data set. The EM algorithm first finds the expected value of the complete-data log-likelihood with respect to the unknown data C given the observed data and the current parameter estimates θ^{i-1}.

$$Q(\theta | \theta^{i-1}) = E\left[\log f(x, c | \theta) | x, \theta^{i-1}\right] \qquad (7.10)$$

Notice that θ is the new parameter that we optimize in order to maximize Q, whereas θ^{i-1} is the current parameter's estimate that we used to evaluate the expectation. The evaluation of this expectation is called the E-step of the algorithm. The second step (the M-step) of the EM algorithm is to maximize the expectation we computed in the first step.

$$\theta^i = \arg\max_\theta Q(\theta | \theta^{i-1}) \qquad (7.11)$$

These two steps are repeated as necessary. Each iteration is guaranteed to increase the log-likelihood, and the algorithm is guaranteed to converge to a local maximum of the likelihood function.

7.4 Linear combination of Gaussians model (LCG1)

For all our previous examples, we have assumed that the observed data are generated from an identical distribution. However, in practice distinct subpopulations can exist in observed data. Early explorations of this idea were by Pearson, who in 1894 tried to model the distribution of the ratio between measurements of forehead and body length of crabs. He used a two-component mixture, and it was hypothesized that the two-component structure was related to the possibility of this particular population of crabs evolving into two new subspecies.

Actually, the mixture model is an alternative to the kernel estimator, where the underlying density is assumed to have the form:

$$\hat{f}(x) = \sum_{j=1}^{k} w_j \varnothing(x | \theta_j), \qquad (7.12)$$

7.4 Linear combination of Gaussians model (LCG1)

where $\emptyset(x|\theta_j)$ is the jth kernel function, W_j is the corresponding weight, and k is the number of components of the mixture. Unlike the kernel estimator where the number of components n is the number of data points, in a mixture the number of components k can be pre-specified based on some *a priori* knowledge about the nature of the subpopulations in the data (dominant modes of the data). The Gaussian function is amongst the most commonly used kernels in the above model; the resulting PDF estimate is known as a linear combination of Gaussians (LCG). The LCG possesses various computational and mathematical characteristics that makes it attractive, in particular its integrability, continuity, and the fact that a well-established suboptimal approach for estimation of the parameters θ_j, $j \in [1, k]$ exists via the EM algorithm (e.g., [7.3] [7.4]).

The parameters of the mixture model can be estimated using the MLE only if the observed data are a complete set. An example of a complete data set is n $\{x_i, C_{i1}, C_{i2}\}$ drawn i.i.d. from two normal distributions, where x_i is the observed value of the ith instance, and C_{i1} and C_{i2} indicate which of two normal distributions was used to generate x_i. Therefore $C_{ij} = 1$ if it was used to generate x_i, and 0 otherwise. However, in practice we do not know the values of C_{ij}. So how can we estimate the parameters given incomplete data (unknown C_{ij})? The answer is the EM algorithm.

The mixture-density parameter estimation problem using EM is described as follows.

$$\Theta = [\omega_1, \ldots, \omega_k, \theta_1, \ldots, \theta_k]$$

$$Q(\Theta \mid \Theta^{i-1}) = \sum_{l=1}^{k} \sum_{j=1}^{n} \log(\omega_l f(x_j \mid \theta_l)) f(l \mid x_j, \Theta^{i-1}) \qquad (7.13)$$

$$f(l \mid x_j, \Theta^{i-1}) = \prod_{j=1}^{n} f(c_j \mid x_j, \Theta^{i-1})$$

Using Bayes' rule, we can compute:

$$f(c_j \mid x_j, \Theta^{i-1}) = \frac{\omega^i_{cj} f(x_j \mid \theta^i_{cj})}{\sum_{l=1}^{k} \omega^i_l f(x_j \mid \theta^i_l)} \qquad (7.14)$$

For some distributions, it is possible to obtain analytical expressions for the distribution parameters. For example, if we assume d-dimensional Gaussian component distributions

$$\mu^i_l = \frac{\sum_{j=1}^{n} x_j f(l \mid x_j, \Theta_l^{i-1})}{\sum_{j=1}^{n} f(l \mid x_j, \Theta_l^{i-1})} \qquad (7.15)$$

$$\Sigma^i_l = \frac{\sum_{j=1}^{n} f(l \mid x_j, \Theta_l^{i-1})(x_j - \mu^i_l)(x_j - \mu^i_l)^T}{\sum_{j=1}^{n} f(k \mid x_j, \Theta_l^{i-1})} \qquad (7.16)$$

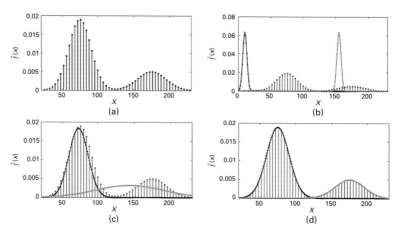

Figure 7.5 Using EM mixture-density estimation. (a) The given data histogram, (b) estimation based on initial values (c) EM estimation after 5 iterations, and (d) EM estimation after 15 iterations.

$$\omega^i{}_l = \frac{1}{n}\sum_{j=1}^{n} f(k \mid x_j, \Theta_l^{i-1}) \qquad (7.17)$$

Example 7.8 A set of n samples is drawn i.i.d. from two 1D normal distributions. The histogram of these samples is shown in Figure 7.5(a). The initial parameters lead to a mixture-density estimation shown in (b), while (c) shows the EM estimation after 5 iterations and (d) shows the EM estimation after 15 iterations.

Approximations of the empirical data using a mixture of positive Gaussians have appeared in many works, e.g. [7.10],[7.11],[[7.12].

7.4.1 Modifications of the linear model (LCG2)

To provide better fitting for the empirical density, we introduced, in [7.13], a modification to the standard linear model above, in which we allowed the weights to take positive and negative values. The new LCG2 model has the following form:

$$\hat{f}(X) = \sum_{i=1}^{k_p} w_{p,i}\emptyset(X|\theta_i) - \sum_{j=1}^{k_n} w_{n,j}\emptyset(X|\theta_j) \qquad (7.18)$$

where k_p and k_n are the number of positive and negative kernels used in the linear model, and $w_{p,i}$ and $w_{n,j}$ are the corresponding weights. In order for the estimate in Eq. (7.18) to be a real density model (i.e. k_p positive and integrates to 1), we imposed a condition on the weights such that:

$$\sum_{i=1}^{k_p} w_{p,i} - \sum_{j=1}^{k_n} w_{n,j} = 1. \qquad (7.19)$$

It has been proven that the new model provides a better fitting for the empirical density [7.13]. Farag et al. [7.13] developed a modified EM algorithm to estimate the parameters of this new LCG model. The model in [7.13] assumes that the number of dominant modes in the LCG model (number of classes in the given multimodal image) is known. To estimate this number, Ali et al. use a technique based on maximizing a new joint likelihood function [7.14].

7.5 Modeling the image intensity/appearance through the linear model

The goal of image modeling is to quantitatively specify visual characteristics of the image in a few parameters, so as to understand natural constraints and general assumptions about the physical world and the imaging process. Random field models can represent prior information about an image, so that the powerful Bayesian decision theory can be applied to solve these problems. Objects of interest in the images are characterized by geometric shapes and visual appearance, although it is very difficult to define these notions formally. The visual appearance is usually characterized by the marginal probability distribution of pixel or voxel intensities, and by spatial interaction between pixels or voxels in each object. Density estimation plays an important role in estimating such marginal probability distributions of pixel intensities. Figure 7.6 provides illustrative examples of medical images and their marginal densities.

To estimate the marginal densities of the original image given the categories or classes found in the image, we assume that this model is an independent random field of gray levels with different gray value distributions:

$$f(\mathbf{I}|1) = \prod_{p \in P} f(I_p|1_p), \qquad (7.20)$$

where $p \in P$, I_p for each pixel I_p is the pixel gray level, and l is the pixel label. To accurately estimate this conditional distribution $P(\mathbf{I}|l)$, we need to approximate the gray-level marginal density of each class $P(I_p|l_p)$.. Approximation of an empirical relative frequency distribution of scalar data with a particular probability density function is widely used to solve segmentation problems, e.g. [7.1][[7.16][[7.17]. Although precise classification cannot be achieved by using only a mixed marginal probability distribution, many important applications (e.g. analysis of images obtained by computer tomography, magnetic resonance imaging, or magnetic resonance angiography) depend on this type of data classification. Since the borders between data classes are usually formed by intersecting tails of the class distributions, classification of the data using distributions created by approximating only the peaks (the modes of the data) of the probability density function is often not enough to give an accurate solution. For more accurate classification, the probability density function approximation should describe the behavior of the function between the peaks.

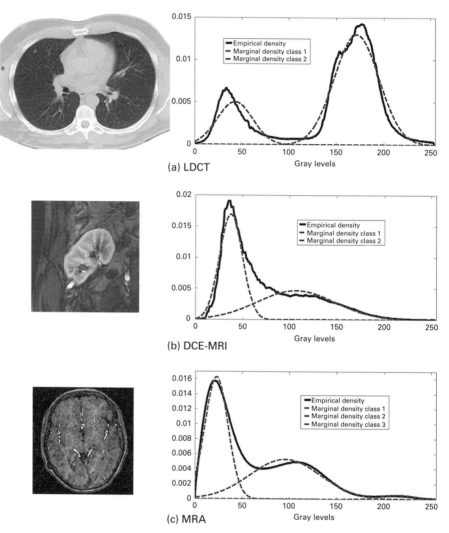

Figure 7.6 Illustrative examples of multimodal images and their empirical and marginal densities. (a) A typical lung slice from LDCT, (b) a typical kidney slice from DCE-MRI, (c) a typical brain slice from MRA. LDCT: low dose computed tomography; DCE-MRI: dynamic contrast enhanced magnetic resonance imaging; MRA: magnetic resonance angiography

7.6 Exercises

7.1 Consider a random sample $D = \{X_1, X_2, \cdots, X_n\}$ drawn from a distribution with exponential density with a single parameter $p(x) = \theta e^{-\theta x} u(x)$, where $u(x)$ is the unit-step function, and $\theta > 0$. Derive the maximum likelihood estimate for θ.

7.2 Consider three coins with probability of head $P_i(h) = \alpha, \beta$, and γ for $i \in [1,3]$. The following experiment is performed: coin 1 is tossed first, and if the outcome is a head then coin 2 is tossed twice; otherwise, coin 3 is tossed twice. Suppose the output of the experiment is as in the following table; estimate the values of α, β, and γ.

Tossed coin	2	3	2	2	3	3
Output	(h,h)	(t,t)	(h,h)	(h,h)	(t,t)	(t,t)

7.3 Complete the proof in Eq. (7.8)

7.4 Prove that the estimator in Eq. (7.9) is unbiased.

7.5 Consider a d-dimensional random sample $D = \{X_1, X_2, \cdots, X_n\}$ drawn from a d-dimensional Gaussian distribution with mean μ and variance Σ. Find the MLE of μ and Σ.

7.6 The formula for the two-parameter probability density function of the log-normal distribution is

$$p(x) = \frac{1}{x\sigma\sqrt{2\pi}} \exp\left(-\frac{1}{2}\left(\frac{\ln\left(\frac{x}{\mu}\right)}{\sigma}\right)^2\right) \qquad x \geq 0;\, \sigma,\, \mu > 0$$

Given n samples $x_1, x_2, \cdots, x_n$ that are drawn independently and identically from a log-normal distribution, derive the maximum likelihood estimate for σ and μ.

7.7 For the two-class 3×4 image given below:

5,c_1	4,c_1	4,c_1	5,c_1
4,c_1	8,c_2	8,c_2	3,c_1
3,c_1	9,c_2	7,c_2	6,?

(a) Estimate $p(6 \mid c_1)$.
(b) Estimate $p(6 \mid c_2)$.
(c) If these pixel values are drawn independently and identically from two different log-normal distributions, estimate $p(6 \mid c_1)$.
(d) If these pixel values are drawn independently and identically from two different log-normal distributions, estimate $p(6 \mid c_2)$.
(e) If these pixel values are drawn independently and identically from two different normal distributions, estimate $p(6 \mid c_1)$.
(f) If these pixel values are drawn independently and identically from two different normal distributions, estimate $p(6 \mid c_2)$.

7.7 Computer laboratory

Task 1 Compute the maximum likelihood estimate for θ for the samples in "data.txt," available online. Plot the maximum likelihood exponential density, overlaid on the histogram of the data.

Task 2 Fit a nonparametric density estimate to the samples in "data.txt" using the Parzen windows approach. You may use the following windows:

(a) $\varphi(x) = \begin{cases} \dfrac{1}{h} & \text{if } |x - x_i| \leq \dfrac{h}{2} \\ 0 & \text{otherwise} \end{cases}$

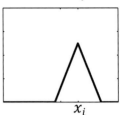

(b) $\varphi(x) = \begin{cases} \dfrac{h + x - x_i}{h^2} & \text{if } x - h \leq x \leq x_i \\ \dfrac{h - x + x_i}{h^2} & \text{if } x_i - x \leq x_i \leq h \\ 0 & \text{otherwise} \end{cases}$

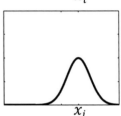

(c) $\varphi(x) = \dfrac{1}{\sqrt{2\pi h^2}} e^{-\dfrac{(x - x_i)^2}{2h^2}}$

i. Using different values of $h = 0.01, 0.1$ and 1, plot the nonparametric density estimates, overlaid on the histogram of the data.

ii. Using the window in (a) find k-NN nonparametric density estimates using different values of $k = 1, 10$, and 30. Plot the nonparametric density estimates, overlaid on the histogram of the data.

Task 3 Consider the K-component Gaussian mixture model with parameters ($K = 3$)

$$\omega_1 = 0.5, \quad \mu_1 = 43, \quad \sigma_1 = 10,$$
$$\omega_2 = 0.2, \quad \mu_2 = 128, \quad \sigma_2 = 10,$$
$$\omega_3 = 0.3, \quad \mu_3 = 170, \quad \sigma_3 = 10,$$

(a) Write a function that takes as input a value for n and returns a $1 \times n$ vector X representing a random sample drawn from this mixture model.
(b) Write a function "EM" that takes X and an integer K and returns the MLE of a Gaussian mixture model with K components, as computed by the EM algorithm.
(c) In the code for the EM algorithm, include commands that show the K different Gaussians components as they are iteratively updated.
(d) Generate a sample from the Gaussian mixture model of size $n = 1000$. Call the EM function with $K = 3$. Report the following:
  i. The estimates of the model parameters and how they compare to the true values;

ii. The effect of initial values and the number of iterations required until convergence;
iii. Plot the log-likelihood as a function of iteration number and verify that it is nondecreasing.

Task 4 Using the EM algorithm, estimate the marginal densities of the classes in the following images, available online:

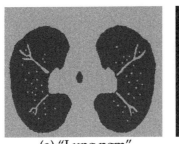 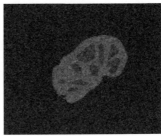

(a) "Lung.pgm"   (b) "Kidney.pgm"

Obtain an initial cluster based on these estimations.

Task 5 Using the EM algorithm, estimate the marginal densities of the classes in the "rose.ppm" image, available online. Obtain an initial segmentation based on these estimations.

References

[7.1] R. O. Duda, P. E. Hart and D. G. Stork, *Pattern Classification*. New York: Wiley (2001).
[7.2] V. N. Vapnik, *Density Estimation for Statistics and Data Analysis*. Chapman and Hall (1986).
[7.3] V. N. Vapnik, *Statistical Learning Theory*. New York: Wiley (1998).
[7.4] K. Fukunaga and R. R. Hayes, The reduced Parzen classifier. *IEEE Trans. Pattern Anal. Machine Intel.* **11** (1989) 423–425.
[7.5] B. W. Silverman, Algorithm, AS176. Kernel density estimation using the fast Fourier transform. *Appl. Stat.* **31** (1982) 93–97.
[7.6] B. W. Jeon and D. A. Landgrebe, Fast Parzen density-estimation using clustering-based branch-and-bound. *IEEE Trans. Pattern Anal. Machine Intel.* **16**(9) (1994) 950–954.
[7.7] M. Girolami and C. He, Probability density estimation from optimally condensed data samples. *IEEE Trans. Pattern Anal. Machine Intel.* **25**(10) (2003) 1253–1264.
[7.8] T. Moon, The expectation-maximization algorithm. *IEEE Signal Proc. Mag.* **11** (1996) 47–60.
[7.9] A. P. Dempster, N. M. Laird and D. B. Rubin, Maximum likelihood from incomplete data via the em algorithm. *J. Roy. Stat. Soc.* **39**B (1977) 1–38.
[7.10] H. W. Sorenson and D. L. Alspach, Recursive Bayesian estimation using Gaussian sums. *Automatica* **7** (1971) 465–479.
[7.11] T. Poggio and F. Girosi, Networks for approximation and learning, *Proc. IEEE* **78** (1990) 1481–1497.

[7.12] A. Goshtasby and W. D. O'Neill, Curve fitting by a sum of Gaussians. *CVGIP Graph. Model Image Proc.* **56** (1999) 281–288.

[7.13] A. A. Farag, A. El-Baz and G. Gimel'farb, Density estimation using modified expectation maximization for a linear combination of Gaussians. *Proc. ICIP* **3** (2004) 1871–1874.

[7.14] A. M. Ali and A. A. Farag, Density estimation using a new AIC-type criterion and the EM algorithm for a linear combination of Gaussians. *Proc. IEEE Int. Conf. Image Proc. (ICIP08)* (2008) 3024–3027.

[7.15] M. P. Wand and M. Jonse, *Kernel Smoothing*. London: Chapman and Hall, (1995).

[7.16] N. R. Pal and S. K. Pal, A review on image segmentation techniques. *Patt. Rec.* **26** (1993) 1277–1294

[7.17] R. C. Dubes and A. K. Jain, Random field models in image analysis. *J. Appl. Stat.* **16** (1989) 131–164.

Part III

Computational geometry

8 Basics of topology and computational geometry

8.1 Introduction

Topology is a branch of mathematics that describes objects using geometry, set theory, and group theory. Geometry deals with primitive figures such as triangles, parallelograms, and polygons. Geometric operations measure lengths, angles and areas of shapes, their congruence, and transformations based on scale, translation, and rotation. These functions are commonly denoted as isometries. Topology deals with such matters as well, but in a more global fashion and with complicated shapes. Computational geometry, a field which started in the 1970s, deals with object models that pertain to computing and visualization. Computational geometry and topology share various terminologies, and both deal with shape modeling.

Advances in data acquisition have enabled reconstruction of high-quality three-dimensional models, on which computational geometry is used for modeling and visualization. Section 8.2 deals with shape representation, as a starting point for geometrical and topological analysis. Section 8.3 deals with topologically equivalent shapes and various entities that define surfaces as manifolds. We consider topological properties of points, curves, and surfaces. We are particularly interested in boundary-based shape representations where the geometrical structure can be described in a parametric form (Section 8.5) or in a piece-wise linear form (Section 8.6). Bézier curves and surfaces are popular parametric surface models. Such models are studied together with polygons, triangles, meshes, curvatures, shape indices, and curvedness.

8.2 Shape representation

Shapes are typically defined as an object, an abstraction, or a representation. An object is something that can be physically felt (seen, touched), such as a ball. An abstraction is a quality separated from an actual example, such as the concept of a ball being a sphere. A representation is a way that a shape is symbolized, for example by representing the ball as an equation for a sphere ($r^2 = x^2 + y^2 + z^2$).

8.2.1 What is shape?

While 3D models of living and man-made objects can be described by their color, texture, and shape information, color and texture may not always be saved in the acquisition technique. Therefore, shape is the lowest common denominator in describing 3D objects, and hence plays an important role in the processing of visual information. Although shape has been studied by many researchers including mathematicians, engineers, and psychologists, it has no universal definition. Kendall [8.1] defines it as follows: "Shape is all the geometrical information that remains when location, scale, and rotation effects are filtered out from an object." In other words, a shape is invariant to Euclidean similarity transformations of scaling, translation, and rotation. Two objects have the same shape if they can be mapped onto each other by translation, rotation, and scaling.

Shapes can be divided into two categories: static or dynamic. Static shapes are rigid shapes that do not change in time by deformation or articulation, for example a model of a ship. On the other hand, dynamic shapes change in time by deformation or articulation. An MRI image of a human brain can be thought of as static, but the changes in the brain that occur over the course of many years from growth and disease can be thought of as dynamic. The human face is a dynamic shape owing to effects of gestures, talking, and expressions. A fluid mechanics model resembling the state of a weather phenomenon is dynamic – and so on.

8.2.2 How should a shape be described?

Unknown shapes are often described with respect to known shapes. For example, "the map of Italy has the shape of a boot." Such a description is not sufficient at the algorithmic level; proper shape analysis requires flexible methods for shape representation and modeling. Shape representation methods aim at providing simplified representations of the original shape while preserving its main characteristics. The simplified representation may be either numeric, such as a feature vector, or non-numeric, such as a graph.

8.2.3 Criteria for shape representation

The quality of a shape representation method depends on the properties of the object and the application. Consistent evaluation criteria still do not exist for shape representation methods, but good shape representations should possess the requirements in Table 8.1 [8.2–8.7].

8.2.4 Data representation of shape

The data of a 3D shape can be represented at different levels of abstraction. The first level is a set of points in 3D space. The second level is the boundary of the shape. Finally, the third level is the volume that the shape occupies. See Figure 8.1 for an example showing a reconstruction of the human colon from abdominal CT.

Point-based representation
The boundary of the object is described by either a cloud of points as shown in Figure 8.1(a) or range images. Range images are similar to intensity images in the sense that they

8.2 Shape representation

Table 8.1 Requirements of good shape representation methods

Requirement	Description
Scope	It must be able to describe all classes of shapes.
Uniqueness	There must be a one-to-one correspondence between the shape and its representation.
Stability	It must be stable to small changes in the shape, i.e. small changes in the shape must result in small changes in its representation.
Sensitivity	It must be able to capture the fine details of the shape, which might contradict the stability criterion.
Hierarchical	It must describe the shape at multiple scales in a similar fashion to a hierarchical structure (i.e. provide coarse to fine levels of detail).
Accessibility	It must be easy to implement.
Efficiency	It must be computationally efficient.

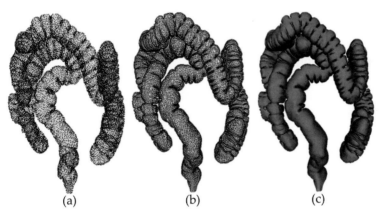

Figure 8.1 Different shape representations of a human colon. (a) Point-based shape representation using cloud of points. (b) Surface-based shape representation using polygonal mesh. (c) Volumetric-based shape representation using grid of voxels (the isosurface (representing points of a constant value) is shown for visualization).

capture the shape from one point of view, except that the color information of the pixel carries the depth information of the surface point from the camera. This representation is generally used in 3D model reconstruction from multiple range images of an object that are acquired using a laser scanner. In general, point-based representation lacks the structure information of a shape but is enough for visualization purposes. Figure 8.1(a) is a recognizable object; as such, point representation still provides recognition of the shape.

Boundary-based representation

A 3D object can be represented in terms of its boundary or surface, which is a common representation in computer-aided design (CAD) and computer graphics. The boundary data can be described by polygonal meshes, as shown in Figure 8.1(b), parametric forms, or implicit (perceived) surfaces. Although local boundary features can be computed efficiently, global shape features such as moments are very difficult to compute. In addition, such methods do not capture the hierarchical structure of the shape, which is an essential requirement for several applications such as object recognition and classification.

Volume-based representation

A 3D shape is represented by the volume it occupies. The volumetric data is described by voxels, as shown in Figure 8.1(c), or solid primitives. A voxel is the minimum 3D unit of a volume. This representation is commonly used in the field of computer vision and medical imaging, owing to the nature of the acquisition process. In constructive solid geometry (CSG), a complex surface or object is composed of simple solid objects, which are glued to each other through Boolean operators on sets such as union, intersection, and difference. Often CSG presents a model or surface that appears visually complex, but is actually little more than cleverly combined or de-combined objects. The simplest solid objects used for the representation are called primitives. Typically they are objects of simple shape: cuboids, cylinders, prisms, pyramids, spheres, and cones.

8.3 Topological equivalence

In topology, we can ignore geometric properties such as lengths and angles since they have already been captured by geometry. Consider two line segments with different lengths: they are said to be topologically equal since we can stretch one of them to turn it into the other. In the same manner, a rectangle has the same topological shape as a square. Keeping all angles equal, we can stretch a square to obtain a rectangle. Moreover, we can straighten one angle to obtain a triangle. As such, as long as there is a continuous deformation between one shape to another without cutting or gluing, we are talking about the same topological shape (see Figure 8.2). Thus topology can be considered as the study of continuity, or "rubber-sheet geometry."

DEFINITION 8.1 *Two objects are topologically identical if there is a continuous deformation (such as bending and stretching) from one to the other.* ∎

An equivalence relation is a relation between objects which plays the role of equality; for example, congruence has the meaning of a geometric equivalence relation between figures.

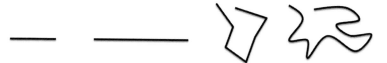

Figure 8.2 Line segments with different lengths are topologically the same shape. If we bend a line segment to obtain the third and fourth shapes, it remains the same topological shape, as long as we have not torn it into parts or glued its ends. Hence we can think of a line segment as a wire which we can shape to give any other form.

8.3 Topological equivalence

DEFINITION 8.2 *An equivalence relation ~ on a set of objects A is a relation on this set such that:*

(1) For each $x \in A$ we have $x \sim x$ (reflexivity).
(2) For $x,y \in A$, if $x \sim y$ then $y \sim x$ (symmetry).
(3) For $x,y,z \in A$, if $x \sim y$ and $y \sim z$, then $x \sim z$ (transitivity). ∎

A geometric equivalence relation has nothing to do with the positioning of the figures; for instance, two congruent triangles can have vertices with different coordinates. Hence congruence only conveys information related to the geometric properties possessed by the figures. Another geometric equivalence relation is similarity, where similar figures have the same angles but proportional sides and areas.

Shapes such as triangles and circles are considered geometrical objects, while topological spaces are the objects of topology.

DEFINITION 8.3 *Let $\mathcal{X}$ be a set and $\mathcal{T}$ a collection of subsets of $\mathcal{X}$. The collection $\mathcal{T}$ is called a topology on $\mathcal{X}$ if:*

(1) The empty set ∅ and $\mathcal{X}$ are in $\mathcal{T}$.
(2) The union of an arbitrary collection of members (sets) of $\mathcal{T}$ is in $\mathcal{T}$.
(3) The intersection of any finite collection of sets in $\mathcal{T}$ is also in $\mathcal{T}$. ∎

The pair $(\mathcal{X}, \mathcal{T})$ is called a topological space.

A topological space might refer to a volume or surface representation of a given class of objects. The equality between objects from the topological viewpoint is formally defined by the topological equivalence relation, which is defined as follows. See Figure 8.3 for illustration.

DEFINITION 8.4 *Let $\mathcal{X}$ and $\mathcal{Y}$ be topological spaces. Then $\mathcal{X}$ is topologically equivalent or homomorphic to $\mathcal{Y}$ if there is a continuous invertible function $f: \mathcal{X} \to \mathcal{Y}$ with continuous inverse $f^{-1}: \mathcal{Y} \to \mathcal{X}$. Such a function f is called a homomorphism.* ∎

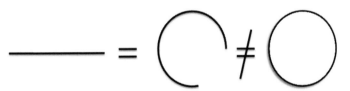

Figure 8.3 A line segment can be bent (deformed) to form a circular arc. Such an operation or function is continuous and has an inverse which involves unbending the arc to form a line segment. However, if we glue together the two end points of the arc, a circle will be formed; this function is not continuous, since we cannot reverse it to form the arc unless we cut the line again. Thus a circular arc is topologically equivalent to a line segment but not topologically equivalent to a circle. You can also view this in reverse: if we cut a circle we will form a circular arc, but this operation is not continuous.

Example 8.1 Let $f(x) = \tan\left(\frac{\pi x}{2}\right)$ which takes the interval $(-1, 1)$ to $(-\infty, \infty)$. This function is continuous and has a continuous inverse $f^{-1}(x) = \frac{2\tan^{-1}x}{\pi}$; thus the interval $(-1,1)$ is topologically equivalent to $(-\infty, \infty) = \mathbf{R}$.

THEOREM 8.1 *Topological equivalence is an equivalence relation.*

Proof Three things must be shown to prove this theorem: reflexivity, symmetry, and transitivity (refer to Definition 8.2); note that we write $A \sim B$ if there is a continuous function $f: A \to B$ with continuous inverse $f^{-1}: B \to A$.

(1) *Reflexivity*: since the identity function $id_A: A \to A$ is continuous and is its own inverse, hence $A \sim A$.
(2) *Symmetry*: since $f^{-1}: B \to A$ is continuous and has continuous inverse $f: A \to B$ then $A \sim B$ implies $B \sim A$.
(3) *Transitivity*: Assume $A \sim B$, i.e. there is a continuous function $f: A \to B$ with continuous inverse $f^{-1}: B \to A$ and $B \sim C$, i.e. there is a continuous function $g: B \to C$ with continuous inverse $g^{-1}: C \to B$. Then the compositions $g \circ f: A \to C$ and $f^{-1} \circ g^{-1}: C \to A$ are continuous, where $\circ$ is the function composition operator (i.e. $g \circ f(.) = g(f(.))$).

Note: We can easily show that these properties hold:

(i) $(f^{-1} \circ g^{-1}) \circ (g \circ f) = f^{-1} \circ (g^{-1} \circ g) \circ f = f^{-1} \circ id_B \circ f = f^{-1} \circ f = id_A$,
(ii) $(g \circ f) \circ (f^{-1} \circ g^{-1}) = gX \circ X(f \circ f^{-1}) \circ g^{-1} = g \circ id_B \circ g^{-1} = g \circ g^{-1} = id_C$.

Hence, $g \circ f$ and $f^{-1} \circ g^{-1}$ are inverses, and thus $g \circ f$ is a homeomorphism from A to C, so $A \sim C$.

This theorem implies that one can use topological equivalence as equality, i.e. topologically equivalent spaces have the same topological shapes.

8.4 Vector spaces

Points – the basic building blocks of Euclidean space – are considered the key ingredient of representing surfaces. In this section we present the notion of points and vectors along with some basic definitions for their manipulation.

Consider point sets which are subsets of the real Euclidean n-space, which is defined as follows.

DEFINITION 8.5 *The real Euclidean n-space is given by* $\mathbf{R}^n = \{\mathbf{x} = (x_1, x_2, \ldots, x_n) \mid x_i \in \mathbf{R}\}$ *where* $\mathbf{x}$ *denotes a point with n coordinates.* ∎

The set $\mathbf{R}^n$ is said to form a vector space since it is closed under addition and scalar multiplication. Moreover, it satisfies the commutative and associative properties, while the zero vector is considered the additive identity of this set.

Here we consider vectors as column vectors. Thus $\mathbf{x}^T$ denotes a row vector where T denotes the transpose. Let $\mathbf{x} = (x_1, x_2, \ldots, x_n)^T$ and $\mathbf{y} = (y_1, y_2, \ldots, y_n)^T$, as such we have the following properties:

1. The scalar product in $\mathbf{R}^n$ is defined as:

$$\langle \mathbf{x}, \mathbf{y} \rangle = \mathbf{x}.\mathbf{y} = \mathbf{x}^T \mathbf{y} = \sum_{i=1}^{n} x_i y_i \tag{8.1}$$

2. Two vectors are said to be perpendicular/normal to each other if $\langle \mathbf{x}, \mathbf{y} \rangle = \mathbf{0}$, e.g. $\mathbf{x} = [1\ 1\ -1]^T$ and $\mathbf{y} = [-1\ 0\ -1]^T$ are perpendicular.

3. The *Euclidean norm* can be defined as:

$$\|\mathbf{x}\| = \sqrt{\langle \mathbf{x}, \mathbf{x} \rangle} = \sqrt{\sum_{i=1}^{n} x_i^2} \tag{8.2}$$

Hence a vector $\mathbf{x}$ is said to be normalized if $\|\mathbf{x}\| = 1$.

4. The Euclidean distance between the vectors $\mathbf{x}$ and $\mathbf{y}$ is then given by:

$$\|\mathbf{x} - \mathbf{y}\| = \sqrt{\langle \mathbf{x} - \mathbf{y}, \mathbf{x} - \mathbf{y} \rangle} = \sqrt{\sum_{i=1}^{n} (x_i - y_i)^2}$$

$$= \sqrt{(x_1 - y_1)^2 + (x_2 - y_2)^2 + \ldots + (x_n - y_n)^2} \tag{8.3}$$

5. The addition of the vectors is given by; $\mathbf{x} + \mathbf{y} = (x_1 + y_1, x_2 + y_2, \ldots, x_n + y_n)^T$.

6. The scalar multiplication the vector $\mathbf{x}$ with a scalar $\alpha \in \mathbf{R}$ is given by $\alpha \mathbf{x} = (\alpha x_1, \alpha x_2, \ldots, \alpha x_n)^T$.

7. The vector multiplication between the vectors $\mathbf{x}$ and $\mathbf{y}$ is defined by

$$\mathbf{x}\mathbf{y}^T = \begin{pmatrix} x_1 \\ x_2 \\ \vdots \\ x_n \end{pmatrix} (y_1\ y_2\ \ldots\ y_n) = \begin{pmatrix} x_1 y_1 & x_1 y_2 & \ldots & x_1 y_n \\ x_2 y_1 & x_2 y_2 & \ldots & x_2 y_n \\ \vdots & \vdots & \ddots & \vdots \\ x_n y_1 & x_n y_2 & \ldots & x_n y_n \end{pmatrix} \tag{8.4}$$

8. The cross product is a binary operation on two vectors in a three-dimensional Euclidean space $\mathbf{R}^3$ that results in another vector which is perpendicular to the plane containing the two input vectors (i.e. is perpendicular to the plane spanned by the two input vectors). It is defined as:

$$\mathbf{x} \times \mathbf{y} = \begin{pmatrix} x_2 y_3 - x_3 y_2 \\ x_3 y_1 - x_1 y_3 \\ x_1 y_2 - x_2 y_1 \end{pmatrix} \tag{8.5}$$

with the following properties:
(a) $\mathbf{x} \times (\mathbf{y} + \mathbf{z}) = \mathbf{x} \times \mathbf{y} + \mathbf{x} \times \mathbf{z}$
(b) $\mathbf{x} \times \mathbf{y} = -\mathbf{y} \times \mathbf{x}$

(c) $\mathbf{x} \times (\mathbf{y} \times \mathbf{z}) + \mathbf{z} \times (\mathbf{x} \times \mathbf{y}) + \mathbf{y} \times (\mathbf{z} \times \mathbf{x}) = 0$ (*Jacobi identity*)
(d) $\mathbf{x} \times (\mathbf{y} \times \mathbf{z}) = (\mathbf{x}.\mathbf{z})\mathbf{y} - (\mathbf{x}.\mathbf{y})\mathbf{z}$ (*vector identity*). ∎

Vectors are directional quantities with magnitude and direction. On the other hand, points represent locations in Cartesian space. While points can be represented as vectors containing the direction and distance from the Cartesian plane origin, the main difference is that points can be moved whereas vectors cannot. For instance, a vector indicating a surface normal is unchanged regardless of the location of the surface point in the Cartesian plane as long as the surface orientation remains constant. In order to differentiate between points and vectors, the homogeneous coordinate system is usually used to embed the vector space $\mathbf{R}^3$ in the vector space $\mathbf{R}^4$, also referred to as *Grassmann* space. This form is beneficial when we define transforms.

DEFINITION 8.6 *Let $x, y, z, w \in \mathbf{R}$ where $w \neq 0$, $(x, y, z, w)^T \in \mathbf{R}^4$ is a homogeneous coordinate representation of the point $\left(\frac{x}{w}, \frac{y}{w}, \frac{z}{w}\right)^T \in \mathbf{R}^3$. A point at infinity is represented by $(x, y, z, 0)^T$* ∎

8.5 Surfaces in parameter space

Parametric representation is the most general approach to specify a surface that can be expressed as a smooth function. In many applications, shape acquisition is limited to a finite number of sampling points and we wish to construct a function which closely fits these points. Surface fitting is useful in these situations. This helps in constructing new points between the known points, i.e. *interpolation*.

We start with concepts of curve parameterization and interpolation, which lends itself directly to surfaces in 3D space. The simplest curve is a line segment which can be defined by its two end points, $\mathbf{x}_0 = (x_0, y_0)$ and $\mathbf{x}_1 = (x_1, y_1)$. There are many ways to define the equation of a line segment. One way is to parameterize the line as follows: imagine that this line represents a road that start at $\mathbf{x}_0$ and ends at $\mathbf{x}_1$, and you need to walk along this road from $\mathbf{x}_0$ to $\mathbf{x}_1$. Let $\mathbf{x}(0) = \mathbf{x}_0$ (i.e. initial location is $\mathbf{x}_0$) and the final location is $\mathbf{x}(1) = \mathbf{x}_1$. Let $t \in [0,1]$ denote the normalized percentage of distance covered between $\mathbf{x}_0$ and $\mathbf{x}_1$, your current position will be defined as follows:

$$\mathbf{x}(t) = \mathbf{x}_0 + t(\mathbf{x}_1 - \mathbf{x}_0) = \mathbf{x}_0 + t\mathbf{x}_1 - t\mathbf{x}_0 = (1-t)\mathbf{x}_0 + t\mathbf{x}_1 \qquad (8.6)$$

Hence, what we have done is to represent any point on the line connecting $\mathbf{x}_0$ and $\mathbf{x}_1$ by a *weighted average* of the two end points. This average is parameterized by one parameter, t. We can re-write (8.6) as:

$$\mathbf{x}(t) = f_0(t)\mathbf{x}_0 + f_1(t)\mathbf{x}_1 \qquad (8.7)$$

where $f_0(t) = 1-t$ and $f_1(t) = t$. Since we are representing a line, the degree of $f_k(t)$ for $k = 0, 1$ is one (i.e. a linear function); hence we only need two points to represent a line segment.

This can be thought of as representing a line segment with *control points* $\mathbf{x}_0$ and $\mathbf{x}_1$ being interpolated with *basis functions* $f_k(t)$. This equation is usually referred to as the *parametric equation of a line*. Let us now generalize this notion to curves and later to surfaces, where curves are represented by non-linear basis functions, and hence we need more control points.

8.5.1 Parametric curves

A curve in R^3 is called a *space curve*, which can be thought of as the intersection of two surfaces. It can be expressed in a parametric form according to the following definition.

DEFINITION 8.7 *Parametric curves are curves defined in the standard 3D Euclidean space R^3 in terms of some parameter, say t. The curve can then be written as: $x(t) = (x(t), y(t), z(t))^T$ where $x(t)$, $y(t)$ and $z(t)$ are continuous functions defined on some interval $t \in [a,b]$ where each value of t defines a point on the curve. The curve is defined to be the set of all such points. In most cases, it is assumed that $x(t)$ can be differentiated at least twice.*

Similar to the parametric form of a line segment, a curve can be expressed in terms of control points and basis functions as in Definition 8.8.

DEFINITION 8.8 *Let $\{x_0, x_1, \ldots, x_n\}$ be a set of points in d-dimensional Euclidean space. A curve can be defined in terms of these points as:*

$$C: \mathbf{x}(t) = f_0(t)\mathbf{x}_0 + f_1(t)\mathbf{x}_1 + \ldots + f_n(t)\mathbf{x}_n = \sum_{k=0}^{n} f_k(t)\mathbf{x}_k \qquad (8.8)$$

*where $f_k(t)$ are continuous functions defined on the interval $t \in [0,1]$. The points $x_0, x_1, \ldots, x_n$ are called **control points** and $f_k(t)$ are called the **basis functions** of the curve C.* ∎

Bézier curves are one of the most popular representations for curves. They can be defined as follows.

DEFINITION 8.9 *Let $x_0, x_1, x_2, \ldots, x_n$ be a set of control points. A **Bézier curve** of degree n is given by:*

$$\mathbf{x}(t) = \sum_{k=0}^{n} B_k^n(t)\mathbf{x}_k \quad t \in [0, 1] \qquad (8.9)$$

where the basis functions $B_k^n(t)$ are the Bernstein polynomials defined by:

$$B_k^n(t) = \binom{n}{k} t^k (1-t)^{n-k} \qquad (8.10)$$

where $\binom{n}{k} = \dfrac{n!}{k!(n-k)!}.$

Bézier curves interpolate their end points; that is, the curve connects the end points in a fashion directed by in-between control points that do not lie on the curve. This is called the end-point interpolation property.

Example 8.2 The most popular Bézier curves are Bézier curves of degree 3. Let the control points be given as: $\mathbf{x}_0 = (1,1)^T$, $\mathbf{x}_1 = (2,3)^T$, $\mathbf{x}_2 = (4,-1)^T$ and $\mathbf{x}_3 = (4.6, 1.5)^T$.

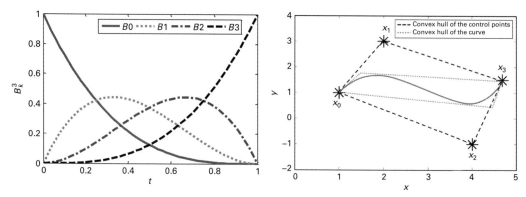

Figure 8.4 Left: Basis functions for Bézier curves of degree 3. Right: Bézier curve of four points, and its convex hull (the smallest continuous surface that encloses the control points).

Now let us define the Bernstein polynomials, i.e. Bézier basis functions with $n = 3$ and $k = 0,1,2,3$.

$$B_0^3(t) = \binom{3}{0} t^0 (1-t)^{3-0} = \frac{3!}{0!(3-0)!}(1-t)^3 = (1-t)^3 = 1 - 3t + 3t^2 - t^3$$

$$B_1^3(t) = \binom{3}{1} t^1 (1-t)^{3-1} = \frac{3!}{1!(3-1)!}t(1-t)^2 = 3t(1-t)^2 = 3t - 6t^2 + 3t^3$$

$$B_2^3(t) = \binom{3}{2} t^2 (1-t)^{3-2} = \frac{3!}{2!(3-2)!}t^2(1-t) = 3t^2(1-t) = 3t^2 - 3t^3$$

$$B_3^3(t) = \binom{3}{3} t^3 (1-t)^{3-3} = \frac{3!}{3!(3-3)!}t^3 = t^3$$

The curve is then defined by (see Figure 8.4):

$$\mathcal{C}: \quad \mathbf{x}(t) = B_0^3(t)\mathbf{x}_0 + B_1^3(t)\mathbf{x}_1 + B_2^3(t)\mathbf{x}_2 + B_3^3(t)\mathbf{x}_3$$
$$= (1 - 3t + 3t^2 - t^3)\mathbf{x}_0 + (3t - 6t^2 + 3t^3)\mathbf{x}_1 + (3t^2 - 3t^3)\mathbf{x}_2 + t^3\mathbf{x}_3$$

For an arbitrary degree n, a Bézier curve can be written as a polynomial (explicit function in the parameter t) instead of a sum of Bernstein polynomials. Binomial theorem can be applied to the definition of the curve followed by rearrangement to yield:

$$\mathbf{x}(t) = \sum_{j=0}^{n} c_j t^j \qquad t \in [0,1] \qquad (8.11)$$

where the coefficients for the expansion of Bernstein polynomials into powers of t are given as follows:

$$c_j = \frac{M!}{(M-j)!} \sum_{i=0}^{j} \frac{(-1)^i \mathbf{x}_{j-i}}{i!(j-i)!} \qquad (8.12)$$

8.5 Surfaces in parameter space

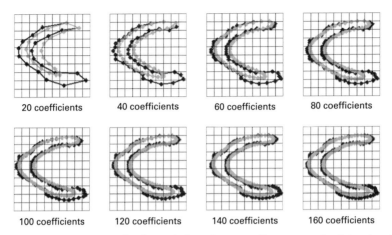

Figure 8.5 Bézier curve reconstruction/interpolation of corpus callosum control points using different numbers of coefficients. The original control curve is shown in dark gray and the reconstruction curve is shown in light gray. The reconstructed points are obtained by sampling the parameter $t \in [0,1]$ at different resolutions; note that the reconstructed curves remain within the convex hull of the control points.

Figure 8.5 illustrates fitting Bézier polynomials to the corpus callosum, using an increasing number of coefficients.

From the implementation viewpoint, a recursive definition of Bézier curves is usually used.

DEFINITION 8.10 A *Bézier curve of degree* n *can be expressed recursively as follows. Let* $\mathbf{x}_{\mathbf{x}_0 \mathbf{x}_1 \ldots \mathbf{x}_n}(t)$ *denote the Bézier curve denoted by the control points* $\mathbf{x}_0, \mathbf{x}_1, \mathbf{x}_2, \ldots, \mathbf{x}_n$, *then:*

$$\mathbf{x}(t) = \mathbf{x}_{\mathbf{x}_0 \mathbf{x}_1 \ldots \mathbf{x}_n}(t) = (1-t)\mathbf{x}_{\mathbf{x}_0 \mathbf{x}_1 \ldots \mathbf{x}_{n-1}}(t) + t\mathbf{x}_{\mathbf{x}_1, \mathbf{x}_2 \ldots, \mathbf{x}_n}(t) \qquad (8.13)$$

Hence, the Bézier curve of degree n is a linear interpolation between two Bézier curves of degree $n-1$. ∎

8.5.2 Parametric surfaces

DEFINITION 8.11 *Consider a set of points, usually in* $\mathbf{R}^3$, *representing a surface. If the surface can be described by a smooth function* $\mathbf{f}$ *such that* $\mathbf{f}(u,v) = [x(u,v)\, y(u,v)\, z(u,v)]^T$, *where* $u, v \in \mathbf{R}$, *we call the surface a parametric surface where x, y, z are differentiable functions in u and v.* ∎

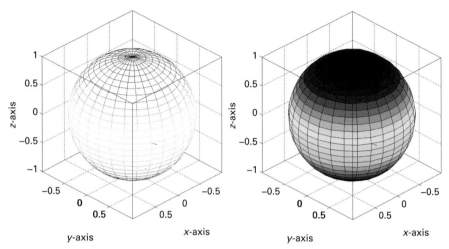

Figure 8.6 The surface defined by the parametric equations of a sphere. Left: polygonal mesh. Right: surface patches being filled.

Example 8.3 Examples of parametric surfaces:
(1) Sphere (Figure 8.6)

$$\mathbf{f}(u, v) = \begin{pmatrix} \sin u \cos v \\ \sin u \sin v \\ \cos u \end{pmatrix} \qquad (8.14)$$

with $0 \leq u \leq \pi$ and $0 \leq v \leq 2\pi$.
(2) Seashell (Figure 8.7)
A parametric seashell surface is such that

$$\mathbf{f}(u, v) = \begin{pmatrix} 2(1 - e^{u/12\pi})\cos u \cos^2\left(\frac{v}{2}\right) \\ 2(-1 + e^{u/12\pi})\sin u \cos^2\left(\frac{v}{2}\right) \\ 1 - e^{u/6\pi} + (-1 + e^{u/12\pi})\sin v \end{pmatrix} \qquad (8.15)$$

with $0 \leq u \leq 12\pi$ and $0 \leq v \leq 2\pi$.

A widely used form of parametric surfaces uses the tensor product of parametric curves to define *tensor product surfaces*. Figure 8.8 is an illustration of surface patches (small regions) defined as the tensor product of parametric curves.

DEFINITION 8.12 *Consider a set of m-parametric curves* $\{\mathbf{x}_j(v)\}$ *each with control points* $\{\mathbf{x}_{j,k}\}$ *defined in terms of basis functions* $f_k^n(v)$ *such that:*

8.5 Surfaces in parameter space

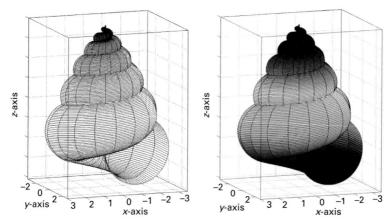

Figure 8.7 The surface defined by the parametric equations of a seashell. Left: polygonal mesh. Right: surface patches being filled.

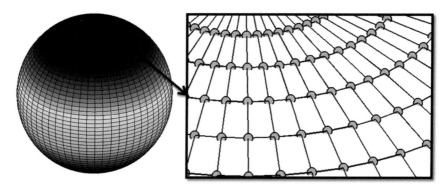

Figure 8.8 Illustration of surface patches defined as the tensor product of parametric curves.

$$\mathbf{x}_j(v) = \sum_{k=1}^{n} f_k^n(v)\mathbf{x}_{j,k} \qquad (8.16)$$

If we choose a particular value for v on each of these curves, then we end up with m points which can be used to construct another curve $\mathbf{x}$. The curve $\mathbf{x}$ is then defined by:

$$\mathcal{S}: \quad \mathbf{x}(u,v) = \sum_{j=1}^{m} f_j^m(u)\mathbf{x}_j(v) = \Sigma_{j=1}^{m} \Sigma_{k=1}^{n} f_j^m(u) f_k^n(v) \mathbf{x}_{j,k} \qquad (8.17)$$

All these curves construct a surface known as a tensor product surface, and the curve of constant v is known as an isocurve. ∎

When defining the basis functions to be Bernstein polynomials, we define what is called a tensor product Bézier surface or *Bézier patch* which is given by:

$$\mathbf{x}(u,v) = \Sigma_{j=0}^{m}\Sigma_{k=0}^{n} B_j^m(u) B_k^n(v)\mathbf{x}_{j,k} \qquad (8.18)$$

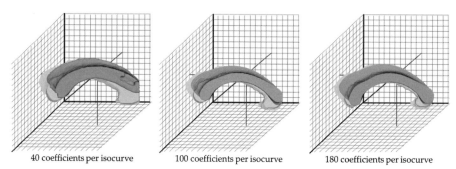

| 40 coefficients per isocurve | 100 coefficients per isocurve | 180 coefficients per isocurve |

Figure 8.9 Bézier surface reconstruction/interpolation of corpus callosum control points using different numbers of coefficients per isocurve for total 10 isocurves. The original control surface is shown in dark gray while the Bézier surface is shown in light gray. Note that using more coefficients makes the Bézier surface approach the original one.

Similar to Bézier curves, the coefficients of the Bezier surface defined by the given control points are given by:

$$\mathbf{x}(u, v) = \sum_{j=0}^{M} \sum_{k=0}^{N} c_{j,k} u^j v^k \qquad u, v \in [0, 1] \qquad (8.19)$$

Using the binomial theorem and the definition of Bernstein polynomials, the coefficients can be given by:

$$c_{\alpha,\beta} = \frac{n!}{(n-\alpha)!} \frac{m!}{(m-\beta)!} \left(\sum_{k=0}^{\alpha} \sum_{l=0}^{\beta} \frac{(-1)^k (-1)^l \mathbf{x}_{(\alpha-k),(\beta-l)}}{k! l! (\alpha-k)! (\beta-l)!} \right) \qquad (8.20)$$

Example 8.4 Representation of the corpus callosum.
The corpus callosum segmented from MRI images of the human brain has a distinctive "banana" shape. Bézier curves may be used to represent the corpus callosum at the contour, surface, or volume levels. Figure 8.9 illustrates Bézier surface reconstruction/interpolation of corpus callosum control points using different numbers of coefficients per isocurve, for a total of 10 isocurves. The original control surface is shown in light gray while the Bézier surface is shown in dark gray. It can be observed that using more coefficients makes the Bézier surface approach the original surface.

8.5.3 Surface curvature

Intuitively, curvature is a measure of how a surface deviates from being flat; that is, it represents local bending of the surface. It can be used to determine how quickly the surface normal changes its direction along the surface points, i.e. the rate of curving. Consider a parametric surface $\mathbf{x}(u,v) = [x(u,v)\ y(u,v)\ z(u,v)]^T$ in 3D space. Two planar

8.5 Surfaces in parameter space

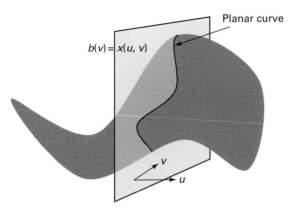

Figure 8.10   Planar curves defined on a surface.

curves are of particular interest, namely $\mathbf{a}(u) = \mathbf{x}(u,v)$ with v constant and $\mathbf{b}(v) = \mathbf{x}(u,v)$ with u constant. See Figure 8.10 for illustration. These curves help us in defining surface local geometries such as principal curvatures.

Let us denote the partial derivatives of $\mathbf{x}$ in terms of u and v as follows:

$$\mathbf{x}_u \equiv \frac{\partial \mathbf{x}(u,v)}{\partial u} \quad , \quad \mathbf{x}_v \equiv \frac{\partial \mathbf{x}(u,v)}{\partial v}$$

$$\mathbf{x}_{uu} \equiv \frac{\partial^2 \mathbf{x}(u,v)}{\partial u^2} \quad , \quad \mathbf{x}_{vv} \equiv \frac{\partial^2 \mathbf{x}(u,v)}{\partial v^2} \quad (8.21)$$

$$\mathbf{x}_{uv} \equiv \frac{\partial^2 \mathbf{x}(u,v)}{\partial u \partial v}$$

DEFINITION 8.13 *The normal to the surface is given by:*

$$\mathbf{n}(u,v) = \frac{\mathbf{x}_u \times \mathbf{x}_v}{\|\mathbf{x}_u \times \mathbf{x}_v\|} \quad (8.22)$$

where $\times$ denotes the cross/vector product and $\|.\|$ denotes the vector norm. ∎

Figure 8.11 shows the normal vectors to the surface of a sphere and a seashell.

DEFINITION 8.14 *The first fundamental forms of the surface are given by:*

$$E \equiv \mathbf{x}_u \cdot \mathbf{x}_u \; , \; F \equiv \mathbf{x}_u \cdot \mathbf{x}_v \; , \; G \equiv \mathbf{x}_v \cdot \mathbf{x}_v \quad (8.23)$$

where $\cdot$ denotes the dot/scalar product. This can be written in matrix form as:

$$\mathbf{I} = \begin{bmatrix} E & F \\ F & G \end{bmatrix} = \begin{bmatrix} \mathbf{x}_u^T \mathbf{x}_u & \mathbf{x}_u^T \mathbf{x}_v \\ \mathbf{x}_u^T \mathbf{x}_v & \mathbf{x}_v^T \mathbf{x}_v \end{bmatrix} \quad (8.24)$$

which defines an inner product on the tangent space of the surface. ∎

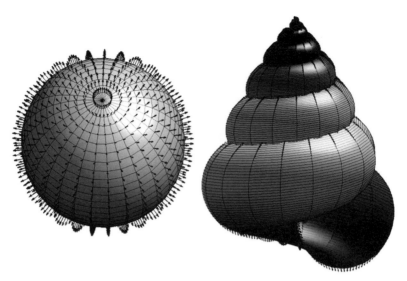

Figure 8.11 Surface normals computed using the parametric form of a sphere (left) and a seashell (right).

DEFINITION 8.15 *The second fundamental forms of the surface are given by:*

$$e \equiv \mathbf{x}_{uu} \cdot \mathbf{n}(u,v) \;,\; f \equiv \mathbf{x}_{uv} \cdot \mathbf{n}(u,v) \;,\; g \equiv \mathbf{x}_{vv} \cdot \mathbf{n}(u,v) \qquad (8.25)$$

where · denotes the dot/scalar product. ∎

We can easily show that the above equation can be written in matrix form as:

$$\mathbf{II} = \begin{bmatrix} e & f \\ f & g \end{bmatrix} = \begin{bmatrix} \mathbf{x}_{uu}^T \mathbf{n} & \mathbf{x}_{uv}^T \mathbf{n} \\ \mathbf{x}_{uv}^T \mathbf{n} & \mathbf{x}_{vv}^T \mathbf{n} \end{bmatrix} \qquad (8.26)$$

DEFINITION 8.16 *The principal curvatures of the surface are given by:*

$$\begin{aligned} \kappa_1(u,v) &\equiv H(u,v) + \sqrt{H^2(u,v) - K(u,v)} \\ \kappa_2(u,v) &\equiv H(u,v) - \sqrt{H^2(u,v) - K(u,v)} \end{aligned} \qquad (8.27)$$

where K(u,v) and H(u,v) are the Gaussian and mean curvatures, respectively, defined as:

$$K(u,v) \equiv \frac{eg - f^2}{EG - F^2} \;,\; H(u,v) = \frac{Eg - 2Ff + Ge}{2(EG - F^2)} \qquad (8.28)$$

Using the principal curvatures, other local geometric features can be derived. For instance, the shape index SI and the curvedness CV are given by [8.8],

$$\text{SI}(u,v) \equiv \frac{1}{2} - \frac{1}{\pi} \arctan \frac{\kappa_1(u,v) + \kappa_2(u,v)}{\kappa_1(u,v) - \kappa_2(u,v)} \qquad (8.29)$$

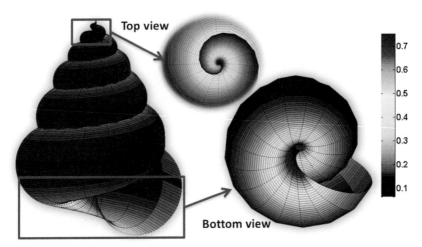

Figure 8.12 Shape index computed using the parametric form of the seashell.

$$\mathrm{CV}(u,v) \equiv \sqrt{\frac{\kappa_1^2(u,v) + \kappa_2^2(u,v)}{2}} \tag{8.30}$$

where $\kappa_1(u,v) \neq \kappa_2(u,v)$. The curvedness represents the magnitude of curvature while the shape index is considered a measure of shape, such that every distinct shape corresponds to a unique shape index value. There are five well-known shape classes, with the following SI values: cup (0.0), rut (0.25), saddle (0.5), ridge (0.75) and cap (1.0).

Figure 8.12 is a shape index, computed using the parametric form of the seashell.

8.6 Surfaces as meshes

A point set can be used to represent most geometric objects by either describing points on the object's surface or being used as control points for parametric surfaces. In order to incorporate the structure information of the underlying shape, polygonal meshes are often used. These describe a set of polygons constructed for the point set. While the position information is stored in the point set, the connectivity information is maintained in a set of faces whose elements encode a set of edges.

8.6.1 Manifolds and surfaces

DEFINITION 8.17 *An* n-*dimensional manifold is a topological space such that the neighborhood of every point is topologically equivalent to an* n-*dimensional open disc* $D^n(\mathbf{x}, r) = \{\mathbf{y} \in \mathbf{R}^n : ||\mathbf{x} - \mathbf{y}|| < r\}$ *with center* $\mathbf{x}$ *and radius* r, *while any two distinct points have disjoint neighborhoods. A 2-manifold is often called a surface.* ∎

An n-manifold is locally n-dimensional. If one imagines oneself as a very small bug living on a 2-manifold, one would not feel the difference between the manifold and the plane.

In a discrete form, a surface (2D manifold) can be represented by a polygonal mesh constructed from a set of vertices embedded in 3D space, where their connectivity information is encoded in the edges and faces connecting them. A formal definition of a polygon can be given as follows.

DEFINITION 8.18 *Let $\mathbf{x}_0, \mathbf{x}_1, \ldots, \mathbf{x}_{n-1}$ be a set of n points in the plane $\mathbf{R}^2$ or embedded in the $\mathbf{R}^3$ space. Here all index arithmetic will be mod n, implying a cyclic ordering of the points, with v_0 following $\mathbf{x}_{n-1}$ since $(n-1)+1 \equiv n \equiv 0 \pmod{n}$.* ∎

Let $e_0 = \mathbf{x}_0\mathbf{x}_1$, $e_1 = \mathbf{x}_1\mathbf{x}_2, \ldots, e_{n-1} = \mathbf{x}_{n-1}\mathbf{x}_0$ be n segments connecting the points. Then these segments bound a polygon (simple closed curve) if and only if:

(1) The intersection of each pair of adjacent segments in the cyclic ordering is the single point shared between them, i.e. $e_i \cap e_{i+1} = \mathbf{x}_{i+1}$, for all $i = 0, 1, 2, \ldots, n-1$.
(2) Nonadjacent segments do not intersect, i.e. $e_i \cap e_j = \phi$, for $j \neq i+1$.

The reason these segments define a curve is that they are connected end to end; the reason the curve is closed is that they form a cycle; the reason the closed curve is simple is that nonadjacent segments do not intersect.

The points $\mathbf{x}_i$ are called vertices of the polygon, and the segments e_i are called its edges. Note that a polygon with n vertices has n edges. A triangle is a special case with $n = 3$. Figure 8.13 is an example of a polyhedral surface.

While 3D modeling programs usually represent a surface as arbitrary polygons, most graphics cards provide hardware for drawing triangles. Thus triangular meshes are usually used for surface representation.

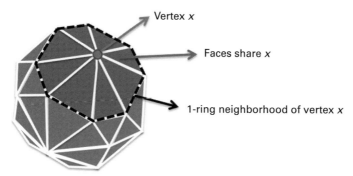

Figure 8.13 An example of a valid polyhedral surface, where the link of a vertex x is defined to be the collection of edges opposite to x in all the triangles incident to x. Thus the link is in a sense the combinatorial neighborhood of x. For a legal triangulated polyhedron, we require that the link of every vertex be a simple, closed polygonal path.

8.6 Surfaces as meshes

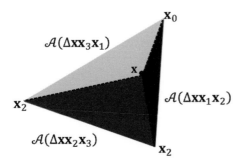

Figure 8.14 Barycentric weights are determined according to the ratio of the smaller triangle formed between the point x and one side, as shown, to the area of the whole triangle.

DEFINITION 8.19 *Let $M = (\mathcal{G}, \mathcal{P})$ be a 2-manifold triangular mesh: $\mathcal{G} = (\mathcal{V}, \mathcal{E}, \mathcal{F})$ is a graph where $\mathcal{V}, \mathcal{E}$ and $\mathcal{F}$ define the vertices, edges, and faces of the mesh respectively; $\mathcal{P}$ is the geometry associated with each vertex in $\mathcal{V}$, where $\mathcal{V} = \{x_0, , x_1, \ldots, x_{n-1}\}$ is a set of n vertices; $\mathcal{F} = \{t_1, t_2, \ldots, t_{n'}\}$ is a set of n' triangular faces, where $t_k = \{x_{k_0}, x_{k_1}, x_{k_2}\}$ is constructed from three vertices with indices k_0, k_1, and k_2. $t_k = \{x_{k_0}, x_{k_1}, x_{k_2}\}$*

8.6.2 Barycentric coordinates

In the barycentric coordinates system, the location of a point inside a triangle is expressed in terms of a weighted combination of the triangle's vertices. Figure 8.14 illustrates the concept: the weights are determined by taking the area of the smaller triangle formed between this point and two corresponding triangle vertices, and calculating the ratio of this area to that of the whole triangle.

DEFINITION 8.20 *Let $t = (x_0, x_1, x_2)$ define a triangle whose vertices are x_0, x_1, and x_2, with $x_i = (x_i, y_i, z_i)^T$. Then the **area** of t can be given by:*

$$A(t) = A(\Delta x_0 x_1 x_2) = \frac{1}{2}|(x_1 - x_0) \times (x_2 - x_0)| \qquad (8.31)$$

where $\times$ is the cross product of two vectors, and $|.|$ denotes the determinant. ∎

DEFINITION 8.21 *Let $t = (x_0, x_1, x_2)$ define a triangle whose vertices are x_0, x_1, and x_2, with $x_i = (x_i, y_i, z_i)^T$. An arbitrary point $x \in t$ can be written as:*

$$v = \alpha x_0 + \beta x_1 + (1 - \alpha - \beta) x_2 \qquad (8.32)$$

where $\alpha = \frac{A(\Delta x x_1 x_2)}{A(\Delta x_0 x_1 x_2)}$ and $\beta = \frac{A(\Delta x x_2 x_0)}{A(\Delta x_0 x_1 x_2)}$ such that $A(abc)$ is the area of the triangle with vertices a, b and c. ∎

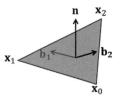

Figure 8.15 Triangle local frame.

8.6.3 Triangle local frame

Although the vertices are embedded in 3D space, the points belonging to a triangle or face constructed by three vertices can be expressed in the 2D domain in terms of the triangle's local frame (coordinate system). Such a frame is formed by a right-hand orthonormal basis which is given by the normal **n** to the triangle, a unit vector parallel to one of its edges b_1 and another unit vector which is orthogonal to both the normal and b_1. See Figure 8.15 for illustration.

DEFINITION 8.22 *Let $t = (x_0, x_1, x_2)$ define a triangle whose vertices are x_0, x_1 and x_2, with $x_i = (x_i, y_i, z_i)^T$. Then the **local frame** (orthonormal basis), also known as the Frenet frame of t, can be defined as the triplet (b_1, b_2, n), forming a right-hand orthonormal basis given by:*

$$n = \frac{(x_1 - x_0) \times (x_2 - x_0)}{\|(x_1 - x_0) \times (x_2 - x_0)\|} \tag{8.33}$$

$$b_1 = \frac{x_1 - x_0}{\|x_1 - x_0\|} \tag{8.34}$$

$$b_2 = \frac{n \times b_1}{\|n \times b_1\|} \tag{8.35}$$

where $\|\cdot\|$ denotes the Euclidean norm, $\times$ is the cross product of two vectors, **n** is the normal vector of the triangle t, b_1 is a unit vector parallel to the edge connecting x_0 and x_1, and b_2 is a unit vector orthogonal to both **n** and b_1. ∎

The vertices of the triangle can now be expressed in terms of this local frame as:

$$x_i' = \mathcal{H}^{-1} x_i \tag{8.36}$$

where $\mathcal{H} = [b_1 | b_2 | n]$ is a square matrix defined in the local frame of the triangle. The three vertices will share the same third component since they are coplanar.

8.6.4 Surface curvature: discrete form

To represent parametric surfaces by curvatures, the surface must be sufficiently differentiable; at the least, the existence of the second derivatives should be guaranteed. In the case of a surface represented by a cloud of points (as in Figure 8.1(a)), where there is no smooth function defining the surface's parametric form, triangular meshes are often considered useful. Yet these meshes are piecewise linear, so it may not be possible to apply the operators of continuous differential geometry in a straightforward manner. Instead, these differential attributes of the underlying surface should be approximated from the mesh vertices. We will follow the notions of Meyer et al. [8.9]. We start by defining the notions of vertex neighborhood from which local geometric attributes can be estimated.

DEFINITION 8.23 *The 1-ring neighborhood faces $\mathcal{F}_x$ of a vertex x on a surface is the list of faces having x as one of their vertices. Hence it can be defined as:*

$$\mathcal{F}_x = \{t = (x_0, x_1, x_2) \subset \mathcal{F} : x \in \{x_0, x_1, x_2\}\} \quad (8.37)$$

DEFINITION 8.24 *The 1-ring neighborhood vertices $\mathcal{V}_x$ of a vertex x on a surface is the list of vertices which are connected to x by an edge. Hence it can be defined as:*

$$\mathcal{V}_x = \{x_i \subset \mathcal{V} : e = xx_i \in \mathcal{E}\} \quad (8.38)$$

DEFINITION 8.25 *The region of influence R_x of a surface point x represents a local part of the surface in the vicinity of x.* ∎

DEFINITION 8.26 *The area $\mathcal{A}_{vor}(t)$ of the Voronoi region of a non-obtuse triangle $t = (x_0, x_1, x_2)$ can be computed as:*

$$\mathcal{A}_{vor}(t) = \frac{1}{8}(\|x_2 - x_0\|\cot\angle x_1 + \|x_1 - x_0\|\cot\angle x_2) \quad (8.39)$$

where $\angle x_i$ is the angle at vertex x_i. ∎

Computation of area of region of influence $\mathcal{A}(\mathcal{R}_x)$

- Initialize $\mathcal{A}(\mathcal{R}_x) = 0$
- For each $t \in \mathcal{F}_x$:
  - If t is a non-obtuse triangle: $\mathcal{A}(\mathcal{R}_x) = \mathcal{A}_{vor}(t)$
  - Else
    - If the angle of t at x is obtuse: $\mathcal{A}(\mathcal{R}_x) = \mathcal{A}(t)/2$
    - Else $\mathcal{A}(\mathcal{R}_x) = \mathcal{A}(t)/4$

DEFINITION 8.27 *The discrete Gaussian curvature can be expressed as:*

$$K(x) = \frac{2\pi - \sum_{t \in \mathcal{F}_x} \theta_x(t)}{\mathcal{A}(\mathcal{R}_x)} \quad (8.40)$$

where $\theta_x(t)$ is the angle of the face t at the vertex x. ∎

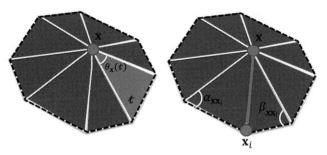

Figure 8.16 Angles used in computing the discrete Gaussian and mean curvatures. Left: $\theta_x(t)$ is the angle of the face t at the vertex x. Right: α_{xx_i} and β_{xx_i} are the angles opposite to the edge xx_i.

DEFINITION 8.28 *The discrete mean curvature can be expressed as:*

$$H(\mathbf{x}) = \frac{1}{4\mathcal{A}(\mathcal{R}_\mathbf{x})} \| \sum_{\mathbf{x}_i \in \mathcal{V}_\mathbf{x}} \left[\cot \alpha_{\mathbf{xx}_i} + \cot \beta_{\mathbf{xx}_i}\right] (\mathbf{x} - \mathbf{x}_i) \| \qquad (8.41)$$

where α_{xx_i} and β_{xx_i} are the angles opposite to the edge xx_i. ∎

Figure 8.16 shows the angles used in computing the discrete Gaussian and mean curvatures.

DEFINITION 8.29 *The discrete principal curvatures of the surface are given by:*

$$\begin{aligned} \kappa_1(\mathbf{x}) &\equiv H(\mathbf{x}) + \sqrt{H^2(\mathbf{x}) - K(\mathbf{x})} \\ \kappa_2(\mathbf{x}) &\equiv H(\mathbf{x}) - \sqrt{H^2(\mathbf{x}) - K(\mathbf{x})} \end{aligned} \qquad (8.42)$$

Example 8.5 Curvatures of complicated biomedical objects.

(a) The human jaw. Figure 8.17 shows a 3D model of the human jaw generated by scanning a mold used in orthodontic measurements and tooth movement planning. Shape indices vary significantly among teeth, which can be used to segment an individual tooth, for example.

(b) Colon object. Figure 8.18 shows a 3D model of the colon illustrating the changes of curvature, especially at haustral folds.

The shape index and curvature are among the features used to study the internal texture of the colon, in order to automatically detect colon polyps.

8.7 Summary

This chapter has introduced the basics of topology and computational geometry for shape modeling. The chapter examined the concept of topologically equivalent shapes and

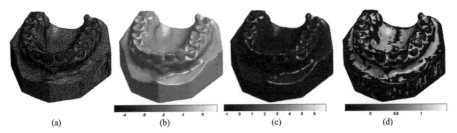

Figure 8.17 Discrete curvatures computed over a triangular mesh representing the shape of a human jaw mold. (a) Triangular mesh, (b) κ_1, (c) κ_2, and (d) shape index. Note the values of these geometric measures for locations where the teeth meet the gum. Hence we can use these curvatures to separate the teeth region from the surface of a human jaw mold.

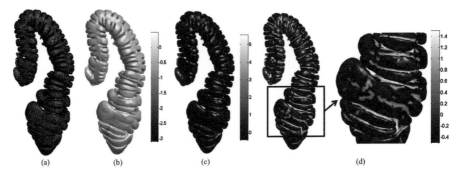

Figure 8.18 Discrete curvatures computed over a triangular mesh representing the shape of a part of a human colon. (a) Triangular mesh, (b) κ_1, (c) κ_2, and (d) shape index. Note the distinct curvature values for the haustral folds. As such, these local measures can be used to localize geometric features on a surface, such as the haustral fold locations in the case of the human colon.

discussed different shape representations, such as boundary-based, parametric surfaces, and triangular meshes. The chapter also examined how geometric local surface features can be extracted using differential geometry. These concepts will be used in the next chapters for further modeling and applications.

8.8 Exercises

8.1 List four attributes needed for a shape representation to be a good one.
8.2 From the figure below,
 (a) Do these objects have the same shape?
 (b) What is meant by a shape? Use your own words.
8.3 Find the equation of the tangent plane to the following parametric surface at the specified control point:

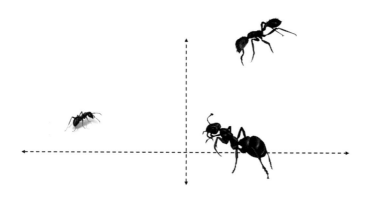

(a) $\mathbf{f}(u, v) = \begin{bmatrix} u+v \\ 3u^2 \\ u-v \end{bmatrix}$ at $(x, y, z) = (2, 3, 0)$

(b) $\mathbf{f}(u, v) = \begin{bmatrix} uv \\ ue^v \\ ve^u \end{bmatrix}$ at $(x, y, z) = (0, 0, 0)$

8.4 Consider the cylinder $x^2 + z^2 = 8$.
  (a) Write down the parametric equation of this cylinder.
  (b) Find a tangent plane to the cylinder using the equations you obtained in (a) at the point (0,4,2).

8.5 Give a complete proof for the following theorem (prove any lemmas you will use in your proof):

THEOREM – AREA OF POLYGON *Let P be a simple polygon (convex or nonconvex), having vertices $\mathbf{x}_0, \mathbf{x}_1, \ldots, \mathbf{x}_{n-1}$ labeled counterclockwise, and let $\mathbf{x}$ be any point in the plane, then*

$$A(P) = A(\mathbf{x}, \mathbf{x}_0, \mathbf{x}_1) + A(\mathbf{x}, \mathbf{x}_1, \mathbf{x}_2) + A(\mathbf{x}, \mathbf{x}_2, \mathbf{x}_3) + \ldots + A(\mathbf{x}, \mathbf{x}_{n-2}, \mathbf{x}_{n-1}) + A(\mathbf{x}, \mathbf{x}_{n-1}, \mathbf{x}_0)$$

Let the coordinates of the ith vertex $\mathbf{x}_i$ be denoted as x_i and y_i; hence twice the area of the polygon P is given by

$$2A(P) = \sum_{i=0}^{n-1}(x_i y_{i+1} - x_{i+1} y_i) = \sum_{i=0}^{n-1}(x_i + x_{i+1})(y_{i+1} - y_i)$$

8.6 Using (5), compute the area of the polygon whose xy-coordinates are given in the following table (show any intermediate results).

x	0	10	12	20	13	10	12	14	8	6	10	7	0	1	3	5	-2	5
y	0	7	3	8	17	12	14	9	10	14	15	18	16	13	15	8	9	5

8.9 Computer laboratory

Codes 8.1 to 8.5 are available online.

Task 1 Extend the class definition in Code 8.1 to define Point3D, which is a class to represent the coordinates of a point in 3D space. Note that you are required to define the implementation details of individual member functions.

Task 2 Build your own graphical user interface (GUI) to allow the user to pick points from the space (2D and 3D) to form their own shapes (e.g. lines, triangles, rectangle, polygons with arbitrary number of points).

Task 3 Extend your GUI to construct a Bézier using the picked control points to allow interactive plotting, noting that for an n degree Bézier curve you will need to have $n+1$ control points. You can construct a class for Bézier curve in 2D and 3D to encapsulate the functionality of such interpolation. Experiment for different degrees ($n = 1,2,3,4,\ldots$); draw the basis functions for each degree and report your results along with your own comments. Implement Bézier curves using the following methods: (1) direct computation of Bernstein polynomials and (2) recursive equations. Use Code 8.2 as your starting point for this task.

Task 4 Extend your GUI to let the user draw 3D parametric surfaces, in particular the following. (Hint: Code 8.3 shows a sample code to generate the surface of a unit sphere.)

(a) $\mathbf{f}(u,v) = \begin{pmatrix} u\cos v \\ u\sin v \\ u \end{pmatrix}$, where $0 \leq u \leq 1$ and $0 \leq v \leq 2\pi$.

(b) $\mathbf{f}(u,v) = \begin{pmatrix} 2(1 - e^{u/6\pi})\cos u \cos^2\left(\frac{v}{2}\right) \\ 2(-1 + e^{u/6\pi})\sin u \cos^2\left(\frac{v}{2}\right) \\ 1 - e^{u/3\pi} + (-1 + e^{u/6\pi})\sin v \end{pmatrix}$,

where $0 \leq u \leq 6\pi$ and $0 \leq v \leq 2\pi$.

(c) $\mathbf{f}(u,v) = \begin{pmatrix} u - \frac{u^3}{3} + uv^2 \\ v - \frac{v^3}{3} + u^2 v \\ u^2 - v^2 \end{pmatrix}$,

where $-1.5 \leq u, v \leq 1.5$. This is known as Enneper's surface.

Task 5 Write a program to compute the first and second fundamental forms of the parametric surfaces in Task 4. Show the principal curvatures, along with the shape index and curvedness, generated a texture on the parametric surface.

Code 8.4 shows how to compute surface derivatives which can be used in your computations.

Task 6 Write a program to compute discrete curvatures of a triangular mesh. Use Code 8.5 to generate a sample surface.

References

[8.1] D. G. Kendall, The diffusion of shape. *Adv. Appl. Prob.* **9** (1977) 428–430.
[8.2] D. Marr and H. K. Nishihara, Representation and recognition of the spatial organization of three-dimensional images. *Proc. Roy. Soc. London B*, **200** (1978) 269–294.
[8.3] R. J. Woodham, Stable representation of shape. *Computational Processes in Human Vision.* New Jersey: Norwood (1987).
[8.4] T. O. Binford, Survey of model-based image analysis systems. *Int. J. Robot. Res.* **1**(1) (1982) 18–64.
[8.5] M. Brady, *Criteria for Representations of Shape in Human and Machine Vision.* London: Academic Press (1983).
[8.6] R. M. Haralick, A. K. Mackworth and S. L. Tanimoto, *Computer Vision Update.* In Barr, A., Cohen, P. R. and Feigenbaum, E. A. (eds.), *The Handbook of Artificial Intelligence* Vol. IV. Reading, MA: Addison-Wesley (1989) 519–582.
[8.7] F. Mokhtarian and A. Mackworth, A theory of multiscale, curvature-based shape representation for planar curves. *IEEE Trans. Pattern Anal. Machine Intel.* **14**(8) (1992) 789–805.
[8.8] C. Dorai and A. K. Jain, Cosmos – a representation scheme for 3d freeform objects. *IEEE Trans. Pattern Anal. Machine Intel.* **19**(10) (1997) 1115–1130.
[8.9] M. Meyer, M. Desbrun, P Schroder and A. H. Barr, Discrete differential-geometry operators for triangulated 2-manifolds. Berlin: VisMath (2002).

Appendix 8.1 Codes

Code 8.1 Point2D class

```
classdef Point2D
    %POINT2D class for points in two-dimensional space
    %  in this class we will define the xy coordinates of a point allowing
    %  for the vector representation of the point

    properties
        x; % the x-coordinate of the point
        y; % the y-coordinate of the point
    end

    methods
        %% the constructor - called when you create an instance of this
        % class
        function obj = Point2D(x,y)
```

```matlab
        if nargin > 0
            obj.x = x;
            obj.y = y;
        else % instance created without initial values
            obj.x = 0;
            obj.y = 0;
        end
    end
    
    %% properties access methods
    % get access methods
    function xval = get.x(obj)
        xval = obj.x;
    end
    
    function yval = get.y(obj)
        yval = obj.y;
    end
    
    % set access methods
    function obj = set.x(obj,xval)
        obj.x = xval;
    end
    
    function obj = set.y(obj,yval)
        obj.y = yval;
    end
    
    %% user-defined functions
    % converting the point into vector representation
    function vec = toVector(obj)
        % TO-DO
    end
    
    %% operators overloading
    function TF = eq(p1,p2)
        % TO-DO
    end
    
    function TF = ne(p1,p2) % not equal to
        % TO-DO
    end
    
    %Binary addition p1+p2
    function p3 = plus(p1,p2)
        % TO-DO
    end
    
    %Binary subtraction p1-p2
    function p3 = minus(p1,p2)
        % TO-DO
    end
```

```
            %Unary minus -p
            function p = uminus(p)
                % TO-DO.
            end

            %Unary plus +p
            function p = uplus(p)
                % TO-DO
            end

            %Element-wise multiplication p1.*p2
            function p3 = times (p1,p2)
                % TO-DO
            end

            % dot product p1*p2
            function res = mtimes(p1,p2)
                % TO-DO
            end

            % divid by scalar
            function p3 = rdivide(p1,alpha)
                % TO-DO
            end

            % power to scalar .^b
            function p3 = power(p1,b)
                % TO-DO
            end

            % compand prompt display
            function display(p)
                % TO-DO
            end
        end
    end
```

Code 8.2 Sample Bezier Curve 2D class

```
        classdef BezierCurve2D
            properties
                control_points % ordered array of control points, for n-degree curve
                                % we need n+1 points
                B_k         % basis functions
                curve_points  % interpolated points calculated using the curve's
                              % parametric equation
            end

            methods
                %%% constructor
```

```matlab
function obj = BezierCurve2D(x,y)
    if nargin < 1
        obj.control_points = {};
        obj.B_k = {};
        obj.curve_points = {};
    else
        if length(x) ~= length(y)
            errordlg('Number of x-coordinates does not match number of y-coordinates ...');
        end

        for i = 1 : length(x)
            obj.control_points{i} = Point2D(x(i),y(i));
        end

        obj = obj.generate_basis_functions();
        obj = obj.generate_curve();
    end
end

%% access functions
% TO-DO

%% generating the basis function
function obj = generate_basis_functions (obj)
    % TO-DO
end

function display_basis_functions (obj,varargin)
    % TO-DO
end

function obj = generate_curve(obj)
    % TO-DO
end

function draw_curve(obj, varargin)
    % TO-DO
end

function draw_control_points(obj, varargin)

    % getting the line points into a suitable structure for display
    for i = 1 : length(obj.control_points)
        obj.control_points{i}.draw(varargin{:});
        hold on;
    end
end
end
end
```

Code 8.3 Sphere parametric form

```
%% sphere surface
Phi        = linspace(0,pi,60);
Theta      = linspace(-pi,pi,60);
[phi,theta] = meshgrid(phi,theta);

x = sin(phi) .* cos(theta);
y = sin(phi) .* sin(theta);
z = cos(phi);

figure('Color','w');
set(gca,'FontWeight','bold','FontSize',12);
surf(x,y,z);
view(135,30);
axis tight;
axis square
box on;
xlabel('x-axis','FontWeight','bold','FontSize',12);
ylabel('y-axis','FontWeight','bold','FontSize',12);
zlabel('z-axis','FontWeight','bold','FontSize',12);
```

Code 8.4 Surface derivatives

```
% Let X,Y,Z be 2D arrays of points on the parametric surface.

% First derivatives
[Xu,Xv] = gradient(X);
[Yu,Yv] = gradient(Y);
[Zu,Zv] = gradient(Z);

% Second derivatives
[Xuu,Xuv] = gradient(Xu);
[Yuu,Yuv] = gradient(Yu);
[Zuu,Zuv] = gradient(Zu);

[Xuv,Xvv] = gradient(Xv);
[Yuv,Yvv] = gradient(Yv);
[Zuv,Zvv] = gradient(Zv);
```

Code 8.5 Sample mesh

```
% Create vertex vectors and a face matrix, then create a triangular surface plot.
[x,y] = meshgrid(1:15,1:15);
faces = delaunay(x,y);
z = peaks(15);
figure, trisurf(faces,x,y,z)
```

9 Geometric features extraction

Objects may be represented by various forms, but robust representations must maintain the features that describe the objects and enable analysis and decision making. As objects may not have a specific geometric description, these features may not be easy to specify. Likewise, known features about an object may be altered in the imaging process. Furthermore, if an object is to be compared with similar ones in a database, it is important that features involved in this comparison be robust (ideally invariant) to changes in scale, rotation, and translation. This chapter deals with feature definitions and characterization through feature descriptors. In the computer vision and image analysis literature, various approaches have been introduced to define, detect, and describe features. Local photometric and geometric features have proven to be very successful in applications such as object recognition, stereo matching, image retrieval, robot localization, video data mining, building panoramas, and recognition of object categories (e.g. [9.1]–[9.5]). This chapter will discuss global and local features, and how to extract corners, edges, contours or salient regions, which are among the common features used in image analysis algorithms. The chapter will describe feature detection and a number of efficient descriptors, including SIFT, ASIFT, and SURF. Good surveys of interest-point detectors and feature descriptors exist in the computer vision literature (e.g. [9.6],[9.7]).

9.1 Introduction

This section will provide basic definitions related to features and descriptors. The previous chapter discussed geometric and topological representations of objects. As much as possible, we will maintain the same terminologies and concepts.

DEFINITION 9.1 *A local feature is a point or pattern in an image that differs from its immediate neighborhood, and is associated with a change in an image property or a number of properties simultaneously.* ∎

The image properties commonly used include intensity, color, and texture. Local features can be points, edges, or small patches on the image.

DEFINITION 9.2 *A feature descriptor is a representation of a feature, or a region around a feature, computed from attributes such as intensity, color, or texture of the feature or the region.* ∎

214 **Geometric features extraction**

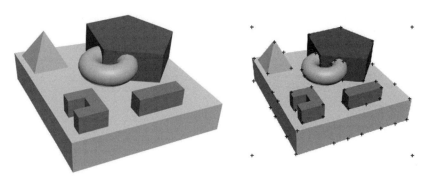

Figure 9.1 A test image with features identified by a corner detector.

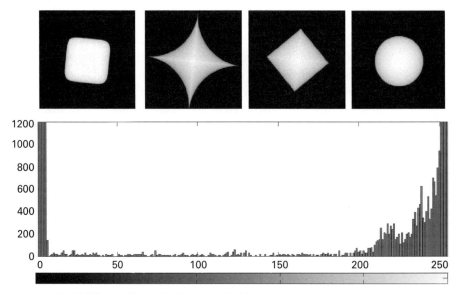

Figure 9.2 An example of different objects that have similar histograms.

Figure 9.1 shows an example of local features extracted by a corner detection technique. This image will be used throughout the chapter to measure effectiveness of various corner detectors and descriptors with respect to rotation and noise.

DEFINITION 9.3 Global features *describe objects as a whole using a single descriptor.*∎

Gray-level histograms, color histograms, texture, shape context, and geometric attributes of an object such as area or perimeter are examples of commonly used global features (e.g. [9.8]–[9.11]). As expected, global features may not be as robust as local features if the objects have complicated topologies. Different objects may have similar gray-level histograms, for example; thus some global features may not provide satisfactory results in image analysis. Figure 9.2 shows an example of four different synthetic images that have similar histograms. It is obvious that using the histogram as a global feature will not provide discrimination between these four objects. In general, global features do not provide the invariance required for such processes as image registration and matching. They may also be less sensitive to occlusion and other uncertainties in the imaging process.

Figure 9.3 shows an object occluded by another object, yet their histograms are not highly distinct. The examples in Fig. 9.2 and 9.3 show that description using global features may fail in extracting distinctive and invariant features in practical situations. A possible improvement in discrimination may result if we divide the objects into subregions and evaluate the global features in those instead of the entire spatial support. This has been especially popular in the context of face detection, and used for recognition of object classes such as pedestrians or cars (e.g. Belongi *et al.* [9.9]).

In contrast to global features, local features describe the object of interest using a set of vectors representing patches around detected features or points of interest. Figure 9.4 illustrates a typical approach to object recognition using local invariant features, which involves three main stages: interest-point detection, descriptor building, and feature matching (or pose estimation).

Several interest-point detectors have been developed in the literature e.g. the Canny edge detector; this provides optimality with respect to edge localization and noise, and can be approximated by the gradient of the Gaussian operator followed by non-maximal suppression of weak edges (e.g. [9.12]). Edge points may be parameterized to form an object model. They may also be used in building models for line segments, corners, roofs, etc. The Harris corner detector, for example, may start at edge points detected by the Canny edge detector [9.13].

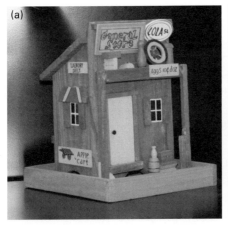 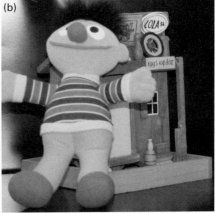

Figure 9.3 Object retrieval using global features fails in the presence of occlusion. (a) Original object; (b) object under occlusion; (c) original object histogram; (d) occluded object histogram. Notice the difference between the features of the non-occluded and occluded objects.

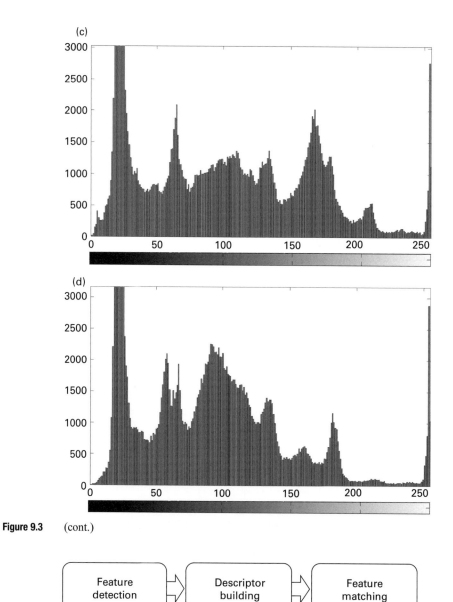

Figure 9.3 (cont.)

Figure 9.4 The three parts of image matching algorithms.

For every detected interest point, a numerical vector called the "feature descriptor" is built to describe that point, or a patch (local neighborhood) around it. Several approaches have been developed for this purpose, e.g. the SIFT, SURF and LBP algorithms, which will be studied later in this chapter. Feature matching may be conducted by various search methods based on a particular similarity or dissimilarity measure. Image registration is a form of matching to find the optimum rotation, translation, and scale among a set of objects that need to be realigned. Recognition of objects in a database is performed by corresponding representations of objects with a candidate object (probe). Robust features are crucial for enhancing the performance of registration and recognition processes. In this chapter we start by studying the notion of invariance in local features, then examine some feature descriptors that have efficient algorithmic implementation to enable incorporation into such image analysis tasks as registration and recognition.

9.2 Edges and corners

Interest points are usually selected at highly informative locations such as edges and corners. Formally, edges and corners are defined as follows.

DEFINITION 9.4 *Edges are the locations in the image at which the variations of the intensity I(x, y) are large along specific direction **d** and are small along the orthogonal direction d_o; that is, $d_o \perp d$.* ■

DEFINITION 9.5 *Corners are the locations in the image at which the variations of the intensity I(x, y) are large along all directions (in practice, large variations along two different directions are sufficient to indicate a corner).* ■

In this section we discus a number of common corner detectors in the image analysis literature. To evaluate these detectors, we created a synthetic image and a set of blurred, scaled, rotated, and noisy versions of this image. Figure 9.5 shows the data set used to test the corner and region detectors.

9.2.1 The Harris detector

The Harris detector [9.13] is based on the second moment matrix, also called the autocorrelation matrix, which describes the gradient distribution in the local neighborhood of a point of interest. The Harris corner detector depends on shifting a window in different directions and tracking the changes in intensities. Corners provide a strong response in all directions, whereas edges give a strong response in a specific direction, and flat regions do not give a strong response at all. The change of intensity $D(\Delta x, \Delta y)$ which result from small shifts Δx and Δy in the x and y directions, respectively, can be represented as follows:

$$D(\Delta x, \Delta y) = \sum_{x,y} w(x,y)[I(x+\Delta x, y+\Delta y) - I(x,y)]^2, \quad (9.1)$$

where $w(x, y)$ is a window function which can be binary or Gaussian, and $I(x, y)$ is the intensity of the pixel at location (x, y). By using small deviations Δx and Δy, $I(x+\Delta x, y+\Delta y) - I(x, y)$ can be approximated by intensity derivatives in the x and y-directions multiplied by $\Delta x, \Delta y$, respectively. Then Eq. (9.1) can be rewritten as follows:

$$D(\Delta x, \Delta y) \cong [\Delta x, \Delta y] \sum_{x,y} w(x,y) \begin{bmatrix} I_x^2 & I_x I_y \\ I_x I_y & I_y^2 \end{bmatrix} \begin{bmatrix} \Delta x \\ \Delta y \end{bmatrix}, \quad (9.2)$$

218 Geometric features extraction

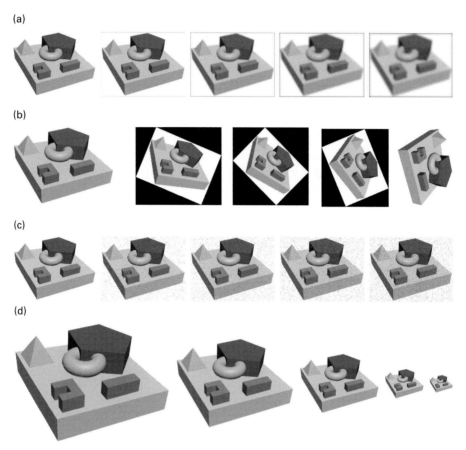

Figure 9.5 Test image at different levels of (a) blur, (b) rotation, (c) noise, and (d) scale. Original image is leftmost.

where $I_x = \dfrac{\partial I}{\partial x}$ and $I_y = \dfrac{\partial I}{\partial y}$. The eigenvalues of the term $M = \sum_{x,y} w(x,y) \begin{bmatrix} I_x^2 & I_x I_y \\ I_x I_y & I_y^2 \end{bmatrix}$ can give a measure of the corner response of the image pixels. The following equation may be used as a measure of the corner response of the image pixels:

$$\rho = \lambda_1 \lambda_2 - C(\lambda_1 + \lambda_2), \qquad (9.3)$$

where C is a constant. The pixels are labeled accordingly as follows:

$$L(x,y) = \begin{cases} \text{Corner} & \rho > \varepsilon \\ \text{Edge} & \rho < -\varepsilon \\ \text{Flat region} & |\rho| < \varepsilon \end{cases} \qquad (9.4)$$

where $\varepsilon \in \mathbf{R}$ is an arbitrary real-valued threshold.

Figure 9.6 shows the performance of the Harris corner on the original test image. In general, this detector is more robust to rotation than scale variations.

9.2 Edges and corners

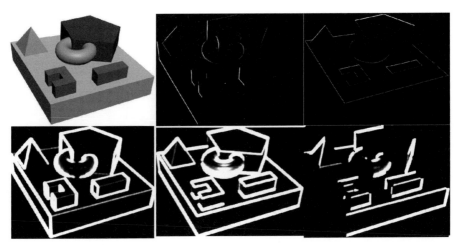

Figure 9.6 Harris corner detector steps. Upper row: the input image, followed by I_x, and I_y. Lower row: I_x^2, I_y^2, and $I_x I_y$.

As shown in Fig. 9.7, a large difference between the eigenvalues (λ_1, λ_2) implies a strong response along one direction and weak response along the orthogonal direction, which means that this pixel may be labelled as an edge point. A small difference between the dominant eigenvalues implies a strong response in all directions, i.e. the pixel is labelled as a corner point. A small difference between the less dominant eigenvalues implies a weak response in all directions, i.e. the pixel may be labelled as a flat-region point.

9.2.2 The SUSAN corner detector

The Smallest Univalue Segment Assimilating Nucleus (SUSAN) corner detector, introduced by Zhang, Smith and Brady [9.16], is illustrated in Fig. 9.8. For each pixel in the image, consider a circular neighborhood of fixed radius around it. The center pixel is referred to as the nucleus, and its intensity value is used as a reference. All other pixels within this circular neighborhood are then partitioned into two categories, depending on whether they have "similar" intensity values to the nucleus or "different" intensity values. In this way, each image point has associated with it a local area of similar brightness, whose relative size contains important information about the structure of the image at that point. The SUSAN corners are detected by segmenting a circular neighborhood into "similar" (gray) and "dissimilar" (white) regions. Corners are located where the relative area of the "similar" region reaches a local minimum below a certain threshold.

9.2.3 Harris–Laplace and Harris–affine corner detectors

Mikolajczyk and Schmid [9.17] developed a scale-invariant corner detector, referred to as Harris–Laplace, and an affine-invariant corner detector, referred to as Harris–affine. Below we briefly describe both detectors.

Geometric features extraction

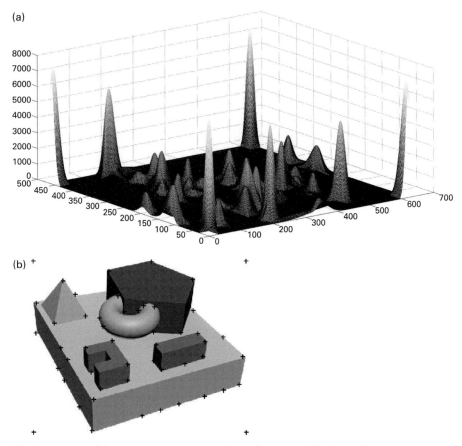

Figure 9.7 Harris corners and detector corner response p in test image, and the detected corners.

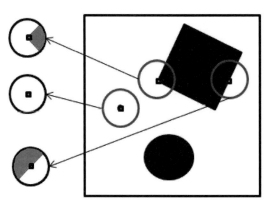

Figure 9.8 SUSAN corners are detected by segmenting a circular neighborhood into similar and dissimilar regions.

Harris–Laplace starts with a multiscale Harris corner detector as initialization in order to determine the location of the local features. The *characteristic scale* is then determined based on scale-space theory (e.g. Lindeberg [9.14]). The characteristic scale is the scale at which there is maximum similarity between the feature detection operator and the local image structure. The idea is to select the *characteristic scale* of a local structure, on which a functional attains an extremum over other scales. The size of the region around points of interest is selected independently of the image resolution for each point. As the name Harris–Laplace suggests, the Laplacian operator is used for scale selection.

Harris–affine: Given a set of initial points extracted at their characteristic scales based on the Harris–Laplace detection scheme, an iterative estimation of elliptical affine regions is used to obtain the affine invariant corners. Instead of circular regions, as used in the Harris–Laplace, the Harris–affine uses ellipses. The procedure consists of the following steps. (1) Detect the initial region with the Harris–Laplace detector. (2) Estimate the affine shape with the second moment matrix. (3) Normalize the affine region to a circular one. (4) Re-detect the new location and new scale in the normalized image. (5) Repeat step 2 if the eigenvalues of the second moment matrix for the new point are not equal to each other (see [9.4]).

Figure 9.9(a) shows the affine-invariant local features obtained by applying the Harris–affine detector, for different images of the same scene related by different transformation changes. The left column shows features detected by a corner detector; the right column shows features picked out by an edge detector. The Harris detector was identified as the most stable one in many independent evaluations (e.g. [9.10]). There are also other multi-scale and affine-invariant extensions of this approach. It is a convenient tool for identifying a large number of features. The SUSAN detector is more efficient, but more sensitive to noise.

Edge-based regions: A technique to obtain affine invariance is to exploit the geometry of the edges that can usually be found in the proximity of a Harris corner. The EBR method was proposed by Tuytelaars and Van Gool [9.2]. It starts from a Harris corner point p and a nearby edge, extracted with the Canny edge detector [9.12]. To increase the robustness to scale changes, these basic features are extracted at multiple scales. More details about this method can be found in [9.2]. Figure 9.9(b) shows the affine-invariant local features obtained by applying the edge-based detector to different images of the same scene related by different transformation changes. Results from the Hessian–affine detector results are shown in Fig. 9.9(c); this detector will be described in the next subsection.

9.2.4 Blob detectors

After corners, the second most important local features are blobs. We will start with a derivative-based method: the Hessian detector. Next, we consider Hessian–Laplace and Hessian–affine detectors.

Hessian detector: The 2×2 matrix Hessian matrix H is constructed from the image intensity function $I(x)$ and is defined as follows:

222 Geometric features extraction

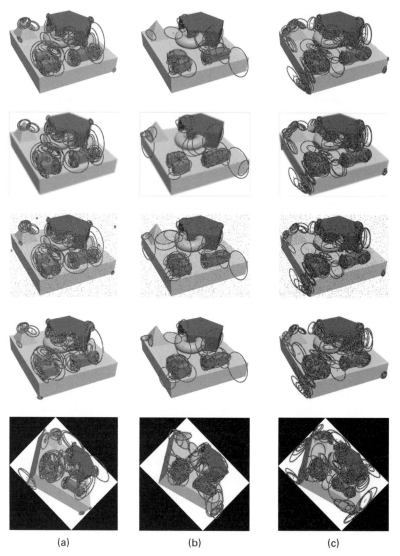

Figure 9.9 Example of Harris–affine and Hessian–affine corner detection under blur, noise, scale, and rotation effects. (a) Corner features; (b) edge features; (c) Hessian–affine features. Upper row shows original features.

$$H = \begin{bmatrix} I_{xx}(x, \sigma_D) & I_{xy}(x, \sigma_D) \\ I_{xy}(x, \sigma_D) & I_{yy}(x, \sigma_D) \end{bmatrix} \quad (9.5)$$

where I_{xx} is second-order derivative of the image after smoothing with a Gaussian filter with standard deviation σ_D. The Laplacian is a separable linear filter and can be approximated efficiently with a difference of Gaussians (DoG) filter. The determinant of the Hessian is used to detect the points of interest. The second-order derivatives give weak responses exactly at the points where the signal change is most significant. Thus, the maxima are localized at blobs for which the size of the Gaussian kernel σ_D matches the size of the blob structure

Hessian–Laplace/affine: The Hessian–Laplace and Hessian–affine detectors are similar in spirit to their Harris-based counterparts, the Harris–Laplace and Harris–affine, except that they start from the determinant of the Hessian rather than the Harris corners. Figure 9.9(c) shows the affine-invariant local features obtained by applying the Hessian detector, for different images of the same scene related by different transformation changes.

9.2.5 Region detectors

We will describe three methods for region detectors: the salient region; intensity-based regions; and maximally stable extremal regions.

Salient regions: Saliency is defined as local complexity or unpredictability, and is measured by the entropy of the probability distribution function of intensity values within a local image region (Kadir and Brady [9.19]). However, looking at entropy alone does not suffice to localize the features accurately over different scales, hence, an additional constraint that measures self-dissimilarity, favoring well-localized complex features in scale-space, is also used. Detection proceeds in two steps: first, at each pixel x the entropy $\mathcal{H}$ of the probability density $p(I,s)$ is evaluated over a range of scales s.

$$\mathcal{H} = -\sum_I p(I,s) \log p(I,s) \tag{9.6}$$

The probability density function $p(I, s)$ is estimated empirically based on the intensity distribution in a circular neighborhood of radius s around x. Local maxima of the entropy are recorded. These are candidate salient regions. Second, for each of the candidate salient regions, the magnitude of the derivative of $p(I, s)$ with respect to scale s is computed as

$$\mathcal{W} = \frac{s^2}{2s-1} \sum_I \left\| \frac{\partial p(I,s)}{\partial s} \right\| \tag{9.7}$$

The saliency $\mathcal{Y}$ is then computed as $\mathcal{Y} = \mathcal{W}\mathcal{H}$ The candidate salient regions over the entire image are ranked by their saliency $\mathcal{Y}$, and the top P ranked regions are retained.

Intensity-based regions: Tuytelaars and Van Gool [9.2] developed a method of detecting affine-invariant regions. It starts from intensity extrema (detected at multiple scales), and explores the image around them in a radial way, delineating regions of arbitrary shape, which are then replaced by ellipses. Given a local extremum in intensity, the intensity function along rays emanating from the extremum is studied. The following function is evaluated along each ray:

$$f(t) = \text{abs}\,(I(t) - I_0) / \max\left(\frac{\int_0^t \text{abs}\,(I(t) - I_0) dt}{t}, d \right) \tag{9.8}$$

where t is an arbitrary parameter along the ray, $I(t)$ the intensity at position t, I_0 the intensity value at the extremum, and d a small number which has been added to prevent division by zero. The point for which this function reaches an extremum is invariant under affine geometric and linear photometric transformations. Typically, a maximum is reached at positions where the intensity suddenly increases or decreases. The function $f(t)$ is in itself already invariant. All points corresponding to maxima of $f(t)$ along rays originating from the same local extremum are linked to enclose an affine-invariant region. This region is replaced by an ellipse having the same shape moments up to second order. This ellipse fitting is an affine covariant construction. An example of regions detected with this method is shown in Fig. 9.10(a).

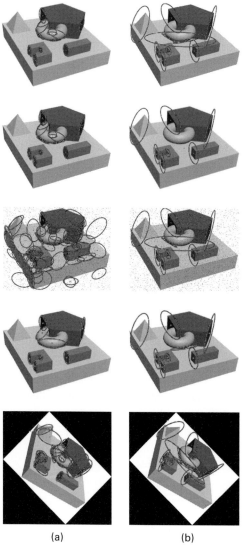

Figure 9.10 (a) Intensity-based regions detection, and (b) maximally stable extremal region detectors for blur, noise, scale, and rotation, respectively. The ellipses show the original size of the detection region.

Maximally stable extremal regions: A maximally stable extremal region (MESR) is a connected component of an appropriately thresholded image (Matas et al. [9.20]). The word "extremal" refers to the property that all pixels inside the MESR have either higher (bright extremal regions) or lower (dark extremal regions) intensity than all the pixels on its outer boundary. The "maximally stable" in MESR describes the property optimized in the threshold selection process. Figure 9.10(b) shows an example of MESR detection. The ellipses show the original size of the detection region. The MSER features typically anchor on region boundaries, so the resulting regions are accurately localized compared with other detectors. The method works best for structured images which can be segmented well.

9.3 Comparative evaluation of interest points

In this section we compare the existing approaches presented before. Using the dataset in Fig. 9.10(b), a comparison between four different detectors is made, and the stability and accuracy of detectors is evaluated using the repeatability criterion introduced in Schmid et al. [9.6]. We also use the average number of corresponding points detected in images under different geometric and photometric transformations.

The repeatability rate and the number of correspondences are shown in Fig. 9.11. Using the test data above, the Hessian–affine detector was most stable, followed by the Harris–affine.

9.3.1 Multi-scale representations

Several multi-scale representations have been developed in the literature. This section presents some examples of early multi-scale representations.

Quad-tree: Klinger [9.21] developed the quad-tree approach as a hierarchical data structure of the image. Consider an image $I = H_I \times W_I$. For simplicity and without loss of generality, let $H_I = W_I = 2^{K_I}$; $K_1 \in R$ is an integer. Let $I^{(k)} \subset I$ and $I^{(K_I)} = I$ be a region in the image. Define the variance σ^2 as the measure of the gray-level variation inside $I^{(k)}$:

$$\sigma^2(I^{(k)}) = E_{I^{(k)}}(I^2) - E^2_{I^{(k)}}(1) \qquad (9.9)$$

where $E_{I^{(k)}}(I)$ is the expected value of the gray-levels of the pixels inside the region $I^{(k)}$. If $\sigma^2(I^{(k)}) > \alpha$, where α is a certain threshold, then split $I^{(k)}$ into P sub-images, $I_j^{(k-1)}$, $j = 1, \ldots, p$ and repeat the process recursively for every subset. Usually, p is set to four. This representation gives a good reduction of images with large homogenous regions. However, for images with strong variations, the worst case occurs when the maximum size of $I_j^{(n)}$, for $n = 1, \ldots, k, j = 1, \ldots, p$, equals one; i.e. only one pixel is assigned to every region. In this case, the representation will be ended by the conventional digital image representation. Image segmentation is another useful application of the quad-tree representation. Using quad-tree, the edges between image regions can

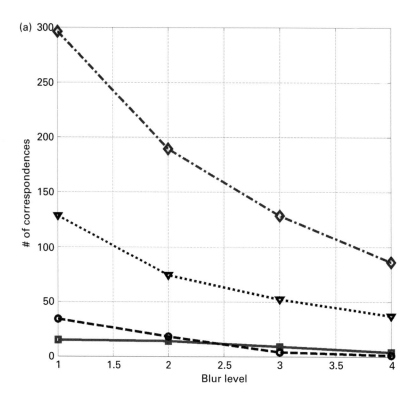

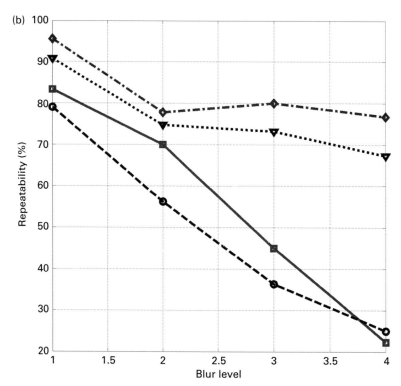

Figure 9.11 The number of correspondences and the repeatability measure under different changes in blurring, noise, rotation, and scale.

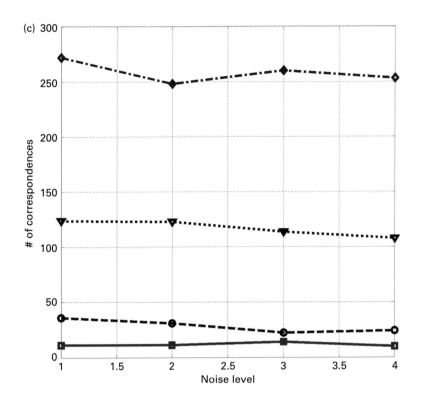
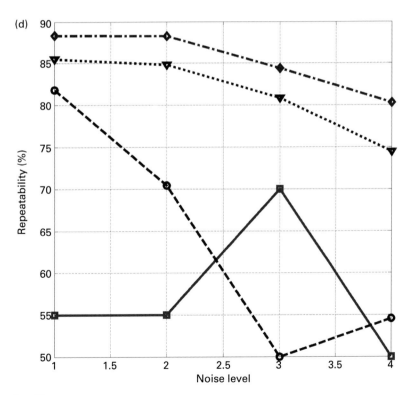

Figure 9.11 (cont.)

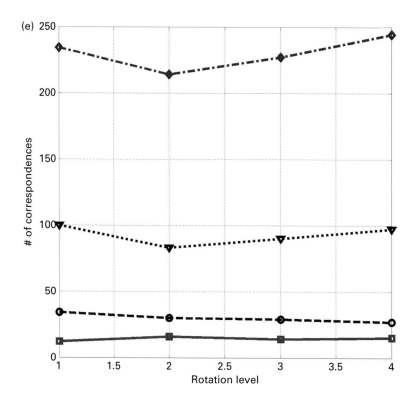

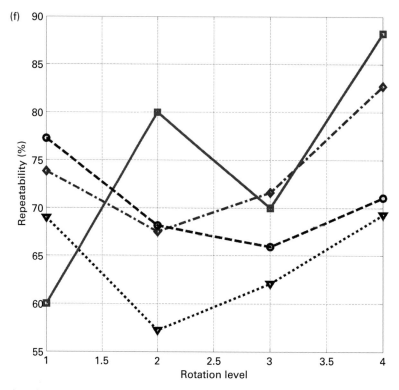

Figure 9.11 (cont.)

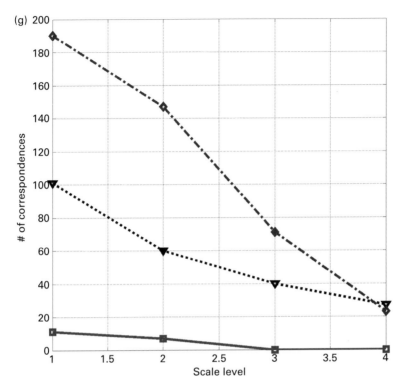

Figure 9.11 (cont.)

be extracted by recursively thinning and connecting the cells with high intensity variations. Quad-tree may also be used in an optimization algorithm to expedite the search process.

Pyramids: Multi-scale representation using pyramids is performed by successively smoothing and sub-sampling the original signal, as shown in Fig. 9.12. For illustration purposes, consider a 2D signal (image) I of size $H_I \times W_I = 2^{K_I} \times 2^{K_I}$; $K_I \in R$ is an integer.

Let $I^{(k_1)} = 1$. To obtain the pyramid representation of I, $I^{(k_1-1)}$ is produced by smoothing and sub-sampling of I as defined below:

$$I^{(k-1)}(x) = \sum_{n=-\infty}^{\infty} c(n) I^{(k)}(2x - n); k = 1 \ldots K, x \in R^2. \quad (9.10)$$

Usually, $c(n)$ are the coefficients of a low-pass kernel.

$$c(n) = 0 \text{ if } |n| > N, \text{ and integer value.} \quad (9.11)$$

$c(n)$ must conform to some constraints [9.17]:

- **Positivity:** $c(n) \geq 0$
- **Unimodality:** $c(|n|) \geq c(|n+1|)$

Geometric features extraction

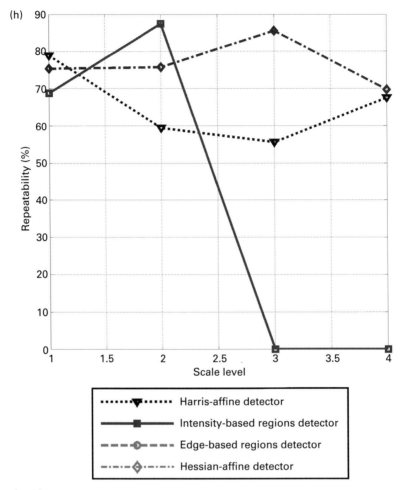

Figure 9.11 (cont.)

- **Symmetry:** $c(n) = c(-n)$
- **Normalization:** $\sum_{n=-\infty}^{\infty} c = (n) = 1$
- **Equal contribution of odd and even-located pixels:** $\sum_{n=-\infty}^{\infty} c(2n) = \sum_{n=-\infty}^{\infty} c(2n+1)$

Figure 9.13 shows an example of generating a pyramid representation of an image by recursively smoothing and resampling the original image.

Wavelets: The wavelet representation is a multi-scale representation of functions introduced by Daubechies [9.22]. Wavelets have found valuable applications in signal and image processing. The wavelets representation involves two indices (time and frequency or scale and translation, etc.) as shown in Eq. (9.12).

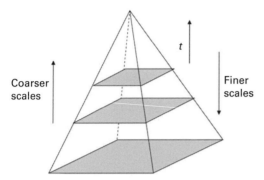

Figure 9.12 Pyramids are generated through a recursive smoothing and resampling process.

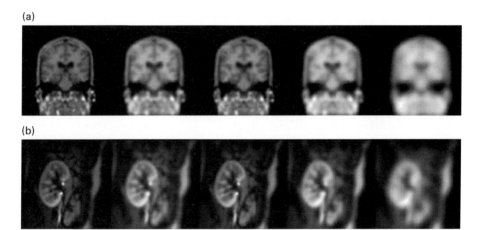

Figure 9.13 Five levels from the pyramid representation of a brian and kidney MRI slices.

$$h_{a,b} = |a|^{-1/2} h\left(\frac{x-b}{a}\right); a, b \in \mathbf{R},\ a \neq 0. \qquad (9.12)$$

Wavelets are the functions $h_{a,b}$ which are derived from a single function $h:\mathbf{R}\to\mathbf{R}$, which must satisfy the admissibility condition:

$$\int_{-\infty}^{\infty} \frac{|H(\omega)|^2}{|\omega|} d\omega < \infty \qquad (9.13)$$

where $H(\omega)$ is the Fourier transform of the function $h(.)$. The continuous wavelet transform (CWT) is given by:

$$(Wf)(a,b) = \ <f, h_{a,b}> \ = |a|^{-1/2} \int_{x \in \mathbf{R}} f(x) h\left(\frac{x-b}{a}\right) dx. \qquad (9.14)$$

9.3.2 Scale-space representation

The scale levels in scale-space representation are described by a single parameter, $t \in \mathbf{R}_+$, of the derived signals [9.23], [9.24]. Given a signal $f(\mathbf{x}): \mathbf{R}^N \to \mathbf{R}$, the scale-space representation $L(\mathbf{x}; t): \mathbf{R}^N \times \mathbf{R}_+ \to \mathbf{R}$ is defined as the convolution of the input signal $f(\mathbf{x})$ with a specific smoothing kernel $g(\mathbf{x};t)$, as shown in Eq. (9.15):

$$L(\mathbf{x}; t) = g(\mathbf{x}; t) * f(\mathbf{x}). \tag{9.15}$$

$$L(\mathbf{x}; t) = \int_{\xi \in \mathbf{R}^N} g(\xi; t) f(\mathbf{x} - \xi) d\xi, \tag{9.16}$$

where $L(\mathbf{x}; 0) = f(\mathbf{x})$ for all $\mathbf{x} \in \mathbf{R}^N$ and $g(\mathbf{x};t)$ is the scale-space kernel. As t increases, the scale-space representation $L(\mathbf{x}; t)$ of the signal tends to coarser scales.

The scale-space representation $L(\mathbf{x};t)$ of a signal $f(\mathbf{x})$ is analogous to evolution of an initial heat distribution f over time t in a homogeneous medium. Hence, fine-scale details will disappear and signals become more diffuse as the scale parameter increases. Therefore, the scale-space representation can equivalently be defined as the solution of the *diffusion equation*, shown in Eq. (9.17), with an initial condition $L(\mathbf{x}; 0) = f(\mathbf{x})$ (see [9.14]).

$$\partial_t L = \frac{1}{2} \nabla^2 L. \tag{9.17}$$

When the scale parameter is increased, the surface levels decrease monotonically. This is referred to as the causality of the scale-space representation (Koenderink [9.24]). Moreover, all spatial points and scale levels must be treated homogeneously. By combining the notions of causality and homogeneity, the scale-space representation of 2D signals can be expressed as follows (Lindeberg [9.14]):

$$\partial_t L = \frac{1}{2} \nabla^2 L = \frac{1}{2(\partial_{xx} + \partial_{yy}) L'} \tag{9.18}$$

where $\partial_{xx}(.)$ and $\partial_{yy}(.)$ are second-order partial derivatives. The scale-space representation of N-dimensional signals will be:

$$\partial_t L = \frac{1}{2} \nabla^2 L = \frac{1}{2} \sum_{i=1}^{N} \partial_{x_i x_i} L. \tag{9.19}$$

The scale-space representation comprises a continuous scale parameter. Moreover, it has the advantage of preserving the same spatial sampling at all scales. Scale-space representation is also causal and scale-invariant. Causality of scale-space means that no new level surface can be created when the scale-parameter is increased. The Gaussian kernel is the unique smoothing kernel that can be used in scale-space kernel representation (see [9.14]).

9.3.3 Scale-space and feature detection

The quality of a detected feature is measured in terms of its invariance to translations, rotations, scalings, affine/projective, and intensity changes. This section studies scale-space representation with respect to these changes.

Differential invariants

Directional derivatives, along certain coordinate directions, have been used to derive "differential invariants" (e.g. [9.25]). The extracted features are guaranteed to be rotation invariant. Moreover, these derivatives are translation invariant. These invariance properties are applicable for both the original image signal f and its scale-space representation L, since this scale-space representation is generated using the rotationally symmetric Gaussian kernel. As stated before, to achieve invariance with respect to rotation, a certain "preferred" direction is assigned to each feature as a local directional reference of this feature, as shown in Fig. 9.14.

One way of choosing the preferred local orthonormal coordinate system (u,v) at any point P_0 is to assign the v and u directions to the gradient direction of the brightness L at P_0 and the perpendicular direction, respectively. This is performed by the following equations:

$$e_v|_{P_0} = \begin{pmatrix} \cos\beta \\ \sin\beta \end{pmatrix} = \frac{1}{\sqrt{L_x^2 + L_y^2}} \begin{pmatrix} L_x \\ L_y \end{pmatrix}\Big|_{P_0} \tag{9.20}$$

$$e_u|_{P_0} = \begin{pmatrix} \sin\beta \\ -\cos\beta \end{pmatrix} = \frac{1}{\sqrt{L_x^2 + L_y^2}} \begin{pmatrix} L_y \\ -L_x \end{pmatrix}\Big|_{P_0} \tag{9.21}$$

Hence, the local directional derivative operators can be calculated in terms of the standard Cartesian coordinates as follows:

$$\partial_{\bar{u}} = \sin\beta\partial_x - \cos\beta\partial_y \tag{9.22}$$

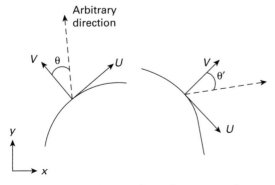

Figure 9.14 Defining a local orthonormal coordinate system for every feature achieves rotation invariance.

$$\partial_{\bar{v}} = \cos\beta\partial_x + \sin\beta\partial_y \qquad (9.23)$$

Another approach is to choose this preferred local orthonormal coordinate system (p,q) such that the mixed second-order derivatives L_{pq} are equal to zero.

Invariance to monotonic intensity transformations

Invariance with respect to monotonic intensity transformations means that any entity that can be calculated from the level curves of the signal will be invariant. For derivatives up to order two, the following irreducible differential expressions are invariant to monotonic intensity transformations (e.g. [9.25]):

$$\kappa = \frac{L_{\bar{u}\bar{u}}}{L_{\bar{v}}} = \frac{L_x^2 L_{yy} + L_y^2 L_{xx} - 2L_x L_y L_{xy}}{(L_x^2 + L_y^2)^{3/2}} \qquad (9.24)$$

$$\mu = \frac{L_{\bar{u}\bar{v}}}{L_{\bar{v}}} = \frac{(L_x^2 - L_y^2)L_{xy} - L_x L_y (L_{yy} - L_{xx})}{(L_x^2 + L_y^2)^{3/2}} \qquad (9.25)$$

where k is the curvature of the level curves of the smoothed signal and μ is the curvature of the flow lines of the gradient vector field. A general scheme to extend this technique to higher-order derivatives is straightforward (e.g. [9.27]).

Invariance with respect to affine intensity transformations

Invariance with respect to affine intensity transformations includes invariance with respect to translations, rotations, and scalings. Invariance with respect to translations and rotations were discussed earlier; a discussion of the invariance with respect to scale changes is presented here. Let $\mathcal{D}L$ be a homogenous differential expression, as shown in Eq. (9.26), and $L'(\mathbf{x}) = L(s\mathbf{x})$ be the smoothed signal response of re-scaled spatial coordinates $(\mathbf{x})$.

$$\mathcal{D}L = \sum_{i=1}^{I} c_j \prod_{j=1}^{J} L_{\bar{u}^{\alpha_{ij}}}, \qquad (9.26)$$

where $L_{\bar{u}^m \bar{v}^n} = L_{\bar{u}^\alpha}$ is a mixed directional derivative of order $|\alpha| = m + n$ and $c \in \mathbf{R}$, $|\alpha_{ij}| > 0$, for all $i = 1, \ldots, I$ and $j=1,\ldots, J$ and $\sum_{j=1}^{J} = |\alpha_{ij}| = N$, for all $i = 1$. Then $\mathcal{D}L'(\mathbf{x}) = \mathcal{D}L(s\mathbf{x}) = s^k \mathcal{D}L$, for some integer value k ([9.14]).

9.3.4 Differential singularities and feature detection

Differential geometric singularities are very important for describing geometric features [9.27]. Singularities, $\mathcal{S}_\mathcal{D}L$, usually denote the zero-crossings of differential expressions, as shown in Eq. (9.27).

$$\mathcal{S}_\mathcal{D}L = \{(\mathbf{x}; t) \in \mathbf{R}^2 \times \mathbf{R}_+ : \mathcal{D}L(\mathbf{x}; t) = 0\}. \qquad (9.27)$$

The absolute invariance with respect to uniform re-scalings of the spatial coordinates is achieved by detecting the features at the singularities of differential expressions of

Eq. (9.25). In other words, the invariant features should be detected at the singularity set $S_D L$ of a differential operator.

For example, consider a junction/corner detection approach using differential singularities. The corners have a high curvature in the gray-level landscape as well as a high intensity gradient. Therefore, a common approach used to detect corners is to multiply the level curvature by the gradient magnitude to suppress the false directions that are obtained in regions of smoothly varying intensity. The level curvature is expressed by:

$$\kappa = \frac{L_x^2 L_{yy} + L_y^2 L_{xx} - 2L_x L_y L_{xy}}{(L_x^2 + L_y^2)^{3/2}} = \frac{L_{\bar{u}\bar{u}}}{L_{\bar{v}}}. \qquad (9.28)$$

By multiplying this curvature by the gradient magnitude raised to an arbitrary power of three, then:

$$\tilde{\kappa} = L_{\bar{v}}^3 \kappa = L_{\bar{v}}^2 L_{\bar{u}\bar{u}} = L_x^2 L_{yy} - 2L_x L_y L_{xy} + L_y^2 L_{xx}. \qquad (9.29)$$

This operator possesses a certain skew-invariance. If scaling factors s_x and s_y are applied to spatial coordinate axes x and y, respectively, then:

$$\tilde{\kappa}' = s_x^2 L_x^2 s_y^2 L_{yy} - 2s_x L_x s_y L_y s_x s_y L_{xy} + s_y^2 L_y^2 s_x^2 L_{xx} = s_x^2 s_y^2 \tilde{\kappa}. \qquad (9.30)$$

Of course, this occurs under the constraint of homogeneity of the derivative terms. According to Eq. (9.30), the maxima of $\tilde{\kappa}$ are exactly similar to those of $\tilde{\kappa}'$. In other words, the singularities of $\partial_{\bar{u}}(\tilde{\kappa})$ and $\partial_{\bar{v}}(\tilde{\kappa})$ are invariant with respect to non-uniform scaling (skew transformations). Hence, the detection of simultaneous zero-crossings of $\partial_{\bar{u}}(\tilde{\kappa})$ and $\partial_{\bar{v}}(\tilde{\kappa})$ is a robust method for junction/corner detection.

9.4 Local descriptors

Image matching algorithms consist of three major parts: feature detector, feature descriptor, and feature matching. This section describes some of the feature detectors and descriptors common in image analysis. Figure 9.15 shows the Shepp and Logan "head phantom," a model image which will be used to test the performance of the feature detectors and descriptors [9.28] (see Appendix 3.1 [3.14]). Different rotation, noise levels, and scales are applied, in order to show the robustness of the feature descriptor.

9.4.1 Scale-invariant feature transform (SIFT)

As detailed in Lowe [9.1], SIFT consists of four main steps: (1) scale-space peak selection, (2) keypoint localization, (3) orientation assignment, (4) keypoint descriptor.

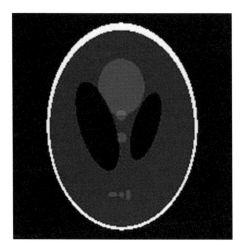

Figure 9.15 Shepp and Logan "head model."

Scale-space reconstruction

The scale space $\mathbf{L}(\mathbf{x}, \sigma_s)$ is constructed by the linear convolution of the image $\mathbf{I}(\mathbf{x})$ with a cylindrical Gaussian kernel $\mathbf{G}(\mathbf{x}, \sigma_s)$ which can be viewed as a stack of 2D Gaussians, one for each band. The scale is discretized as $\sigma_s \in \{k^s\}$ where $k = 2^{1/3}$ and $s = \left\{-1, 0, 1, 2, \ldots, \frac{\log(s_{\max})}{(1/3)\log 2}\right\}$. Scale-space extrema detection is performed by searching over all scales σ_s and image locations $\mathbf{x} = \{(x,y)\}$, in order to identify potential interest points which are invariant to scale and orientation. This can be efficiently implemented using difference-of-Gaussians $\mathbf{D}(\mathbf{x}, \sigma_s)$ which takes the difference between consecutive scales, i.e. $\mathbf{D}(\mathbf{x}, \sigma_s) = \mathbf{L}(\mathbf{x}, \sigma_s) - \mathbf{L}(\mathbf{x}, \sigma_{s-1})$, where for a spectral band b, a point $\mathbf{x}$ is selected to be a candidate interest point if it is larger or smaller than its 3×3×3 neighborhood system defined on $\{D(\mathbf{x}, \sigma_{s-1}; b), D(\mathbf{x}, \sigma_s; b), D(\mathbf{x}, \sigma_{s+1}; b)\}$, where σ_s is marked to be the scale of the point $\mathbf{x}$. This process leads to too many points, some of which are unstable (sensitive to noise); hence points with low contrast and points that are localized along edges are removed. Examples of keypoint detection using the SIFT detector are shown in Fig. 9.16 for the Shepp and Logan model under moderate rotation and noise.

Figure 9.17 shows the keypoint detection using the SIFT detector for our test image showing the effects of rotation and blur.

Keypoint localization

In order to obtain a point descriptor which is invariant to orientation, a consistent orientation should be assigned to each detected interest point based on the gradient of its local image patch. Considering a small window surrounding x, the gradient magnitude and orientation can be computed using finite differences. The orientation of the local image patch is then weighted by the corresponding magnitude and Gaussian

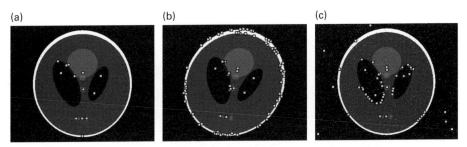

Figure 9.16 Examples of keypoint detection using the SIFT detector with moderate rotation and noise.

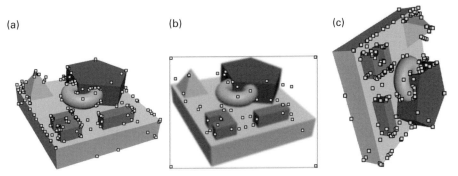

Figure 9.17 Examples of keypoint detection using the SIFT detector with moderate rotation and blurring.

window. Finally the orientation is selected to be the peak of the weighted orientation histogram.

Building a point descriptor: The process of building a descriptor around a keypoint is similar to orientation assignment. A 16 × 16 image window surrounding the interest point **x** is divided into sixteen 4 × 4 sub-windows. An 8-bin weighted orientation histogram is computed for each sub-window; hence we end up with 16 × 8= 128 descriptors for each interest point. Thus each detected interest point can now be defined by location, specific scale, orientation θ and a descriptor vector, as $\mathbf{x} = \{x, y, \sigma, \theta, \mathbf{d}\}$. Figure 9.18 shows plots of the 128 values of the SIFT descriptor under different blur, noise, rotation, and scale levels, each for the same selected point on the transformed images in Fig. 9.17.

Interest point matching: Interest point matching is performed to provide correspondences between two or more given images. Two points $\mathbf{x}_i^t$ and $\mathbf{x}_j^{t+1}$ with SIFT descriptors $\mathbf{d}_i^t$ and $\mathbf{d}_j^{t+1}$ are said to be in correspondence if $d_{L_2}(\mathbf{x}_i^t, \mathbf{x}_j^{t+1}) = \sqrt{||\mathbf{d}_i^t - \mathbf{d}_j^{t+1}||^2}$ is minimum. This measure is computed as: $d_{L_2}(\mathbf{x}_i^t, \mathbf{x}_j^{t+1}) = \left(\sum_{k=1}^{128} |d_{ik}^t - d_{jk}^{t+1}|^2\right)^{1/2}$. Examples of matched feature pairs using SIFT are shown in Fig. 9.19 on the Shepp and Logan head phantom, and in Fig. 9.20 on the test image used throughout this chapter.

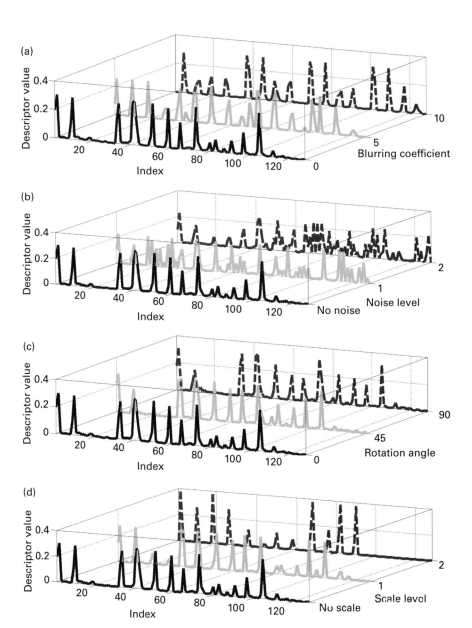

Figure 9.18 Plot of the SIFT descriptor under different blur, noise, rotation, and scale levels at the same selected point on transformed images.

9.4.2 Case study: Descriptors of small-size lung nodules in chest CT

Farag et al. [9.35] used the SIFT algorithm for classification of small-size nodules that appear in low-dose CT (LDCT) scanning of the human chest for early detection of lung cancer. Figure 9.21 shows four slices containing nodules <1 cm in size. The SIFT algorithm was applied to the four nodule types (well-circumscribed, vascular,

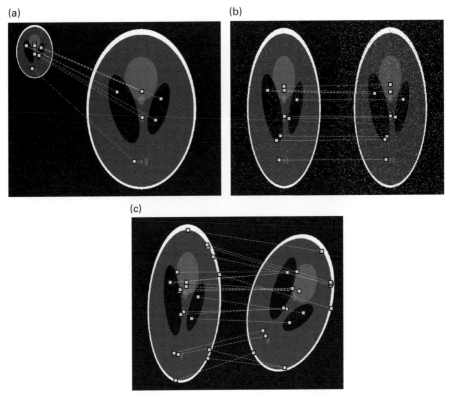

Figure 9.19 Matched feature pairs using SIFT on the Shepp and Logan head phantom. (a) Scale; (b) noise; and (c) rotation effects.

juxta-pleural, and pleural-tails) and the resulting descriptors were used to classify the nodules after a detection step, in order to reduce false positives. Small-size nodules lack textural distinction, but the shapes are distinct. Figure 9.22 shows the construction and values of the SIFT algorithm for the four nodule types. The values of the SIFT descriptor show decent discrimination among the nodules.

9.4.3 Extensions to the SIFT algorithm

A modification to the SIFT algorithm, known as ASIFT and introduced by Morel and Yu [9.29], results in a fully affine descriptor. The ASIFT algorithm simulates all image views that can be obtained by varying the latitude and longitude angles of the imaging sensor. Then the SIFT is used to simulate the scale and normalize the rotation and the translation. A two-resolution scheme further reduces the ASIFT complexity to about twice that of SIFT. Examples of keypoint detection using the ASIFT detector are shown in Fig. 9.23, and examples of matched feature pairs using ASIFT are shown in Fig. 9.24. The ASIFT algorithm provides more keypoint detection and better matching rate than the SIFT algorithm, but at the cost of slower execution time.

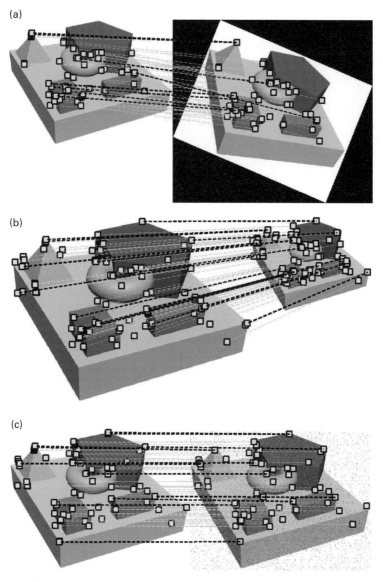

Figure 9.20 Matched feature pairs using SIFT on the test image. (a) Rotation; (b) scale effects.

Abdelhakim and Farag [9.30] extended the SIFT algorithm to color. Their C-SIFT algorithm has been very efficient for color object categorization, recognition, and registration. The same approach has been extended to multi-spectral imaging (e.g. the M-SIFT algorithm of Brown and Süsstrunk [9.31]). As expected, not all keypoints are significant. The computer vision and machine learning literature has a number of approaches to reduce "false positives." The Random Sample Consensus (RANSAC), introduced by Fischler and Bolles [9.30], is among the most efficient algorithms for false positive reductions.

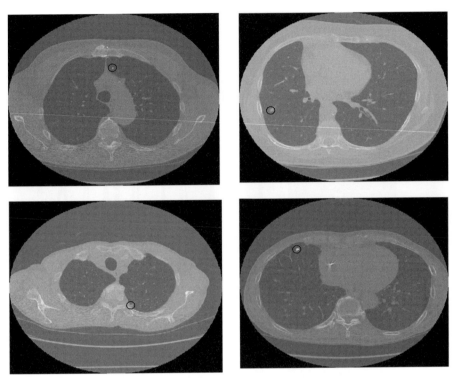

Figure 9.21 Small-size lung nodules from LDCT scans. Upper left (well-circumscribed); upper right (vascular); lower left (juxta-pleural); lower right (pleural-tail). Nodules are marked by a circle.

9.4.4 Speeded-up robust features (SURF)

The SURF descriptor (Bay *et al.* [9.33]) is a distribution of Haar-wavelet responses within the neighborhood of interest. The detector is based on the Hessian matrix (Eq. (9.5)) and relies on integral images to reduce computation time.

The SURF descriptor consists of several steps: a square region is constructed around the interest point and oriented either in a rotation-invariant method, where the Haar-wavelet response in the x- and y- directions are computed and weighted with a Gaussian centered at the interest point, or a non-rotation-invariant method. The wavelet responses in both directions are then summed over each sub-region. The total number of descriptors for each point is 64.

SURF uses mainly the texture information concentrated around interest points. Principal component analysis (PCA) and linear discriminant analysis (LDA) are used to project the extracted SURF descriptors to a low-dimensional subspace where noise is filtered out. We show the plot of the 64 values of the SURF descriptor under different blur, noise, rotation, and scale levels at the same selected point on transformed images in Fig. 9.25.

9.4.5 Multi-resolution local binary pattern (LBP)

The local binary pattern (Ojala *et al.* [9.34]) is an operator invariant to monotonic changes in grayscale and can resist illumination variations as long as the absolute

242 **Geometric features extraction**

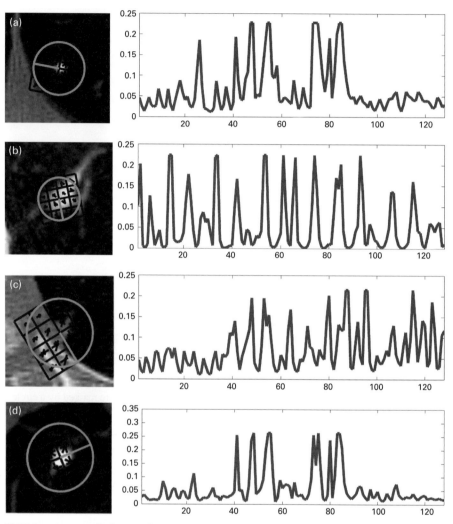

Figure 9.22 SIFT descriptor applied to small-size nodule types in LDCT of the human chest. From top to bottom: well-circumscribed, vascular, juxta-pleural, and pleural-tail nodule types.

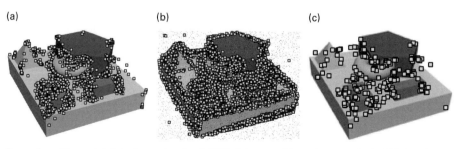

Figure 9.23 Examples of keypoint detection using the ASIFT detector with moderate scale (middle) and noise (right).

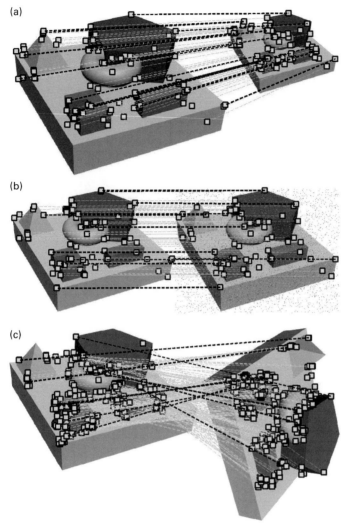

Figure 9.24 Matched feature pairs using ASIFT. Scale (upper); noise (middle); and rotation (bottom) effects.

gray-level value differences are not badly affected. The original operator labeled the pixels of an image by thresholding the 3 × 3 neighborhood of each pixel with the center value and considered the result as a binary number. At a given pixel position (x_c, y_c), the decimal form of the resulting 8-bit word is given by the following equation:

$$\text{LBP}(x_c, y_c) = \sum_{i=0}^{7} s(I_i - I_c) 2^i \qquad (9.31)$$

where I_c corresponds to the center pixel (x_c, y_c), I_i to gray level values of the eight surrounding pixels, and function $s(\cdot)$ is a unit-step function.

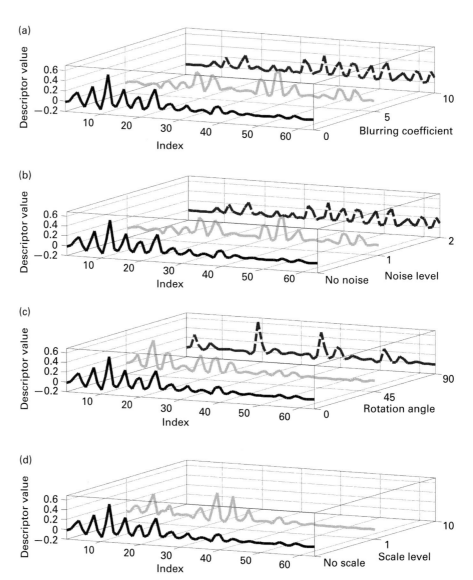

Figure 9.25 The plot of the SURF descriptor under different blur, noise, rotation, and scale levels at the same selected point on transformed images.

The LBP operator was extended to a circular neighborhood of different radius size to overcome the limitation of the small original 3 × 3 neighborhood size in failing to capture large-scale structures. Each instance is denoted as (P, R), where P refers to equally spaced pixels on a circle of radius R. The parameter P controls the quantization of the angular space, and R determines the spatial resolution of the operator.

An LBP pattern is considered uniform if it contains at most two bitwise transitions from 0 to 1 and vice versa, when the binary string is circular. The reason for using uniform patterns is that they contain most of the texture information and mainly represent

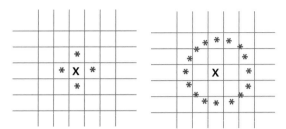

Figure 9.26 Circularly symmetric neighbor sets for different values of (**P**, **R**); left (a) **P** = 4, **R** = 10; right **P** = 16, **R** = 2.0.

texture primitives. The operator is derived on a circularly symmetric neighbor set of P members on a circle of radius R and is denoted as LBP_{PR}^{u2}.

Figure 9.26 illustrates examples of circularly symmetric neighbor sets for various (P, R). The LBP operator can be further enhanced by combining it with a rotation invariant measure $\text{VAR}_{P, R}$, which characterizes the contrast of local image texture. The combination of the LBP_{PR}^{u2} operator and the variance measure produces a powerful operator that is rotation and gray-scale invariant.

In the multi-resolution analysis the responses of multiple operators realized with different (P, R) are combined together and an aggregate dissimilarity is defined as the sum of individual log-likelihoods computed from the responses of individual operators. The notation LBP_{PR}^{u2} used in this chapter refers to the extended LBP operator in a (P, R) neighborhood, with only uniform patterns considered. Figure 9.27 illustrates the formation of the LBP descriptors for lung nodules in low-dose CT (LDCT) scanning of the chest (e.g. Amal Farag [9.36]).

As we did for the SIFT descriptor, we show in Fig. 9.28 readings of the LBP for some keypoints on the test image in Fig. 9.1 under the effect of blur, noise, rotation, and scale. In general, the LBP descriptor works well when the neighborhood around the keypoints has reasonable texture content.

To test the performance of the three descriptor (SIFT, SURF, and LBP) we used the test images in Fig. 9.5, we manually selected a set of 46 points on the original image. Figure 9.29 shows these feature points. The ground truth locations of these points are calculated on every transformed image based on the transformation applied to generate this image.

The descriptors are calculated at these points for all the images and the numbers of correctly matched points are used as an evaluation criteria. The results are shown in Fig. 9.30. The LBP showed a more robust performance with respect to noise, while the SIFT was more robust to rotation.

9.4.6 Image stitching

In order to illustrate the concepts in this chapter, we apply the descriptors to estimate the parameters of affine transformation used to stitch segments of overlapping images together, in order to form a panoramic view. Stitching, in the sense of removing

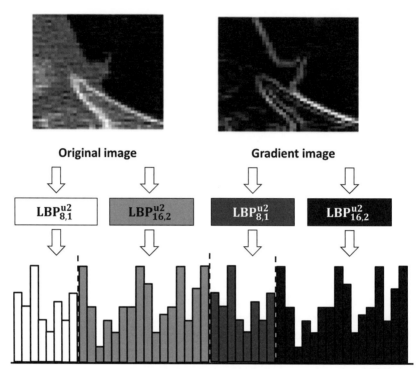

Figure 9.27 Block diagram for generating the LBP for a juxta-pleural nodule. The equation for this picture is: $\mathbf{LBP}_{8,1}^{u2} + \mathbf{LBP}_{16,2}^{u2} + \mathbf{LBP}_{8,1}^{u2} + \mathbf{LBP}_{16,2}^{u2}$, where the first two terms represent the original image and the last two terms represent the gradient image.

overlapping regions, is essentially a rigid registration process, which will be detailed in the next chapter.

Registering two image segments is performed by mapping point correspondences, in order to estimate the rotation, translation, and scaling that relate a source and a target image. A point in the source image (e.g. in the first of a pair of overlapping segments) is related to its corresponding target position (in the second overlapping segment) by a projective transformation. In practice, the overlap between the two segments results, for instance, from imaging a segment of the jaw at two different camera positions. Registration is a well-studied process in image analysis and computer vision. We will dedicate two chapters in this book to this important subject matter. Here, we scratch the surface by providing a direct example of geometric object descriptors for image stitching.

Given a set of K homogeneous image point correspondences $C_l^s \in R^d$ (in the original/source image) and $C_l^t \in R^d$ (in the target image), where d is the dimension of the data ($d = 2$ for images and $d = 3$ for three-dimensional data, etc.) and $l \in 1, 2, \ldots, K$, we want to estimate a projective transformation $\mathbf{H}_{3\times 3}$ to map a point in the source image to its corresponding position in the target image using the relationship (e.g. [9.38]):

9.4 Local descriptors

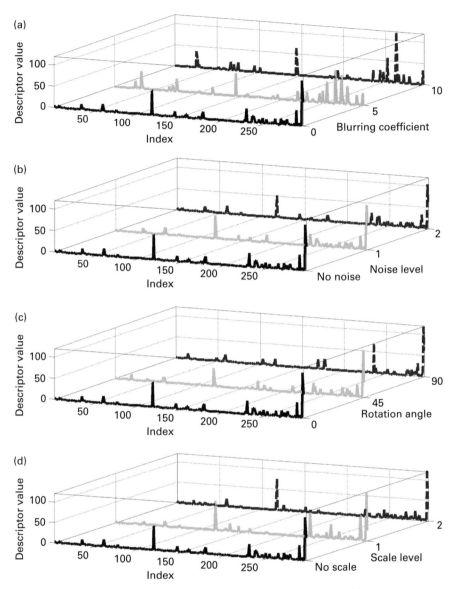

Figure 9.28 Plot of the LBP descriptor performance on the test image under different blur, noise, rotation, and scale levels at the same selected point on transformed images.

$$\alpha \begin{bmatrix} x_l^t \\ y_l^t \\ 1 \end{bmatrix} = \begin{bmatrix} h_{11} & h_{12} & h_{13} \\ h_{21} & h_{22} & h_{23} \\ h_{31} & h_{32} & h_{33} \end{bmatrix} \begin{bmatrix} x_l^s \\ y_l^s \\ 1 \end{bmatrix} \qquad (9.32)$$

where α is a scaling coefficient for the projective transformation. This equation can be expressed as follows:

248 Geometric features extraction

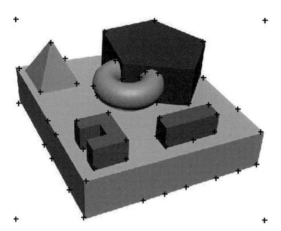

Figure 9.29 Manually selected corners.

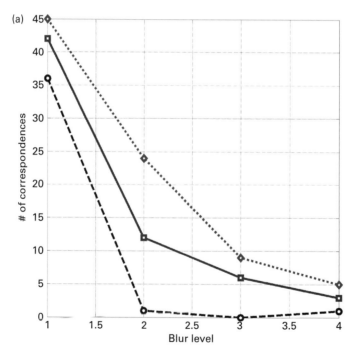

Figure 9.30 The number of correspondences under different blur, noise, rotation, and scale levels for the SIFT (solid curves), SURF (dashed curves), and LBP (dotted curves) descriptors.

9.4 Local descriptors

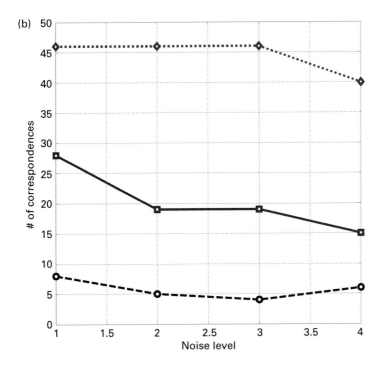

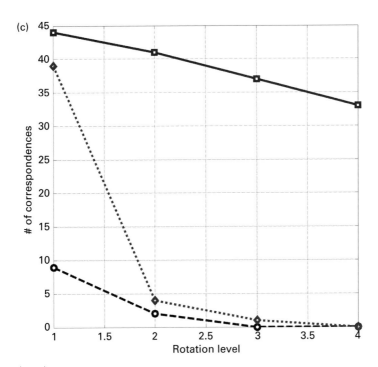

Figure 9.30 (cont.)

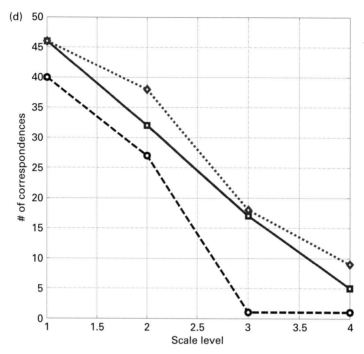

Figure 9.30 (cont.)

$$\alpha C_l^t = H C_l^s \qquad (9.33)$$

The equation may be decomposed into two linear equations:

$$h_{11}x_l^s + h_{12}y_l^s + h_{13} - h_{31}x_l^t x_l^s - h_{32}x_l^t y_l^s - h_{33}x_l^t = 0$$
$$h_{21}x_l^s + h_{22}y_l^s + h_{23} - h_{31}y_l^t x_l^s - h_{32}y_l^t y_l^s - h_{33}y_l^t = 0 \qquad (9.34)$$

where (x, y) are the coordinates of the point. Using the treatment in [9.38], we can construct a linear system of equations $\Psi\Theta = 0$, where $\Theta = [h_{11}\ h_{12}...h_{33}]$ is the parameters column of the projective transformation H, and Ψ is the coefficients matrix. We can estimate the projective transformation parameters by solving this linear system using the singular value decomposition (SVD) approach. If the point correspondence is accurate, the overall difference between the source and target images vanishes when fused together. This approach depends on proper selection of the source and target point correspondences.

For the registration approach described above, only four points are required to estimate the transformation. Using the resulting point correspondences, a projective transformation is computed and applied to the source image, in order to perform the desired stitching.

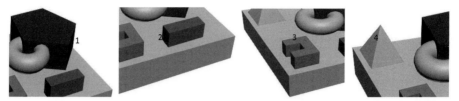

Figure 9.31 A sequence of overlapped images from the test image.

Numerical example

We use the test image in this chapter to illustrate image stitching. We cut the test images into a sequence of four images as shown in Fig. 9.31.

Figure 9.32 shows the four segments in Fig. 9.31 paired into three pairs of overlapping segments covering the whole image, and are used to construct a panoramic view of the image using stitching. Keypoints are selected manually, and then correspondences are used to estimate the affine transformation parameters, in order to perform the stitching. The pair-wise transformations are as follows:

$$T = \begin{bmatrix} \cos\theta & -\sin\theta & t_x \\ \sin\theta & \cos\theta & t_y \\ 0 & 0 & 1 \end{bmatrix} \quad (9.35)$$

where θ is the rotation angle, t_x is the translation in the x-direction and t_y is the translation in the y-direction.

We selected 24 points as ground truth from the original image. The correspondences between the sequence of four overlapping images were used to estimate the transformations. The transformations are shown in Fig. 9.35 for each overlapping pair. The last row in Fig. 9.32 shows the original and stitched image.

Table 9.1 contains the original locations of the keypoints and the estimated correspondences in the stitched image. We note that the error in correspondence is minimal; thus the rigid registration (involving only rotation and translation) is quite successful in this case.

Dental application

We use a similar approach to the above example for stitching a sequence of images of the oral cavity, in order to construct the human jaw. In this application, intra-oral cameras may only be able to capture small segments of the jaw; stitching these segments, while maintaining the geometry of the jaw, provides a panoramic view of the entire jaw. The broader context of this application is described in the author's long-standing research on the Jaw Project at the CVIP Lab, which aims at using non-ionizing radiation for orthodontic, educational, and interventional dental studies and practices (e.g. [9.39]–[9.43]).

Geometric features extraction

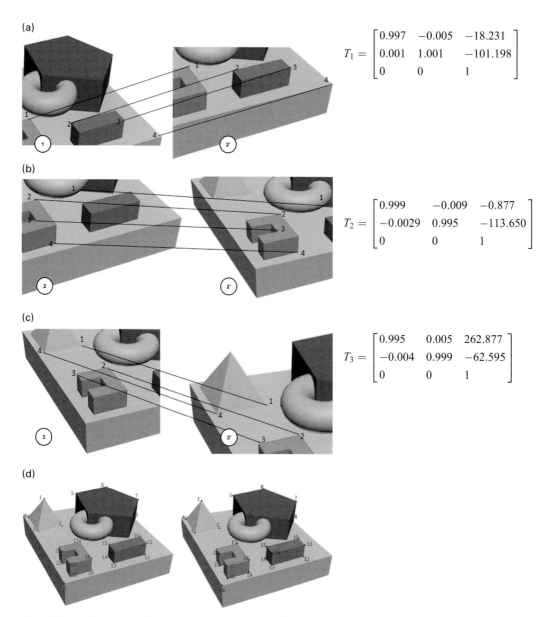

Figure 9.32 Calculation of correspondences for the stitching process.

The example below is simplistic; we have a known ground truth, where the image of the entire shape and jaw are provided, and we cut that image into overlapping pairs. As with the previous example, we chose keypoints between pairs, in order to estimate the transformation for the stitching. Figure 9.33 shows eight overlapping segments, which generate seven pairs for the stitching process, shown in Fig. 9.34. The entire process is shown in Table 9.2 and Fig. 9.35, where the keypoints and the transformation parameters are shown. Figure 9.34 illustrates the acquisition of the source and target image segments.

9.4 Local descriptors

Table 9.1 A set of 24 keypoints from the original image and their corresponding points from the stitched image.

Point number	Original image		Reconstructed image		Errors (in pixels)	
	x_i	y_i	x'_i	y'_i	$x_i - x'_i$	$y_i - y'_i$
1	92	50	93	52	−1	−2
2	165	154	165	155	0	−1
3	66	174	66	173	0	1
4	28	119	27	121	1	−2
5	221	31	220	32	1	−1
6	343	6	344	7	−1	−1
7	471	54	473	54	−2	0
8	446	118	447	118	−1	0
9	271	103	271	105	0	−2
10	481	194	482	193	−1	1
11	506	218	508	218	−2	0
12	500	262	502	261	−2	1
13	374	294	376	293	−2	1
14	351	270	352	269	−1	1
15	353	224	355	224	−2	0
16	377	250	380	249	−3	1
17	235	213	236	212	−1	1
18	284	277	285	275	−1	2
19	283	323	284	322	−1	1
20	197	345	198	346	−1	−1
21	197	299	196	298	1	1
22	166	297	168	296	−2	1
23	164	253	165	252	−1	1
24	174	371	175	371	−1	0

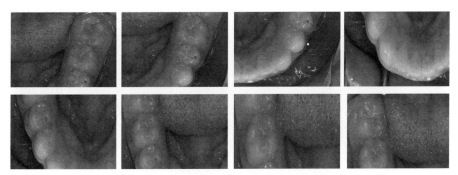

Figure 9.33 Original eight pairs of segments covering the entire jaw.

Since the overlapping images were controlled, the rotation was small; scaling was virtually non-existent; hence, only translation was significant between segments. Therefore, the transformation matrices T_1 to T_7 are identical, and they only have values at t_x and t_y. The overall segmentation of the jaw and the reconstruction is shown in Fig. 9.36.

Table 9.2 The locations of keypoints in the corresponding pairs.

Pair	Location	$X = [(x, y)_1, (x, y)_2, \ldots, (x, y)_N]^t$				
P1	(x, y)	(52,203)	(24,248)	(108,228)	(93,178)	(142,226)
	(x', y')	(153,219)	(127,271)	(209,247)	(193,200)	(244,246)
P2	(x, y)	(29,222)	(18,195)	(44,176)	(105,153)	
	(x', y')	(89,307)	(106,287)	(65,341)	(81,378)	
P3	(x, y)	(89,307)	(106,287)	(65,341)	(81,378)	(84,291)
	(x', y')	(154,44)	(168,23)	(125,77)	(142,114)	(145,25)
P4	(x, y)	(19,137)	(57,127)	(41,87)	(51,182)	(65,227)
	(x', y')	(117,139)	(154,127)	(137,84)	(151,185)	(161,226)
P5	(x, y)	(59,128)	(16,120)	(27,77)	(48,113)	
	(x', y')	(185,130)	(138,118)	(151,76)	(175,113)	
P6	(x, y)	(72,95)	(35,83)	(123,114)	(39,57)	
	(x', y')	(89,99)	(47,91)	(137,117)	(58,60)	
P7	(x, y)	(152,97)	(111,90)	(98,28)	(166,32)	
	(x', y')	(75,95)	(33,87)	(18,26)	(87,33)	

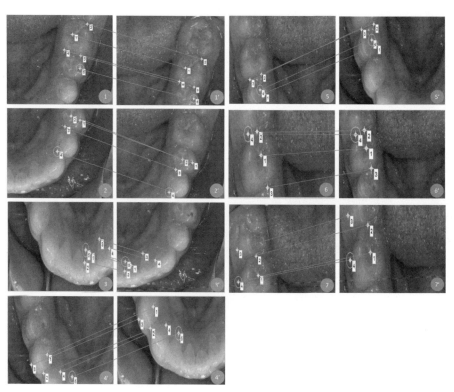

Figure 9.34 Keypoint selection for the pairs used in stitching the human jaw. The eight segments are paired into seven pairs of overlapping segments covering the human jaw, and are stitched to construct a panoramic view of the jaw. Key points are selected manually, and correspondences are used to estimate the affine transformation parameters, in order to perform the stitching.

9.4 Local descriptors

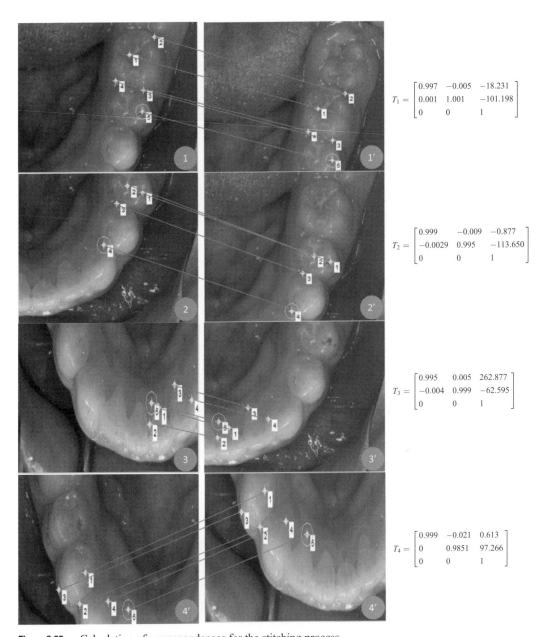

Figure 9.35 Calculation of correspondences for the stitching process.

In practice, the keypoints in the source segments and the corresponding points on the target image are obtained by a SIFT-like descriptor followed by RANSAC, in order to reduce the false correspondences (false positives).

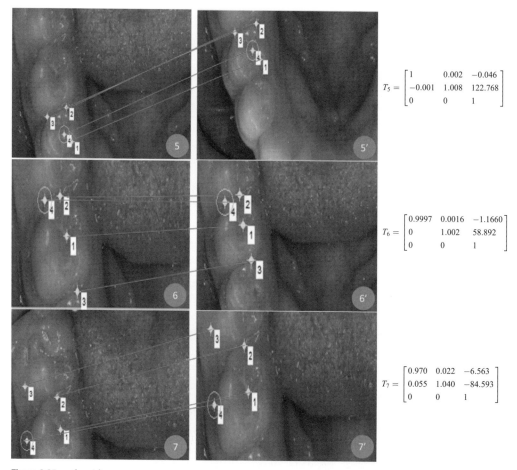

Figure 9.35 (cont.)

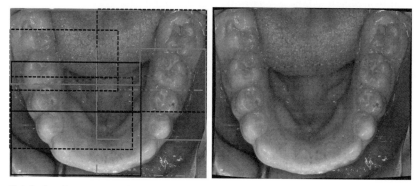

Figure 9.36 Original and reconstructed jaw image by stitching procedure.

Practical implementation of stitching for jaw reconstruction
Below we discuss a complete example of how features and their descriptors may be used to reconstruct a 3D estimate of the human jaw from a series of calibrated images, obtained by an intra-oral camera. Local features extracted from these images are used to estimate an affine transformation to register these images together, in order to build a panoramic view of the jaw. Then a shape from shading (SFS) algorithm can be used to build a 3D model from the panoramic image. Of course, SFS can be implemented over the segments and the stitching can be performed in 3D as well, although it will be rather complicated.

Figure 9.37 shows the matched features between pairs of images that span the oral cavity. Using the matching from the SIFT algorithm, the rotation components were estimated and used to register the image pairs. Figure 9.38 shows pairs of images, with variable intensities, after registration. The process is used to create a 3D estimate of the jaw, shown in Fig. 9.39. Details of this work have been reported elsewhere (e.g., Abdelrahim et al. [9.43]).

9.5 Three-dimensional local invariant feature descriptors

The bottleneck in several medical imaging applications, such as volume registration problems, is finding robust features and correspondence in two 3D volumes. Most feature-based registration approaches depend on relatively primitive feature extractors with a low degree of robustness against variations in the imaging conditions. Furthermore, the diversity and irregularity of the deformable 3D objects of biomedical images make matching using global or fixed features and regions a difficult task for 3D medical applications.

Previously, local invariant features have been used successfully in 2D medical imaging applications (e.g., Farag et al. [9.36]). Below, we discuss some aspects of feature detection and matching that are useful for biomedical image registration. The subject of registration will be further examined in several chapters to follow.

9.5.1 Interest point detection

As shown before, scale-space enables robust feature detection and representation. Although scale-space theory is extendable to higher dimensions (e.g. Koenderink [9.24]), most existing object description approaches use scale-space theory in 2D spaces. This section deals with some 3D extensions. Scale-space representation is formed by an iterative convolution with 3D Gaussian filters, as shown in Eq. (9.36).

$$L(\mathbf{x};t) = g(\mathbf{x};t) * f(\mathbf{x}), \mathbf{x} \in \mathbf{R}^3, \tag{9.36}$$

258   **Geometric features extraction**

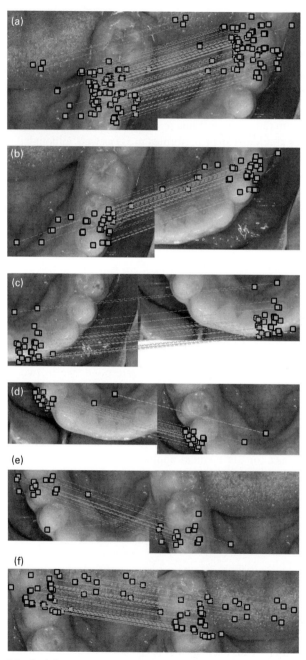

Figure 9.37 Matched features from regions around key points using modified version of the SIFT algorithm.

9.5 Three-dimensional local invariant feature descriptors

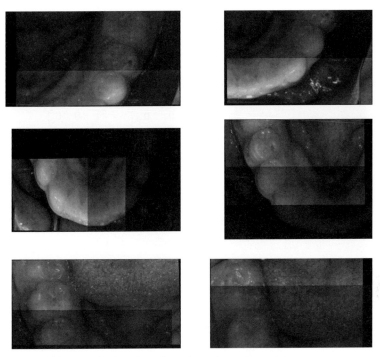

Figure 9.38   Registered image pairs based on the estimated transformation.

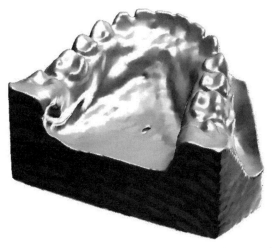

Figure 9.39   3D reconstructed jaw model from the stitched images. The SFS was applied to the stitched images in order to estimate the shape.

$$g(\mathbf{x}; \Sigma) = \frac{1}{\sqrt{2\pi \det(\Sigma)}} e^{\frac{-1}{2}\mathbf{x}^T \Sigma^{-1} \mathbf{x}}, \qquad (9.37)$$

where $g(\mathbf{x}; \Sigma)$ is a Gaussian filter. The covariance matrix is given by:

$$\Sigma = \text{diag}(\sigma^2) = \begin{bmatrix} \sigma^2 & 0 & 0 \\ 0 & \sigma^2 & 0 \\ 0 & 0 & \sigma^2 \end{bmatrix} = \begin{bmatrix} t & 0 & 0 \\ 0 & t & 0 \\ 0 & 0 & t \end{bmatrix}. \qquad (9.38)$$

Then:

$$g(\mathbf{x}; t) = \frac{1}{\sqrt{2\pi t}} e^{\frac{-\|\mathbf{x}\|^2}{2t}}, \qquad (9.39)$$

where $g(\mathbf{x}; t)$ is a Gaussian filter with diagonal covariance matrix.

Figure 9.40 shows a virtual visualization of scale-space representation in 3D space. The process of detecting scale-space differential singularities is performed in a similar way to that used in 2D spaces. Each point in the scale-space representation of the input 3D volume is checked. If it is a local extremum in its hyper-pyramid level, it is checked versus the corresponding neighborhoods of the upper and lower levels. If it is still an extremum, it is selected as an interest point. The detected interest points are collected in a set, as shown in Eq. (9.40):

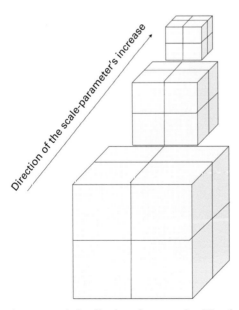

Figure 9.40 A conceptual visualization of representing 3D volumes in scale-space as 4D Laplacian-of-Gaussian hyper-pyramids.

$$\mathcal{P}^3 = \{\mathbf{x} : L(\mathbf{x};t) \lessgtr (\mathbf{x}';t') \forall \mathbf{x}' \in [\mathbf{x}-1, \mathbf{x}+1], t' \in [t_-, t_+], (\mathbf{x}', t') \neq (\mathbf{x}, t)\}, \qquad (9.40)$$

where $\mathcal{P}$ is the set of the detected interest points.

For each voxel $(\mathbf{x}; t)$ in the 4D hyper-pyramid, check its 3×3×3 neighborhood for the same t. $L(\mathbf{x}; t)$ is a local maximum or local minimum if $L(\mathbf{x}; t) >$ maximum of 3×3×3 neighborhood of $(\mathbf{x}; t_+)$ OR $L(\mathbf{x}; t) <$ minimum of 3×3×3 neighborhood of $(\mathbf{x}; t_+)$.

If $L(\mathbf{x}; t) >$ maximum of 3×3×3 neighborhood of $(\mathbf{x}; t_-)$
OR
$L(\mathbf{x}; t) <$ minimum of 3×3×3 neighborhood of $(\mathbf{x}; t_-)$ then add $(\mathbf{x}; t)$ to $\mathcal{P}_3$.

The 3D quadratic fitting of the scale-space Laplacian is shown below:

$$L(\mathbf{x}_t) = L + \frac{\partial L^T}{\partial \mathbf{x}_t}\mathbf{x}_t + 0.5 \mathbf{x}_t^T \frac{\partial^2 L}{\partial \mathbf{x}_t^2} \mathbf{x}_t. \qquad (9.41)$$

In the 3D case, $\mathbf{x}_t = (x, y, z, t)$. The subvoxel/subscale is taken as the extremum of this quadratic:

$$\hat{\mathbf{x}}_t = -\frac{\partial^2 L^{-1}}{\partial \mathbf{x}_t^2} \frac{\partial L}{\partial \mathbf{x}_t}$$

Figure 9.41 illustrates feature detection on 3D models of individual human teeth.

9.5.2 3D descriptor building

The scale-space-based local invariant features can be readily extended to 3D as follows. The gradient magnitude r of each voxel in the neighborhood of an interest point is calculated as follows:

$$r = \sqrt{G_x^2 + G_y^2 + G_z^2}, \qquad (9.42)$$

where G_x, G_y and G_z are the gradient components in the x, y and z directions, respectively. Figure 9.42 illustrates the relation between θ, ϕ and the gradient components.

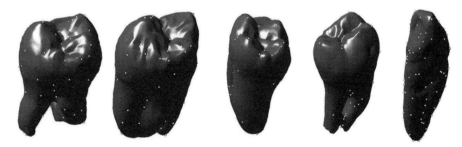

Figure 9.41 Interest point detection in individual 3D human teeth.

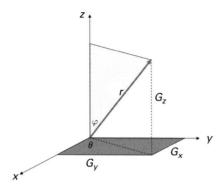

Figure 9.42 Calculation of θ and ϕ using the 3D gradient components.

$$\theta = \tan^{-1} \frac{G_y}{G_x} \qquad (9.43)$$

$$\phi = \sin^{-1} \frac{\sqrt{G_x^2 + G_y^2}}{r} = \cos^{-1} \frac{G_z}{r} \qquad (9.44)$$

Like in the 2D cases, in order to describe the neighborhood of an interest point successfully, the closer voxels should have a larger influence on the descriptor's entries. Therefore, Gaussian weights are assigned to every voxel in the neighborhood of the interest point. Using these Gaussian weights with their mean located at the interest point itself guarantees a distance-weighted contribution to the gradient orientation histogram. Gradient orientations are weighted by the gradient magnitude to reduce the contribution of small-gradient voxels to the histogram.

In order to achieve rotation invariance, a canonical orientation is assigned to each interest point. The canonical orientation is set to the dominant gradient orientation in the neighborhood of the interest point. This dominant gradient orientation is set to the histogram bin with the maximum value. All the descriptor entries are set relative to this canonical orientation. Therefore, the 3D histogram bin (ϕ_i, θ_i) for the ith feature is updated by adding the term $r(x_i, y_i, z_i) g(x_i, y_i, z_i, \sigma)$. The bin to be updated is calculated as follows:

$$\theta_r = \theta - \theta_c \qquad (9.45)$$

$$\phi_r = \phi - \phi_c \qquad (9.46)$$

where θ_c, ϕ_c are the components of the canonical orientation of the interest point and θ, ϕ are the components of the gradient orientation referred to as the zero-axes of the coordinate system, as calculated in Eq. (9.43) and Eq. (9.44). The final descriptor is built as illustrated in Fig. 9.43. This way of describing the gradient orientations of the neighboring voxels guarantees its invariance to rotation changes.

9.5 Three-dimensional local invariant feature descriptors

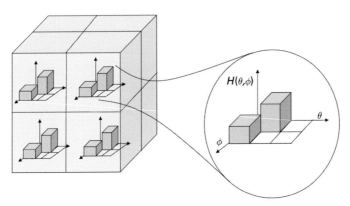

Figure 9.43 The structure of the 3D feature descriptor. Only eight neighboring cells and six histogram bins are shown in the figure for illustration purposes.

In order to prove the rotation invariance property of this descriptor, consider a volume $\mathcal{V}$ with K features, $F(\vec{x_i}) : i \to K$. Let a rotation be applied to the volume. For simplicity, consider the two components of the rotation transformation as $\Delta\theta$ and $\Delta\phi$. Then the canonical orientations of the features become:

$$\theta'_c(x_i) = \theta_c(x_i) + \Delta\theta \tag{9.47}$$

$$\phi'_c(x_i) = \phi_c(x_i) + \Delta\phi \tag{9.48}$$

Similarly, all the gradient orientations of the neighborhood of the interest points are shifted by $\Delta\theta$ and $\Delta\phi$. Then Eq. (9.47) will be:

$$\theta'_i = \theta' - \theta'_c = (\theta + \Delta\theta) - (\theta_c + \Delta\theta) = \theta - \theta_c = \theta_i \tag{9.49}$$

$$\phi'_i = \phi' - \phi'_c = (\phi + \Delta\phi) - (\phi_c + \Delta\phi) = \phi - \phi_c = \phi_i \tag{9.50}$$

Hence, the proposed descriptor is invariant to rotation transformations.

Translation invariance is achieved because every feature descriptor is built using the local neighborhood of its interest point and is independent of the point location. Therefore, translation changes do not affect the descriptor structure.

To prove the illumination intensity invariance, assume a constant intensity change, a bias ΔI, on the images of the volume. Now,

$$I'(\mathbf{x}) = I(\mathbf{x}) + \Delta I. \tag{9.51}$$

The gradients are evaluated as follows:

$$G'_x = \left(I'(x + \Delta x, y, z) - I'(x, y, z)\right)/\Delta x \tag{9.52}$$

$$= \left(9\left[I(x + \Delta x, y, z) + \Delta I\right] - 9\left[I(x, y, z) + \Delta I\right]\right)/\Delta x = G_x \tag{9.53}$$

Similarly, G'_y and G'_z are equal to G_y and G_z, respectively. We note that the gradient orientation and magnitude calculations are not affected by bias. Thus, the feature descriptor is invariant to uniform intensity bias. To reduce the effect of linear intensity changes, the final feature vector is normalized. Furthermore, thresholding the values in the normalized feature vector reduces the influence of large gradient magnitudes.

9.5.3 Descriptor matching

There are several approaches to matching feature descriptors, e.g. the Mahalanobis distance, the Euclidean distance, and the nearest neighborhood matching (e.g. [9.14]). The Euclidean distance is defined as follows:

$$D(F_1, F_2) = ||F_1 - F_2|| = \sqrt{\sum_{i=1}^{M} [9F_1(i) - F_2(i)]^2}, \quad (9.54)$$

where M is the descriptor length, and F_1, F_2 are two features from the first and the second volumes, respectively. Feature F_1 is matched with feature F_2 if:

$$r_D = \frac{D(F_1, F_2)}{\min(D(F_1, F'_2))} < \text{Threshold} < 1 \text{ for all } F'_2 \neq F_2, \quad (9.55)$$

where r_D indicates the matching reliability. As r_D decreases, the matching reliability becomes stronger. We may use $1 - r_D$ as a quantitative matching score.

Examples of matched feature pairs using the 3D SIFT are shown in Fig. 9.44 on 3D models of teeth. The matched points can be used to estimate a transformation between the two 3D models in order to achieve a global registration for the two models. Such techniques will be studied later on in the book.

Feature matching can be also considered on complicated objects that have folds and extreme deformations. For example, Fig. 9.45 shows feature correspondence on segments of the human colon reconstructed from abdominal CT. These correspondences may be used to develop the registration of supine and prone scans (e.g., Hassouna and Farag, [9.44] and Chen et al. [9.45]).

Applications of feature descriptors are abundant in object modeling, categorization, and recognition. Various applications and use of these features will be shown in the following chapter.

9.6 Summary

This chapter has studied feature definition and descriptors as basic ingredients for object modeling. Many of these concepts will be used in the upcoming chapters as we study segmentation and registration. Biomedical objects rarely have a well-defined topology; therefore the robustness of various image analysis methods depends on accurate feature detection and representation (description). The reader should consult the computer vision literature for various details and algorithms on the subject of

9.6 Summary

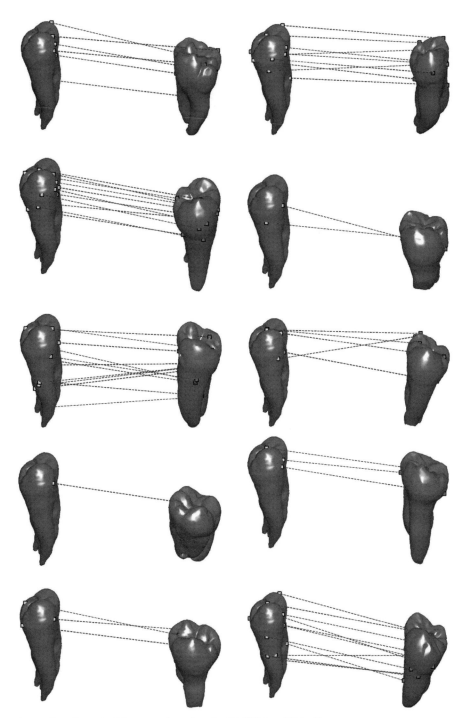

Figure 9.44 Examples of matched feature pairs using the 3D SIFT on 3D teeth.

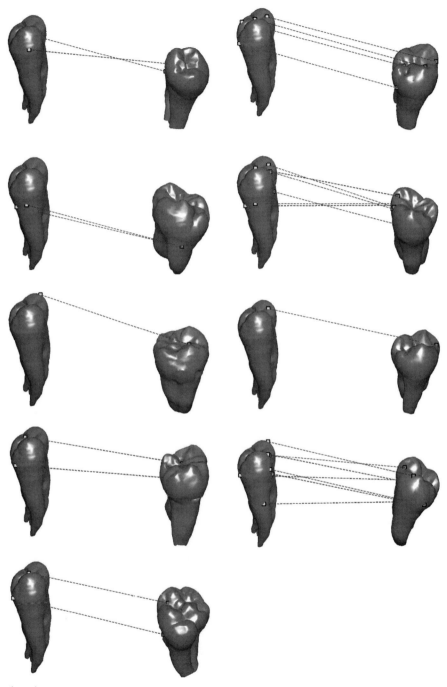

Figure 9.44 (cont.)

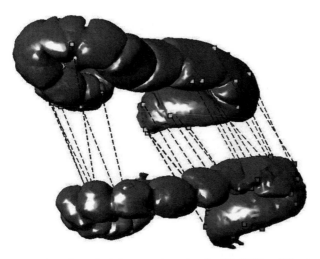

Figure 9.45 Examples of matched feature pairs using the 3D SIFT on 3D colon parts.

feature extraction and description. There are various open-source implementations available for a number of efficient methods on this subject.

9.7 Exercises

9.1 Define the following terms with the help of an example:
(a) Corner, edge, and flat region from the point of view of the Harris approach.
(b) Scale-invariant transformation.
(c) Rotation-invariant transformation.

9.8 Computer laboratory

Task 1 Implementation of edge and corner detection.
(a) Use the MATLAB function "edge" to find the edges of any image with different methods (e.g. Sobel, Marr–Hildreth, Canny).
(b) The Harris corner detector finds corners in an image. Conceptually, corner detection can be thought of as an auto-correlation of an image patch. Consider a window which slides over an image patch. If the image patch is constant or "flat," then there will be little to no intensity change in the window. If the image patch has an edge, then there will be no intensity changes in the window along the direction of the edge. If a corner is present, however, then there will be strong intensity changes in the window regardless of the direction. Implement a Harris corner detector. A helping code that can be used to get the corners is provided below. You can call this function **harris** (imag,2.5,10,10,1);

```
function [cim, r, c] = harris(im, sigma, thresh, radius, disp)
  dx = [-1 0 1; -1 0 1; -1 0 1];           % Derivative masks
  dy = dx';
  Ix = conv2 (im, dx, 'same');             % Image derivatives
  Iy = conv2 (im, dy, 'same');
  g = fspecial ('gaussian', max(1,fix (6*sigma)), sigma);
  Ix2 = conv2 (Ix. ^2, g, 'same');         % Smoothed squared image derivatives
  Iy2 = conv2 (Iy. ^2, g, 'same');
  Ixy = conv2(Ix.*Iy, g, 'same');
  cim = (Ix2. *Iy2–Ixy.^2). / (Ix2 + Iy2 + eps);   % My preferred measure.
```

(c) Generate a set of rotated and resized images (10 images) to test the performance of the Harris detector and then answer these questions. Is it scale-invariant? Is it rotation-invariant?

Task 2 This problem aims at studying the concepts of feature definition and correspondence.

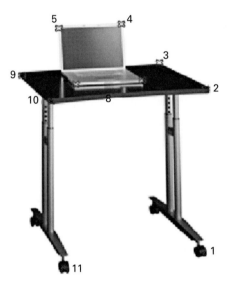

(a) Construct an object using a table and laptop as illustrated.
(b) Use two cameras and perform passive camera calibration. Describe the process briefly and use a suitable calibration pattern.
(c) Construct a stereo imaging mechanism, such that the object will be in the field of view of the two cameras (already calibrated in (b)).
(d) Manually determine the coordinates of the 12 corner points in your images.
(e) Calculate the corners by the Harris corner detector. Compare the position of the corner with the ground truth.

(f) Construct the 12 feature descriptors using the SIFT, ASIFT, and SURF approaches. You may use any available software.

(g) Do you obtain different numbers of features for each method?

(h) Are there parameters leading to similar results for all three methods?

(i) Are the feature points located in the same regions?

(j) Use the different images provided. Can you still detect the same feature points?

(k) Write a code to match interest points.

(l) Reduce the matches based on the best score you have found. Search for the best score and keep only matches with at most twice the best score.

(m) Display the best matches for different thresholds. Can you obtain only correct matches?

Task 3 Use the RANSAC algorithm on the image in the previous task to obtain the following:

(a) Choose *three* matches (at random or all combinations) and calculate an affine transformation from the book to the library image.

(b) Calculate inliers as points transformed from the book image to the library images, that lie within a given pixel distance (use 10 or 20 pixels).

(c) Select the affine transformation with the most inliers and draw all matches of inliers.

(d) Use the affine transformation you found and warp the left image to the right image. Does it work for all images? If not, what may be the reason?

References

[9.1] D. G. Lowe, Distinctive image features from scale-invariant keypoints. *Int. J. Computer Vision*, **60**(2) (2004) 91–110.

[9.2] T. Tuytelaars and L. Van Gool, Matching widely separated views based on affine invariant regions, *Int. J. Computer Vision*, **1**(59) (2004) 61–85.

[9.3] C. Schmid and R. Mohr, Local grayvalue invariants for image retrieval. *IEEE Trans. Pattern Anal. Machine Intel.* **19**(5) (1997) 530–535.

[9.4] K. Mikolajczyk, T. Tuytelaars, C. Schmid *et al.*, A comparison of affine region detectors. *Int. J. Computer Vision* **65**(1/2) (2005) 43–72.

[9.5] M. Brown and D. Lowe, Recognising panoramas, *Proc. Ninth Int. Conf. Computer Vision* (2003) 1218–1227.

[9.6] C. Schmid, R. Mohr and C. Bauckhage, Evaluation of interest point detectors. *Int. J. Computer Vision* **37**(2) (2000) 151–172.

[9.7] K. Mikolajczyk and C. Schmid, A performance evaluation of local descriptors. *IEEE Trans. Pattern Anal. Machine Intel.* **27**(10) (2005) 1615–1630.

[9.8] J. Hafner, H. S. Sawhney, W. Equitz *et al.*, Efficient color histogram indexing for quadratic form distance functions. *IEEE Trans. Pattern Anal Machine Intel.* **17**(7) (1995) 729–736.

[9.9] S. Belongie, J. Malik and J. Puzicha, Shape matching and object recognition using shape contexts. *IEEE Trans. Pattern Anal. Machine Intel* **24**(4) (2002) 509–522.

[9.10] S. Nayar and R. Bolle, Reflectance based object recognition. *Int. J. Computer Vision* **17**(3) (1996) 219–240.

[9.11] A. Pentland, R. W. Picard and S. Sclaroff, Photobook: content-based manipulation of image databases. *Int. J. Computer Vision* **18**(3) (1996) 233–254.

[9.12] J. Canny, A computational approach to edge detection. *IEEE Trans. Pattern Anal. Machine Intel* **8**(6) (1986) 679–698.

[9.13] C. Harris and M. Stephens, A combined corner and edge detector. *Proc. Fourth Alvey Vision Conf.* (1988) 147–152.

[9.14] T. Lindeberg, *Scale-Space Theory in Computer Vision*. Norwell, MA: Kluwer Academic (1994).

[9.15] S. Belongie, J. Malik and J. Puzicha, Shape context: a new descriptor for shape matching and object recognition. In Leen, T. K., Dietterich, T. G. and Tresp, V. (eds.) *Advances in Neural Information Processing Systems 13*. MIT Press (2001) 831–837.

[9.16] Y. Zhang, M. Brady and S. Smith, Segmentation of brain MR images through a hidden Markov random field model and the expectation maximization algorithm. *IEEE Trans. Medical Imaging* **20**(1) (2001) 45–57.

[9.17] K. Mikolajczyk and C. Schmid, An affine invariant interest point detector. *Proc. 7th Eur. Conf. Computer Vision-Part I (ECCV '02)*. Copenhagen: Springer (2002) 128–142.

[9.18] K. Mikolajczyk and C. Schmid, Scale and affine invariant interest point detectors. *Int. J. Computer Vision* **60**(1) (2004) 63–86.

[9.19] T. Kadir and M. Brady, Scale, saliency and image description. *Int. J. Computer Vision* **45**(2) (2001). 83–105.

[9.20] J. Matas, O. Chum, M. Urban and T. Pajdla, Robust wide-baseline stereo from maximally stable extremal regions. In *Proc. British Machine Vision Conf.Cardiff, UK* (2002) 384–393.

[9.21] A. Klinger, Pattern and search statistics. In J. S. Rustagi (ed.) *Optimizing Methods in Statistics*. New York: Academic Press (1971).

[9.22] I. Daubechies, Orthonormal bases of compactly supported wavelets. *Comm. Pure Appl. Math.* **41** (1988) 909–996.

[9.23] A. Witkin, Scale-space filtering. *Int. Joint Conf. Artificial Intelligence, Karlsruhe, Germany* (1983) 1019–1022.

[9.24] J. Koenderink, The structure of images. *Biol. Cybernet.* **50** (1984) 363–370.

[9.25] K. Kanatani, *Group Theoretical Methods in Image Understanding*. Secaucus, NJ: Springer (1990).

[9.26] L. Florack, B. Haar Romeny, J. Koenderink and M. Viergever, Cartesian differential invariants in scale-space. *J. Math. Imaging Vision* **3**(4) (1993). 327–348.

[9.27] J. Bruce and P. Giblin, *Curves and Singularities*. Cambridge: Cambridge University Press (1984).

[9.28] L. A. Shepp and B. F. Logan, The Fourier reconstruction of a head section. *IEEE Trans. Nucl. Sci.* (**21**) (1974) 21–43.

[9.29] J. M. Morel and G. Yu, ASIFT: A new framework for fully affine invariant image comparison. *SIAM J. Imaging Sci.* **2**(2) (2009) 438–469.

[9.30] A. Abdel-Hakim and A. Farag, CSIFT: A SIFT descriptor with color invariant characteristics. *IEEE Conf. Computer Vision and Pattern Recognition (CVPR06)*, New York City, 17–22 June (2006). 1978–1983.

[9.31] M. Brown and S. Süsstrunk, Multispectral SIFT for Scene Category Recognition. *Proc. IEEE Int. Conf. Computer Vision and Pattern Recognition (CVPR2011), Colorado Springs* (2011) 177–184.

[9.32] M. A. Fischler and R. C. Bolles, Random sample consensus: a paradigm for model fitting with applications to image analysis and automated cartography. *Comm. ACM* **24**(6) (1981) 381–395.

[9.33] H. Bay, A. Ess, T. Tuytelaars and L. Van Gool, Speeded-Up Robust Features (SURF), *Computer Vision Image Understand.* **110** (3) (2008) 346–359.

[9.34] T. Ojala, M. Pietikainen and T. Maenpaa, Multiresolution gray-scale and rotation invariant texture classification with local binary patterns. *IEEE Trans. Pattern Anal. Machine Intel.* **24** (2002) 971–987.

[9.35] Amal Farag, S. Elhabian, J. Graham, Aly Farag and R. Falk, Toward precise pulmonary nodule descriptors for nodule type classification. *Proc. 13th Int. Conf. Medical Image Computing and Computer Assisted Intervention (MICCAI), Beijing, China* (2010) 626–633.

[9.36] Amal Farag, Modeling small size objects under uncertainty: novel algorithms and applications. Unpublished Ph.D. dissertation, CVIP Lab., University of Louisville, May 2012.

[9.37] A. Farag, A. El-Baz, G. Gimel'farb and A. Abdel-Hakim, Robust image registration based on Markov–Gibbs appearance model. In *IEEE Int. Conf. Pattern Recognition ICPR06, Hong Kong, August 20–24* (2006) 1204–1207.

[9.38] R. Hartley and A. Zisserman, *Multiple View Geometry in Computer Vision.* Cambridge: Cambridge University Press (2003).

[9.39] M. N. Ahmed, S. M. Yamany, E. E. Hemayed and A. A. Farag, 3D reconstruction of the human jaw from a sequence of images, *IEEE Int. Conf. Computer Vision and Pattern Recognition (CVPR'97), Puerto Rico* (1997) 646–653.

[9.40] S. M. Yamany, A. A. Farag, D. Tasman and A. G. Farman, Robust 3-D modeling of the human jaw using sequence of intra-oral images. *IEEE Trans. Med. Imaging* **19**(5) (2000) 538–547.

[9.41] A. Farag and A. Eid, Video reconstructions in dentistry, *Orthod Craniofacial Res.* **6** (Suppl. 1) (2003) 108–116.

[9.42] A. Farag, S. Yamany and D. Tasman, US Patent 7084868: System and method for 3-D digital reconstruction of an oral cavity from sequence of 2-D images. Issued 8/1/2006.

[9.43] A. Abdelrahim, M. Abderahman, H. Abdelmunim, A. Farag and M. Miller, Novel image-based 3D reconstruction of the human jaw using shape from shading and feature descriptors, *22nd British Machine Vision Conf. (BMVC)*, **41** (2011) 1–11.

[9.44] M. Sabry Hassouna and A. Farag, PDE-based three dimensional path planning for virtual endoscopy. *Proc. Information Processing in Medical Imaging (IPMI), Glenwood Springs, CO, July 11–15* (2005) 529–540.

[9.45] D. Chen, A. Farag, R. Falk and G. Dryden, Variational approach based image pre-processing techniques for virtual colonoscopy. In Gonzalez, F. and Romero, E. (eds.) *Biomedical Image Analysis and Machine Learning Technologies: Application and Techniques*, Hershey, PA: Medical Information Science Reference (2009) Chapter 4.

Part IV

Variational approaches and level sets

10 Variational approaches and level sets

Objects captured in a scene may intersect and occlude each other in the field of view of an imaging sensor, and may suffer from uncertainties in the imaging process. The object shape may be described by its outline (contour). There exists a rich image analysis literature on approaches to extract the contours of objects. This chapter will focus on deformable models and *level set* methods to extract object contours. Active contours are curves that deform within an object representation (e.g., a digital image) in order to recover the object shape. They are classified as *parametric* or *geometric*, according to their representation and implementation. In particular, *parametric active contours* are represented explicitly in terms of parameterized curves in a *Lagrangian* formulation (e.g. [10.1],[10.2]). On the other hand, *geometric active contours* are represented implicitly as level sets of 2D distance functions, which evolve according to an *Eulerian* formulation. They are based on the theory of curve evolution implemented via level set techniques. Parametric active contours are the older of the two formulations.

Geometric active contours, also known as level set methods (LSM), handle topological changes during curve evolution (e.g. [10.3]). They describe an object contour by considering it as a slice through a higher-dimensional object known as the level set function. The contour intersects the level set function at the x–y plane, which is known as the zero-level set. Contour motion normal to the level set is given by a *Hamilton–Jacobi* partial differential equation (PDE). This chapter discusses the mathematical foundation of classical deformable models and level sets. LSM can be used for 2D or 3D object representations, and can address various topological and geometrical characteristics of the objects. These methods lead to solutions in the continuous domain [10.4][10.5]. Deformable models and LSM have been successful in image analysis, especially image segmentation and registration [10.6–10.11].

10.1 Calculus of variation and Euler equation

The variational formulation of level sets is based on finding a variable or function that minimizes a given energy. The Euler–Lagrange equation is the basic formulation for solving this problem [10.4][10.5]. Given an energy E, finding the function $\phi: \mathbf{R} \to \mathbf{R}$ that minimizes E can be expressed as:

$$E(\phi) = \int_\Omega F d\Omega \tag{10.1}$$

$$\phi = \arg\min_\phi E(\phi) \tag{10.2}$$

where F is integrable over the domain Ω and is a function of Ω and ϕ. In this context, we will next look at the derivation of the Euler–Lagrange equation for different cases.

10.1.1 Euler–Lagrange equation for one independent variable

Let us define an energy functional as a definite integral of a scalar function $F(x, \phi, \phi_x)$:

$$E = \int_a^b F(x, \phi, \phi_x) dx \tag{10.3}$$

where $\phi_x = \dfrac{d\phi}{dx}$ and $a, b \in \boldsymbol{R}$ are scalars. To find an extremal value for E, the Taylor series expansion is used around the value $\bar{\phi}$:

$$E(\phi + \Delta\phi) = E(\phi) + \Delta\phi\, \delta E(\phi) + \cdots. \tag{10.4}$$

We note that ϕ is a function, not a variable, which contradicts the use of the Taylor's series expansion. The problem can be resolved for a 1D case as follows. If $\bar{\phi} = \bar{\phi}(x)$ minimizes E, then the following condition has to be achieved:

$$\delta E(\bar{\phi}) = 0 \tag{10.5}$$

Assume the variations of ϕ around $\bar{\phi}$ can be written as:

$$\phi(x) = \bar{\phi}(x) + \varepsilon\eta(x) \tag{10.6}$$

where ε is a small arbitrary constant and η is an arbitrary function with the constraint $\eta(a) = \eta(b) = 0$. The derivative can be written as:

$$\phi_x(x) = \bar{\phi}_x(x) + \varepsilon\eta_x(x) \tag{10.7}$$

The use of η converts the problem into an infinite-dimensional problem (taking infinite points around $\bar{\phi}$). The zero derivative condition can be written as:

$$\delta E(\bar{\phi}) = \frac{d}{d\varepsilon} E(\bar{\phi} + \varepsilon\eta)\bigg|_{\varepsilon=0} = 0. \tag{10.8}$$

The variables x, a, and b are independent of ε. Using Leibnitz's rule, the derivative can be moved inside the integral sign, resulting in:

$$\delta E(\bar{\phi}) = \int_a^b \left(\frac{\partial F}{\partial \phi} \frac{\partial \phi}{\partial \varepsilon} + \frac{\partial F}{\partial \phi_x} \frac{\partial \phi_x}{\partial \varepsilon} \right) dx. \tag{10.9}$$

and by integration by parts and setting $\eta = \dfrac{\partial \varphi}{\partial \varepsilon}$, the above equation can be rewritten in the form:

$$\int_a^b \left(\frac{\partial F}{\partial \phi} - \frac{d}{dx} \frac{\partial F}{\partial \phi_x} \right) \eta(x) dx + \eta(x) \frac{\partial F}{\partial \phi_x} \bigg|_a^b = 0 \qquad (10.10)$$

Taking into consideration that $\eta(a) = \eta(b) = 0$, the following relation is achieved:

$$\int_a^b \left(\frac{\partial F}{\partial \phi} - \frac{d}{dx} \frac{\partial F}{\partial \phi_x} \right) \eta(x) dx = 0 \qquad (10.11)$$

and the following condition must be satisfied:

$$\frac{\partial F}{\partial \phi} - \frac{d}{dx} \frac{\partial F}{\partial \phi_x} = 0 \qquad (10.12)$$

The above equation is the Euler–Lagrange equation for the 1D problem.

10.1.2 Euler–Lagrange equation for multiple independent variables

In this case the dependent variable $\phi: R^n \to R$, where n is the space dimension. The function F will have a more complicated expression:

$$F = F(x_i, \phi, \phi_{x_i}, \phi_{x_i x_j}), \quad \forall \ i, j \in [1, n] \qquad (10.13)$$

We can write the extremal condition as follows:

$$\int_{a_1}^{b_1} \cdots \int_{a_n}^{b_n} \left(\frac{\partial F}{\partial \phi} \frac{\partial \phi}{\partial \varepsilon} + \sum_{i=1}^n \frac{\partial F}{\partial \phi_{x_i}} \frac{\partial \phi_{x_i}}{\partial \varepsilon} + \sum_{i=1}^n \sum_{j=1}^n \frac{\partial F}{\partial \phi_{x_i x_j}} \frac{\partial \phi_{x_i x_j}}{\partial \varepsilon} \right) dx_1 \ldots dx_n = 0 \qquad (10.14)$$

The first-order derivative term k can be replaced by integration by parts, resulting in:

$$\int_{a_1}^{b_1} \cdots \int_{a_n}^{b_n} \left(\frac{\partial F}{\partial \phi_{x_k}} \frac{\partial \phi_{x_k}}{\partial \varepsilon} \right) dx_1 \ldots = -\int_{a_1}^{b_1} \cdots \int_{a_n}^{b_n} \left(\frac{d}{dx_k} \frac{\partial F}{\partial \phi_{x_k}} \right) \frac{\partial \phi}{\partial \varepsilon} dx_1 \ldots dx_n \qquad (10.15)$$

The second derivative term $k \geq h$ ($h \in [1,n]$) is also replaced as follows:

$$\int_{a_1}^{b_1} \cdots \int_{a_n}^{b_n} \left(\frac{\partial F}{\partial \phi_{x_h x_k}} \frac{\partial \phi_{x_h x_k}}{\partial \varepsilon} \right) dx_1 \ldots = -\int_{a_1}^{b_1} \cdots \int_{a_n}^{b_n} \left(\frac{d}{dx_h} \frac{\partial F}{\partial \phi_{x_h x_k}} \right) \frac{\partial \phi_{x_k}}{\partial \varepsilon} dx_1 \ldots dx_n$$

$$= \int_{a_1}^{b_1} \cdots \int_{a_n}^{b_n} \left(\frac{d^2}{dx_h dx_k} \frac{\partial F}{\partial \phi_{x_h x_k}} \right) \frac{\partial \phi}{\partial \varepsilon} dx_1 \ldots dx_n \qquad (10.16)$$

taking into consideration that $\eta(a_1,\ldots,a_n) = \eta(b_1,\ldots,b_n) = 0$ and $\eta_{x_i}(a_1,\ldots,a_n) = \eta_{x_i}(b_1,\ldots,b_n) = 0$ for all $i \in [1, n]$.

Gathering the above equations will lead to the following Euler–Lagrange equation:

$$\frac{\partial F}{\partial \phi} - \sum_{i=1}^{n} \frac{d}{dx_i} \frac{\partial F}{\partial \phi_{x_i}} + \sum_{i=1}^{n} \sum_{j=1}^{n} \frac{d^2}{dx_i dx_j} \frac{\partial F}{\partial \phi_{x_i x_j}} = 0 \qquad (10.17)$$

In the case of more than one dependent variable in the form of $\Phi : R^n \to R^m$ or in a vector form $\Phi = [\phi_1 \ldots \phi_m]^T$, the above equation can be directly transformed to the following vector equation:

$$\frac{\partial F}{\partial \Phi} - \sum_{i=1}^{n} \frac{d}{dx_i} \frac{\partial F}{\partial \Phi_{x_i}} + \sum_{i=1}^{n} \sum_{j=1}^{n} \frac{d^2}{dx_i dx_j} \frac{\partial F}{\partial \Phi_{x_i x_j}} = 0 \qquad (10.18)$$

where

$$\frac{\partial F}{\partial \Phi} = \left[\frac{\partial F}{\partial \phi_1} \ldots \frac{\partial F}{\partial \phi_m} \right]^T \qquad (10.19)$$

In case of adding constraints, the restriction is put into the form of an equation (e.g., $\int U dx_1 \ldots dx_n = \alpha$, where α is an arbitrary constant). The condition is added to the original function using a mixing parameter λ to form a new energy as follows:

$$\hat{E} = E + \lambda \left(\int U dx_1 \ldots dx_n - \alpha \right)^2 \qquad (10.20)$$

10.1.3 Euler–Lagrange and the gradient descent flow

The Euler–Lagrange equations lead to the derivative of the energy E with respect to a set of variables (unknowns) $\mathbf{P} = [P_1 \ldots P_m]^T$:

$$\frac{\partial E}{\partial \mathbf{P}} = \mathbf{0} \qquad (10.21)$$

In limited situations, these unknowns have a closed form solution. One general technique to solve this problem is gradient descent flow by adding the time parameter to drive the change of the unknown towards the extremal point:

$$\frac{\partial \mathbf{P}}{\partial t} = -\frac{\partial E}{\partial \mathbf{P}} \qquad (10.22)$$

where the minus sign is for the minimum point. The variables/functions change with time starting with $\mathbf{P}_0$ (initial values) to reach the point where $\frac{\partial E}{\partial \mathbf{P}} = 0$ at steady state, and a solution for the Euler–Lagrange is obtained. The solution of the given PDE is unique when the objective energy function is convex. If the function is non-convex, more than one solution is obtained depending on the initialization $\mathbf{P}_0$.

10.2 Curve/surface evolution via classical deformable models

10.2.1 Curves and planar differential geometry

We start with a few basic definitions related to curves and surfaces [10.5].

DEFINITION 10.1 *A planar curve is defined in parametric form as* $\mathbf{C}(p): [0,1] \to \mathbf{R}^2$. *This vector represents the coordinates of each point as functions of p.*

DEFINITION 10.2 *The curve is* self intersecting *when* $\mathbf{C}(p_1) = \mathbf{C}(p_2)$ *and* $p_1 \neq p_2$. *Otherwise it is said to be* simple. *The curve is said to be* closed *if the start and end points are identical, i.e.* $\mathbf{C}(0) = \mathbf{C}(1)$.

DEFINITION 10.3 *The* tangent vector *is the derivative vector with respect to the parameter p, and is defined as closed if* $\frac{\partial}{\partial p}\mathbf{C} = \mathbf{C}_p$. *The unit tangent vector can be written as* $\hat{\mathbf{T}} = [x_p \ y_p]^T / \sqrt{x_p^2 + y_p^2}$. *The normal is* $\hat{\mathbf{N}} = [y_p \ -x_p]^T / \sqrt{x_p^2 + y_p^2}$. ∎

DEFINITION 10.4 *The Euclidean* arc-length *measured from the starting point of the curve is calculated by:*

$$s(p) = \int_0^p \sqrt{x_p^2 + y_p^2}\,dp. \blacksquare \tag{10.23}$$

The Euclidean arc-length does not change on rotation and translation of the planar curve. Changing the parameterization from p to s results in $\mathbf{C}_s = \mathbf{C}_p \frac{dp}{ds} = \hat{\mathbf{T}}$ and $|\mathbf{C}_s| = 1$, which means that the point vector moves with a unit velocity magnitude in the arc-length direction. The vector derivative is intrinsic and geometric.

DEFINITION 10.5 *The* curvature $\kappa = \kappa(s)$ *meaures the directional changes of a curve or surface in terms of its first and second directional derivatives at a point s.* ∎

The curvature of a curve is the rate at which that curve turns. Since the tangent line or the velocity vector shows the direction of the curve, this means that the curvature is the rate at which the tangent line or velocity vector is turning. For example, a circle has a constant curvature because it is always turning at the same rate; a smaller circle has a higher constant curvature because it turns faster.

DEFINITION 10.6 *The second derivative is defined as follows:*

$$\mathbf{C}_{ss} = \left(\frac{\partial}{\partial p}\frac{\mathbf{C}_p}{|\mathbf{C}_p|}\right)\frac{dp}{ds} = \kappa \hat{\mathbf{N}}. \blacksquare \tag{10.24}$$

The second derivative of the point vector is along the normal direction, and it depends on the curvature at the given point, defined as follows:

$$\kappa = \frac{(\mathbf{C}_p, \mathbf{C}_{pp})}{|\mathbf{C}_p|^3} \tag{10.25}$$

where $([a\ b]^T, [c\ d]^T) = ad - bc$, which represents the area of the parallelogram formed by the two vectors (magnitude of their vector product). This representation is affected when a transformation is applied to the curve with different scales, rotation, and translation. The relation $|(\mathbf{C}_s, \mathbf{C}_{ss})| = |\kappa|$ holds and is affected when an affine transformation with scales changes the curve.

If the arc-length s is replaced by the relation $z = z(u,v)$ in order to obtain an *equi-affine* representation, then the first derivative with respect to s will be:

$$\frac{dv}{ds} = |(\mathbf{C}_s, \mathbf{C}_{ss})|^{1/3} \qquad (10.26)$$
$$= |\kappa|^{1/3}$$

The affine tangent will be $\mathbf{C}_v = |\kappa|^{-1/3}\hat{\mathbf{T}}$. Therefore,

$$\begin{aligned}
\mathbf{C}_{vv} &= \frac{\partial}{\partial v}\left(\mathbf{C}_s \frac{\partial s}{\partial v}\right) \\
&= \mathbf{C}_{ss}\left(\frac{\partial s}{\partial v}\right)^2 + \mathbf{C}_s \frac{\partial^2 s}{\partial v^2} \qquad (10.27) \\
&= |\kappa|^{1/3}\hat{\mathbf{N}} + \frac{\partial^2 s}{\partial v^2}\hat{\mathbf{T}}
\end{aligned}$$

As a result of this representation the relation $|(\mathbf{C}_v, \mathbf{C}_{vv})| = 1$ is obtained, which does not depend on the curve properties. We note that the Euclidean *arc-length* and the *curvature* are considered unique signatures.

10.2.2 Geometry of surfaces

Curves can be embedded in surfaces as a higher-dimensional representation, and surfaces can also be embedded into higher-dimensional functions. Consider a regular surface $\mathbf{S}(u, v): R^2 \to R^3$, where $(u, v) \in [0, 1] \times [0, 1]$. $\mathbf{S}$ can be written in vector form as $\mathbf{S}(u, v) = [x\ y\ z]^T$. Note that each coordinate projection is a function of the two parameters (u, v), i.e. $x = x(u, v)$, $y = y(u, v)$, and $z = z(u, v)$. The surface is assumed to have derivatives with respect to the parameters; i.e.

$$\frac{\partial}{\partial \mathbf{P}}\mathbf{S} = \begin{pmatrix} x_u & x_v \\ y_u & y_v \\ z_u & z_v \end{pmatrix} \qquad (10.28)$$

where $\mathbf{P} = [u\ v]^T$. The vectors $\mathbf{S}_u$ and $\mathbf{S}_v$ are in the tangent plane. The *surface area*, which is an intrinsic quantity, can be calculated as follows:

$$A = \int_0^1 \int_0^1 |\mathbf{S}_u \times \mathbf{S}_v|\ du dv, \qquad (10.29)$$

where $\mathbf{S}_u \times \mathbf{S}_v$ is the surface normal vector.

10.2.3 Geodesic curvature

Consider a parameterized curve $\mathbf{C}(s)$, embedded into the parameterized surface $\mathbf{S}$. The acceleration vector $\mathbf{C}_{ss}$ can be put into the following form:

$$\mathbf{C}_{ss} = \kappa_g \hat{\mathbf{T}}_1 + \kappa_n \hat{\mathbf{N}} \tag{10.30}$$

where in this case $\hat{\mathbf{N}} = \dfrac{\mathbf{S}_u \times \mathbf{S}_v}{|\mathbf{S}_u \times \mathbf{S}_v|}$ is the unit normal vector to the surface, and $\hat{\mathbf{T}}_1$ is the unit surface tangential vector which lies in the same plane of $\mathbf{C}_{ss}$ and the surface normal. The tangential component is called the *geodesic curvature* κ_g and the other component is called the *normal curvature* κ_n. All curves with the condition $\kappa_g = 0$ are called *geodesics*.

10.2.4 Principal curvatures

Principal curvatures are the maximum and minimum normal curvatures κ_1 and κ_2 at any point on the surface. They measure the amount of bending of the surface. The *Gaussian curvature* K is the product of the maximum and minimum curvatures, whereas the *mean curvature* H is their arithmetic mean; that is,

$$K = \kappa_1 \kappa_2 \tag{10.31}$$

$$H = \frac{1}{2}(\kappa_1 + \kappa_2) \tag{10.32}$$

The above two equations can be solved together to obtain expressions for the maximum and minimum curvatures:

$$\kappa_1 = H + \sqrt{H^2 - K}, \tag{10.33}$$

$$\kappa_2 = H - \sqrt{H^2 - K}. \tag{10.34}$$

10.2.5 Planar curves and surface normal

Consider the planar curve resulting from intersection of the surface $\mathbf{S}$ with the x–y plane. The surface is parameterized as defined above, and its height has the relation $z = \phi(x, y)$. The curve may be described as $\mathbf{C} = \{[x\, y]^T : \phi(x\, y) = 0\}$. The normal vector resulting from the vector product of the two tangential vectors in the u and v directions has the following expression:

$$\mathbf{N} = \mathbf{S}_u \times \mathbf{S}_v = \begin{pmatrix} y_u z_v - y_v z_u \\ x_v z_u - x_u z_v \\ x_u y_v - x_v y_u \end{pmatrix}. \tag{10.35}$$

Substituting for $z_u = \phi_x x_u + \phi_y y_u$ and $z_v = \phi_x x_v + \phi_y y_v$, results in:

$$\mathbf{N} = (x_u y_v - x_v y_u) \begin{pmatrix} \phi_x \\ \phi_y \\ -1 \end{pmatrix} \tag{10.36}$$

and the unit surface normal will be:

$$\hat{\mathbf{N}} = \frac{\text{sgn}(x_u y_v - x_v y_u)}{\sqrt{\phi_x^2 + \phi_y^2 + 1}} \begin{pmatrix} \phi_x \\ \phi_y \\ -1 \end{pmatrix}, \tag{10.37}$$

where sgn(.) is the sign function. The projection of the above vector in the x–y plane will also be normal to the associated implicit planar curve. The unit normal vector in the plane can be calculated in terms of the implicit function gradient and its magnitude as follows:

$$\hat{\mathbf{n}} = \frac{1}{\sqrt{\phi_x^2 + \phi_y^2}} \begin{pmatrix} \phi_x \\ \phi_y \end{pmatrix} \tag{10.38}$$

which is directly equivalent to:

$$\hat{\mathbf{n}} = \frac{\nabla \phi}{|\nabla \phi|} \tag{10.39}$$

We can show that the curvature of any point on the planar curve is related to the unit normal by the divergence operator as follows:

$$\kappa = \text{div}(\hat{\mathbf{n}}) \tag{10.40}$$

The representation in Equation (10.40) is also applicable for implicit surfaces in higher dimensions.

10.2.6 Curve/surface evolution as a variational problem

A deformable model (often known as a snake) is defined as a parametric contour embedded in the image plane (x,y) [10.2]. The contour is required to evolve so that it covers the desired object in the image $I(x, y)$ and minimizes a certain energy function defined as follows:

$$E(\mathbf{C}) = E_{\text{internal}}(\mathbf{C}) + E_{\text{external}}(\mathbf{C}). \tag{10.41}$$

The first term is defined as the internal energy which characterizes the deformation of the contour and may be expressed as follows:

10.2 Curve/surface evolution via classical deformable models

$$E_{\text{internal}}(\mathbf{C}) = \frac{1}{2}\int_0^1 \left(w_1(p)|\mathbf{C}_p|^2 + w_2(p)|\mathbf{C}_{pp}|^2 \right) dp. \tag{10.42}$$

The non-negative values w_1, w_2 have an important role in controlling the stretching and bending of the contour. The length of the contour is reduced by increasing w_1 which removes the ripples and loops. Larger values of w_2 increase the bending and make the contour smoother.

The external energy term is the force that drives the contour towards the object boundaries. The edge is one of the object features that is used to design that term. Using the calculus of variations, the contour evolves according to the following vector-valued PDE:

$$\mathbf{C}_t = \left(-\frac{\partial}{\partial p}(w_1 \mathbf{C}_p) - \frac{\partial}{\partial p}(w_2 \mathbf{C}_{pp}) \right) - \nabla_\mathbf{C} E_{\text{external}}. \tag{10.43}$$

The above energy function is redefined for a deformable surface as follows:

$$E_{\text{internal}}(\mathbf{S}) = \frac{1}{2}\int_0^1 \int_0^1 (w_{10}(u,v)|\mathbf{S}_u|^2 + w_{01}(u,v)|\mathbf{S}_v|^2 \\ + w_{20}(u,v)|\mathbf{S}_{uu}|^2 + 2w_{11}(u,v)|\mathbf{S}_{uv}|^2 + w_{02}(u,v)|\mathbf{S}_{vv}|^2) du dv. \tag{10.44}$$

This functional is the natural 2D generalization of the snake energy. The physical parameters w_{ij} control the tension and rigidity of the deformable surface [10.3, 10.7].

10.2.7 Discretization and numerical simulation of snakes

Discretization of the energy is required to obtain the minimum, or to calculate how the unknown vectors change with time. The conventional approach is to express the vector $\mathbf{C}$ in terms of support functions. Finite elements and finite differences can be used. The continuous vector $\mathbf{C}$ is represented by $\mathbf{v}$ (essentially the velocity of changes in $\mathbf{C}$) with shape parameters associated with the basis functions. The energy can be written in the form:

$$E(\mathbf{v}) = \frac{1}{2}\mathbf{v}^T \mathbf{K} \mathbf{v} + E_{\text{external}} \tag{10.45}$$

where $\mathbf{K}$ is called the stiffness matrix. The solution of the system results from setting the gradient of the above equation to 0 as follows:

$$\mathbf{K}\mathbf{v} + \nabla E_{\text{external}} = 0 \tag{10.46}$$

Then the problem is transformed to an algebraic equation form. Applying the finite differences to Eq. (10.45), we will have nodes $\mathbf{v}_i = \mathbf{C}(ih)\ \forall\ i = 0, \ldots N-1$ where $h = 1/(N-1)$, $\mathbf{C}_p = (\mathbf{v}_{i+1} - \mathbf{v}_i)/h$, and $\mathbf{C}_{pp} = (\mathbf{v}_{i+1} - 2\mathbf{v}_i + \mathbf{v}_{i-1})/h^2$. The stiffness matrix will be:

$$\mathbf{K} = \begin{pmatrix} a_0 & b_0 & c_0 & & & & c_{N-2} & b_{N-1} \\ b_0 & a_1 & b_1 & c_1 & & & & c_{N-1} \\ c_0 & b_1 & a_2 & b_2 & c_2 & & & \\ & c_1 & b_2 & a_3 & b_3 & c_3 & & \\ & & \cdot & \cdot & \cdot & \cdot & \cdot & \\ & & & \cdot & \cdot & \cdot & \cdot & \\ b_{N-1} & c_{N-1} & & & & b_{N-1} & a_{N-1} \end{pmatrix} \qquad (10.47)$$

The contour is assumed to be closed, and the matrix element can be calculated by:

$$a_i = (w_{1i-1} + w_{1i})/h^2 + (w_{2i-1} + 4w_{2i} + w_{2i+1})/h^4 \qquad (10.48)$$

$$b_i = -w_{1i}/h^2 - 2(w_{2i} + w_{2i+1})/h^4 \qquad (10.49)$$

$$c_i = w_{2i+1}/h^4 \qquad (10.50)$$

The parametric deformable models are used efficiently in many applications (e.g. [10.7]). However, they have many disadvantages. The model depends on the parameterization, which causes problems with topology changes. Also, the initialization needs to be near the steady state solution, which represents a big problem in 3D.

10.3 Level sets

The level set representation was proposed by Osher and Sethian (e.g. [10.3]) to overcome the problems of classical deformable models. Topology changes, such as merging and splitting, are handled naturally without the need for parameterization. Efficient and stable numerical schemes have been developed for implementation of the level set method (LSM) both in 2D and 3D. The LSM has found appreciation in various image analysis applications (e.g. [10.6]–[10.11]). In this section, we will study the definition of the level set function, ϕ, and numerical simulation of the curve/surface evolution problem.

10.3.1 Implicit representation and the evolution PDE

Consider a curve Γ that can be embedded into a higher-dimensional function ϕ as $\Gamma = \{\mathbf{X} : \phi(\mathbf{X}) = 0\}$; this curve is defined as the zero level of the function. When dealing with evolving curves (fronts), we need to add time as another variable, so the function changes to $\phi = \phi(\mathbf{X}, t)$. For a unimodal object Γ, the size of the zero-level set changes as $\phi(\mathbf{X}, t)$ changes with t. For example, as shown in Fig. 10.1, the circles (ellipses) describing the zero-level set change in diameter as t changes. In general, $\phi(\mathbf{X}, t)$ captures the topology of the propagating front as t changes. In this way, the merging/splitting problem can be

10.3 Level sets

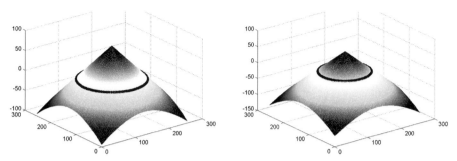

Figure 10.1 The figure illustrates how level-set representation captures the contraction of a surface of a unimodal object.

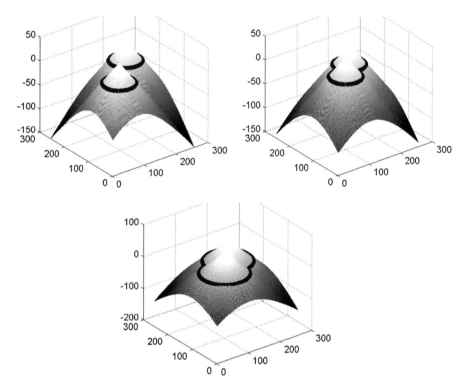

Figure 10.2 Topology changes are captured by level-set representation. A curve containing two parts (circles) is represented on the left. The merger of the two circles is represented in the middle.

addressed naturally, as shown in Fig. 10.2, where we see the behavior of the two circles with time.

The surface function ϕ evolves with time, and the associated front is always represented as the zero level. The zero-level set contour (which represents the shape at $t = 0$) is obtained by solving the following equation.

$$\phi(\mathbf{X}, t) = 0 \tag{10.51}$$

To quantify the process of front propagation, various ideas have been introduced. Many have been borrowed from fluid mechanics and heat equations. We provide the basic derivations below. Taking the derivative of $\phi(\mathbf{X}, t)$ in Eq. (10.51) with respect to t, we obtain

$$\phi_t(\mathbf{X}, t) + \nabla \phi(\mathbf{X}, t) \cdot \mathbf{V} = 0 \tag{10.52}$$

where $\mathbf{V} = \dfrac{d\mathbf{X}}{dt}$ is the velocity vector which can be set in terms of the tangent and normal vectors as $\mathbf{V} = V_T \hat{\mathbf{T}} + V_N \hat{\mathbf{N}}$. This leads to the following:

$$\phi_t(\mathbf{X}, t) + \nabla \phi(\mathbf{X}, t)(V_T \hat{\mathbf{T}} + V_N \hat{\mathbf{N}}) = 0 \tag{10.53}$$

Substituting for $\nabla \phi(\mathbf{X}, t) = |\nabla \phi(\mathbf{X}, t)| \hat{N}$ gives:

$$\phi_t(\mathbf{X}, t) + V_N |\nabla \phi(\mathbf{X}, t)| = 0 \tag{10.54}$$

Equation (10.54) shows that the tangential component of the velocity has no effect on the change of the implicit surface, since the gradient is along the normal direction. The above formulation, called the Eulerian formulation, is parameter free, unlike the classical deformable models (e.g., [10.2][10.3]).

10.3.2 Level-set calculus

Tracking the front, or the evolving curve, requires the calculation of some quantities. The Heaviside function and its derivative have proven to be important to the treatment of the level-set methods. Below is a slightly modified version, suitable for the desired analysis:

$$H_\alpha(\phi) = \begin{cases} \dfrac{1}{2}\left(1 + \dfrac{\phi}{\alpha} + \dfrac{\sin\left(\dfrac{\pi \phi}{\alpha}\right)}{\pi}\right) & \text{if } |\phi| \le \alpha \\ 1 & \text{if } \phi > \alpha \\ 0 & \text{otherwise} \end{cases} \tag{10.55}$$

$$\delta_\alpha(\phi) = \left(1 + \cos(\pi \phi / \alpha)\right)/(2\alpha), \quad |\phi| \le \alpha \tag{10.56}$$

The area or volume enclosed by the front can be calculated by the following relation:

$$A = \int_\Omega H_\alpha(\phi) d\Omega \tag{10.57}$$

while the length of the front, or the surface area, can be calculated by:

$$A = \int_\Omega \delta_\alpha(\phi) |\nabla \phi| d\Omega \tag{10.58}$$

Derivation of the above equations is straightforward and will be left as an exercise to the reader.

As mentioned before, the curvature can be calculated as the divergence of the unit normal to the curve at any point. If the explicit representation $\mathbf{C}=\phi^{-1}(0)$ is considered and s is taken as the usual arc length, the following derivatives exist with respect to s (if time is fixed):

$$(\nabla\phi)^T \mathbf{C}_s = 0 \qquad (10.59)$$

and the second derivative will be:

$$(\nabla\phi)^T \mathbf{C}_{ss} + \mathbf{C}_s^T \nabla(\nabla\phi)\mathbf{C}_s = 0 \qquad (10.60)$$

Substituting for $\mathbf{C}_{ss} = \kappa\hat{\mathbf{N}} = \dfrac{\nabla\phi}{|\nabla\phi|}$ and $\mathbf{C}_s = \dfrac{[\phi_y \ -\phi_x]}{|\nabla\phi|}$ will give the following expression that relates the curvature and the level-set function:

$$\kappa|\nabla\phi|^3 + (\phi_y \ -\phi_x)\begin{pmatrix}\phi_{xx} & \phi_{xy} \\ \phi_{xy} & \phi_{yy}\end{pmatrix}\begin{pmatrix}\phi_y \\ -\phi_x\end{pmatrix} = 0. \qquad (10.61)$$

10.4 Numerical methods for level sets

10.4.1 Conservation law and weak solutions

The conservation law states that the rate of change of a material contained in a domain Ω is equal to the flux across the boundary:

$$\frac{d}{dt}\int_{\partial\Omega} u d\mathbf{X} = -\int_{\partial\Omega} \mathbf{f} d\mathbf{A} \qquad (10.62)$$

where u is the amount of material, $\mathbf{f}$ is the flux, $d\mathbf{A}$ is the differential surface area vector, and $\partial\Omega$ is surface area. Applying the divergence theorem and taking the derivative with respect to time into the integration, we obtain:

$$u_t + \text{div}(\mathbf{f}) = 0 \qquad (10.63)$$

which is called the differential conservation law. If f is a function of u or $\mathbf{f} = \mathbf{H}(u)$, it is called the *Hamilton–Jacobi* equation. Consider a 1D case: the integration over time is calculated as follows:

$$\int_{x_0}^{x_1}[u(x,t_1) - u(x,t_0)]dx + \int_{t_0}^{t_1}[f(x_1,t) - f(x_0,t)]dt = 0 \qquad (10.64)$$

Variational approaches and level sets

and for $f_x = (H(u))_x$, a weak solution for the above equation will be:

$$\frac{d}{dt}\int_{x_0}^{x_1} u(x,t)dx = H(u(x_0,t)) - H(u(x_1,t)) \tag{10.65}$$

The weak solution is very useful especially when dealing with non-smooth signals. The function u does not need to be differentiable in order to satisfy the above equation. The weak solution is not unique; hence, the choice of a suitable weak solution will be based on adding physical constraints to the problem.

In two dimensions, the Hamilton–Jacobi equation has the following form:

$$\phi_t + H(\phi_x, \phi_y) = 0 \tag{10.66}$$

It is clear that the level-set evolution equation is of the same type as the above equation.

10.4.2 Entropy condition and viscosity solutions

Adding a condition to get a physically realizable weak solution is referred to as the entropy condition. The following version of the conservation law

$$u_t + (H(u))_x = \varepsilon u_{xx} \tag{10.67}$$

is called the "viscous" conservation law. The effect of the viscosity term εu_{xx} is to smear discontinuities [10.5] so that a unique smooth solution is achieved. The equation type is transformed from hyperbolic to parabolic, where there is always a unique smooth solution. In the case that $\varepsilon \to 0$, this is referred to as vanishing viscosity.

10.4.3 Upwind direction and discontinuous solutions

Using the classical finite difference method to obtain a numerical solution is not always possible. Different numerical schemes have been suggested to solve the conservation law for the Hamilton–Jacobi equations: the forward, centered, and backward schemes are used to remedy the difficulties with the finite difference method. The method of selecting an appropriate scheme is the key to the smoothness and accuracy of the solution. Consider the following equation:

$$u_t + a(x)u_x = 0 \tag{10.68}$$

The speed a depends on the position x. A numerical solution is built to select the correct upwind direction (forward or backward) depending on the sign of the speed as follows:

$$u_i^{n+1} = u_i^n - \Delta t[\max(0, a_i)D^{-x}u_i^n + \min(0, a_i)D^{+x}u_i^n] \tag{10.69}$$

The interpretation is the following: if the speed is negative, the forward scheme is used. Otherwise the backward difference is selected, where the differences are defined as follows:

$$D^{+x} = (u_{i+1}^n - u_i^n)/(\Delta x) \tag{10.70}$$

$$D^{-x} = (u_i^n - u_{i-1}^n)/(\Delta x) \tag{10.71}$$

$$D^{0x} = (u_{i+1}^n - u_{i-1}^n)/(2\Delta x) \tag{10.72}$$

10.4.4 The Eulerian formulation and the hyperbolic conservation law

Assume that the front is a curve (graph) in the plane defined as $\mathbf{C} = [x \; y(x)]^T$. The unit tangent and unit normal vectors are calculated directly as follows:

$$\hat{\mathbf{T}} = \frac{[1 \; \gamma_x]}{\sqrt{1 + \gamma_x^2}} \tag{10.73}$$

$$\hat{\mathbf{N}} = \frac{[-\gamma_x \; 1]}{\sqrt{1 + \gamma_x^2}} \tag{10.74}$$

where x is considered as the parameter instead of the conventional parameterizations p. The evolving curve moves according to the equation $\mathbf{C}_t = \beta(\kappa)\hat{\mathbf{N}}$ as shown before, which results in the following relation:

$$\gamma_t = \beta(\kappa)\sqrt{1 + \gamma_x^2} \tag{10.75}$$

by comparing the vector components of both sides one by one. Restricting the velocity to the form $\beta = 1 + \varepsilon\kappa$ (equivalent to V_N) and evaluating the curvature taking into consideration that $x = p$, the above equation will be:

$$\gamma_t = (1 + \gamma_x^2)^{\frac{1}{2}} + \varepsilon \frac{\gamma_{xx}}{1 + \gamma_x^2} \tag{10.76}$$

Differentiating both sides with respect to x leads to the form:

$$(\gamma_x)_t = \left[(1 + \gamma_x^2)^{\frac{1}{2}}\right]_x + \varepsilon\left[\frac{\gamma_{xx}}{1 + \gamma_x^2}\right]_x \tag{10.77}$$

which can be reformulated to the following equation:

$$(\gamma_x)_t + [H(\gamma_x)]_x = 0. \tag{10.78}$$

Hence, the evolution of the function γ_x is the hyperbolic conservation law with viscosity that interprets the selection of the velocity β in Eq. (10.71); thus, Eq. (10.78) has two parts, the Hamilton–Jacobi and the viscosity terms. If $\varepsilon > 0$, the parabolic part diffuses steep gradients and enforces smoothness in the evolution of the front.

10.5 Numerical algorithm

This section presents the solution for the level set evolution equation $\phi_t + F|\nabla\phi| = 0$ and $F = V_N$. The basic scheme used for the initial value problem is as described in Sethian [10.3]. Numerical schemes are constructed in order to calculate the function at any time. The aim is to present a scheme based on the link with the Hamilton–Jacobi equations and hyperbolic conservation laws.

It is straightforward to show that for a second-order convex space, the solution will be:

$$\phi_{ijk}^{n+1} = \phi_{ijk}^n - \Delta t (\nabla^+ \ \nabla^-) \begin{pmatrix} \max(F_{ijk}, 0) \\ \min(F_{ijk}, 0) \end{pmatrix} \quad (10.79)$$

where

$$\nabla^+ = \left[\max(A,0)^2 + \min(B,0)^2 + \max(C,0)^2 + \min(D,0)^2 + \max(E,0)^2 + \min(F,0)^2 \right]^{0.5} \quad (10.80)$$

$$\nabla^- = \left[\min(A,0)^2 + \max(B,0)^2 + \min(C,0)^2 + \max(D,0)^2 + \min(E,0)^2 + \max(F,0)^2 \right]^{0.5} \quad (10.81)$$

$$A = D_{ijk}^{-x}\phi + \frac{\Delta x}{2} m(D_{ijk}^{-x-x}\phi, D_{ijk}^{+x-x}\phi) \quad (10.82)$$

$$B = D_{ijk}^{+x}\phi - \frac{\Delta x}{2} m(D_{ijk}^{+x+x}\phi, D_{ijk}^{+x-x}\phi) \quad (10.83)$$

$$C_p = D_{ijk}^{-y}\phi + \frac{\Delta y}{2} m(D_{ijk}^{-y-y}\phi, D_{ijk}^{+y-y}\phi) \quad (10.84)$$

$$D = D_{ijk}^{+y}\phi - \frac{\Delta y}{2} m(D_{ijk}^{+y+y}\phi, D_{ijk}^{+y-y}\phi) \quad (10.85)$$

$$E = D_{ijk}^{-z}\phi + \frac{\Delta z}{2} m(D_{ijk}^{-z-z}\phi, D_{ijk}^{+z-z}\phi) \quad (10.86)$$

$$F = D_{ijk}^{+z}\phi - \frac{\Delta z}{2} m(D_{ijk}^{+z+z}\phi, D_{ijk}^{+z-z}\phi) \quad (10.87)$$

$$F_{ijk} = v + \varepsilon \kappa_{ijk} \quad (10.88)$$

The switching function m is given by:

$$m(a,b) = \begin{cases} aH(ab) & \text{if } |a| \leq |b| \\ bH(ab) & \text{if } |a| > |b| \end{cases} \quad (10.89)$$

A number of topologies for curve/surface evolution are given in Figs. 10.3, 10.4, and 10.5.

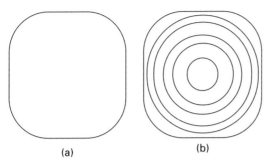

Figure 10.3 Curvature flow of a synthetic shape. Note that the straight sides have zero curvature and do not move until the top and the bottom sides (with negative curvature) collapse the contour to a circle. Initial shape is given in (a), and evolution steps are demonstrated in (b). The contour shrinks to a circle then disappears.

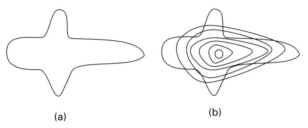

Figure 10.4 Curvature flow of a synthetic shape. Note that different parts have different curvature signs, and hence they move in opposite directions until the shape contour deforms to a circle. Initial shape is given in (a), and evolution steps are demonstrated in (b). The contour shrinks to a circle then disappears.

10.5.1 Need for reinitialization and the distance function

The level-set function is defined as the signed distance function. The value is the distance to the nearest point on the front which is positive inside and negative outside (and, of course, zero on the boundaries). The numerical scheme is implemented only within this narrow band, which saves a lot of time. The existence of the front means that the signed distance level-set function has positive and negative parts. This property should be kept throughout the iterations in order not to lose the front. There are several approaches (e.g. [10.12]) in the literature for the reinitialization of the level-set function (to avoid breaking the contours into infinite islands). The level-set function is updated by the following equation:

$$\phi_t = \text{sgn}(\phi)(1 - |\nabla \phi|) \qquad (10.90)$$

Repeatedly solving this equation keeps the function with a gradient magnitude equal to one at the steady state ($|\nabla \phi| = 1$). The above equation adds positive values to the change of the level-set function with time when it is positive, and the rate will be negative on the

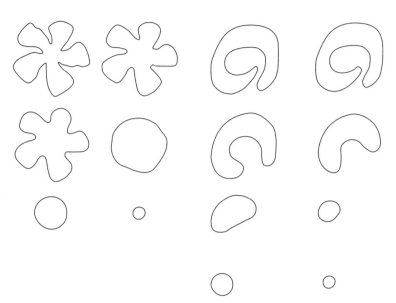

Figure 10.5 Curvature flow of different shapes. (a) Flower, and (b) ring shape. Note that different parts have different curvature signs, and hence they move in opposite directions until the shape contour deforms to a circle.

other side of the front. This process will maintain the function surface around the evolving contour.

10.5.2 Front evolution without reinitialization

As mentioned before, the problem is formulated as energy minimization which includes image information in addition to front evolution characteristics. To keep the signed distance map property, an extra term should be added which minimizes the distance between $\nabla\phi$ and 1 (see [10.13]). After adding a new term, the total energy becomes:

$$E = E_{\text{conv}} + \frac{1}{2}\lambda \int_\Omega (|\nabla\phi| - 1)^2 d\Omega \qquad (10.91)$$

Using calculus of variation, the Euler–Lagrange equation is used with the gradient descent flow to obtain the change of the level-set function with time:

$$\frac{\partial}{\partial t}\phi = -\frac{\partial}{\partial t}E_{\text{conv}} - \lambda \text{div}\left(\nabla\phi - \frac{\nabla\phi}{\|\nabla\phi\|}\right) \qquad (10.92)$$

and by substituting for the curvature, the equation becomes:

$$\frac{\partial}{\partial t}\phi = -\frac{\partial}{\partial t}E_{\text{conv}} - \lambda(\Delta\phi - \kappa) \qquad (10.93)$$

10.6 Exercises

10.1 Given an ellipsoid represented by the equation $\frac{x^2}{a^2} + \frac{y^2}{b^2} + \frac{z^2}{c^2} = 1$, suggest a suitable parameterization (θ, ϕ) for this surface.

Derive a formula for the surface unit normal vector at any arbitrary point on the surface of the ellipsoid.

Derive and compute the Gaussian and mean curvatures at the point $(0, 0, c)^T$.

10.2 Given a planar curve C, represented by a level-set function Φ, prove that the curvature is equal to the divergence of the unit normal to the contour.

10.3 Give an example from medical imaging analysis in which it would be appropriate to use Gaussian and mean curvatures. Write a short paragraph and also add images for illustration.

10.4 Derive the gradient descent flow for the energy defined by $E = \int_{\Omega} F(\phi, \phi_x, \phi_y, \phi_z, \phi_{xz}) d\Omega$ where $\phi: R^3 \to R$ and $F: R^5 \to R$.

10.5 Given a linear transformation A that moves a point from Ω_1 to Ω_2, derive the gradient descent equations for the given transformation parameters with the energy equation $E = \int_{\Omega} r^T r d\Omega$ where $r = \Phi_1 - \Phi_2(A)$ and $\Phi: R^2 \to R^2$. ϕ.

10.6 Derive the vector-valued PDEs that guide the deformation of an evolving explicitly represented surface.

10.7 Show that for a distance transform ϕ, the magnitude of its gradient is always equal to unity ($||\nabla \phi|| = 1$).

10.7 Computer laboratory

Task 1 Implement a fast algorithm for computing the distance transform. You are required to implement it for 2D and 3D shapes. Your results must be accompanied by the exact execution time for both 2D and 3D. Compare this method with classical methods for computing the distance transform.

Task 2 Write a program to compute the curvature of a curve or a surface using implicit representations. Test your program using the signed distance map representation of a circle and a sphere of different radii. Use suitable resolutions.

Task 3 Implement the curve evolution process using the implicit representation (level sets). The process needs to handle the actions of expanding, shrinking, splitting, and merging of the curve. You can also simulate the curvature flow process. Implement your method without need for reinitialization.

References

[10.1] M. Kass, A. Witkin and D. Terzopoulos, Snakes: active contour models. *Int. J. Comp. Vis.* **1** (1987) 321–331.

[10.2] T. McInerney and D. Terzopoulos, Deformable models in medical image analysis: a survey. *Med. Image Anal.* **1**(2) (1996) 91–109.

[10.3] J. A. Sethian, *Level Set Methods and Fast Marching Methods*. Cambridge: Cambridge University Press (1999).

[10.4] G. Sapiro, *Geometric Partial Differential Equations and Image Analysis*. Cambridge: Cambridge University Press (2001).

[10.5] R. Kimmel, *Numerical Geometry of Images: Theory, Algorithms, and Applications*. Berlin: Springer (2004).

[10.6] ,R. Malladi, J. Sethian and B. Vemuri, Shape modeling with front propagation: a level set approach. *IEEE Trans. Pattern Anal. Mach. Intel.* **17**(2) (1995) 158–175.

[10.7] S. Osher and N. Paragios, *Geometric Level Set Methods in Imaging, Vision, and Graphics*. Berlin: Springer (2003).

[10.8] A. A. Farag, H. Hassan, R. Falk and S. G. Hushek, 3D volume segmentation of MRA data sets using level sets. *Acad. J. Radiol.* **5** (2004) 419–435.

[10.9] I. Ben Ayed, A. Mitiche and Z. Belhadj, Polarimetric image segmentation via maximum-likelihood approximation and efficient multiphase level-sets. *IEEE Trans. Pattern Anal. Mach. Intel.* **28**(9) (2006) 1493–1500.

[10.10] A. M. Yip, C. Ding and T. F. Chan, Dynamic cluster formation using level set methods. *IEEE Trans. Pattern Anal. Mach. Intel.* **28**(6) (2006) 877–889.

[10.11] C. Vazquez, A. Mitiche and A. R. Laganiere, Joint multiregion segmentation and parametric estimation of image motion by basis function representation and level set evolution. *IEEE Trans. Pattern Anal. Mach. Intel.*, **28**(5) (2006) 782–793.

[10.12] M. Sussman, P. Smereka and S. Osher, A level set approach for computing solutions to incompressible two-phase flow. *J. Comput. Phys.* **114** (1994) 146–159.

[10.13] L Chunming, X Chenyang, G. Changfeng and M. D. Fox, Level set evolution without re-initialization: a new variational formulation. *Proc. IEEE Computer Soc. Conf. Computer Vision and Pattern Recognition CVPR'05* (2005) 430–436.

Part V
Image analysis tools

11 Segmentation: statistical approach

11.1 Introduction

Segmentation is a fundamental step in understanding images. As image formation involves various sensor types, and objects vary in complexities of shape, spatial support, texture, and color, and the circumstances of the scenes may not be fully understood in advance, various approaches and algorithms for image segmentation have evolved over the years. In this book we address the basic issues in image segmentation: this chapter and the next will consider statistical and variational calculus approaches for segmentation. The focus will be on general frameworks which can be altered according to the specifics of the objects in the image, and the models used.

This chapter describes an unsupervised maximum-*a-posteriori* (MAP) based segmentation framework of N-dimensional multimodal images, in which objects occupy distinct, albeit overlapping, domains in the intensity histogram. The input image and its desired map (labeled image) are described by a joint Markov–Gibbs random field (MGRF) model of independent image signals and interdependent region labels. These models were discussed in Chapter 6. We deploy the kernel approach of Chapter 7 to model the joint and marginal probability densities of objects from the gray-level histogram, which incorporates a generalized linear combination of Gaussians (LCG), where the weights of the kernels may take positive and negative values, while maintaining the positivity and integrability constraints. The number of classes is estimated using a maximum likelihood approach applied to the LCG model. An approach is devised for MGRF model identification based on region characteristics. The segmentation process is conducted by using the LCG-model to provide an initial segmentation (pre-labeled image), and then a subsequent algorithm iteratively refines the labeled image using the MGRF. The convergence of the algorithm is examined, and a sensitivity analysis is performed to quantify its robustness with respect to initialization, improper estimation of the number of classes, and discontinuities in the objects. We illustrate the effectiveness of this approach for modeling and segmentation of objects (structures) in synthetic and biomedical images.

The class of images described above, in which the objects occupy distinct albeit overlapping domains in the gray-level histograms, has been the subject of extensive research in the literature. Such a class of images appears in several practical applications of computer vision and biomedical imaging analysis. For example, in a quality control system to check proper packaging or labeling, a camera may take snapshots of the object in a controlled environment, in order to facilitate automatic decision making. Likewise, in CT scanning of the chest, a typical CT slice would contain portions of the lung tissues, the surrounding ribs, and portions of the chest cavity. In CT or MRI angiography, a slice would contain bright spots, representing blood vessels, and a homogenous background representing the surrounding tissues, etc. Images of this sort will have a set of peaks (modes) in the gray-level histogram, which provides a good clue to the number of objects in the image and their gray-level intensity distributions. Figure 11.1 provides illustrative examples of the images in question.

The bimodal nature of the class of images considered in this chapter (e.g. Figure 11.1) may suggest at first sight that a straightforward segmentation, such as thresholding or deterministic region growing, is possible. Unfortunately, uncertainties in the nature of the objects as well as the image formation process preclude a robust segmentation using

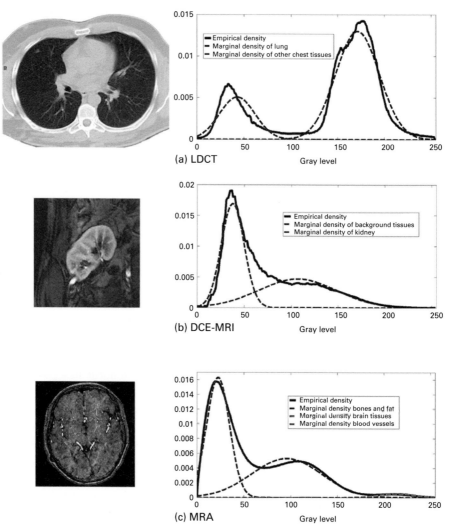

Figure 11.1 Illustrative examples of multimodal images and their empirical and marginal densities. (a) A slice from a low-dose CT (LDCT) scan of the lung. (b) A slice from a dynamic contrast-enhanced MRI (DCE-MRI) scan of the kidney. (c) A typical slice from magnetic resonance angiography (MRA) of the human brain.

simple approaches. Such uncertainties include overlapping characteristics of objects, such as texture, spatial supports, and colors. Image formation adds uncertainties in the imaging process. For example, if the sensor is a camera, then the viewing angle, the light source, and the movement of the camera and the objects affect the quality of the resulting image. The objects of interest may suffer from occlusion, motion artifacts, etc. In an MRI imaging system, uncertainties due to subject movement, partial volume effects, and bias field errors all affect the quality of the image. In a CT image, the X-ray absorption of unrelated objects may carry similar characteristics, leading to ambiguity in object classification. These are just examples of the challenges of image segmentation, even if one has a degree of prior knowledge about what is in the scene. The problem takes on another scale of difficulty when segmentation is performed without *a priori* information.

This chapter is confined to segmenting objects in which the image formation process is rather deterministic, and the uncertainties of the imaging system can be neglected or corrected with great certainty, for example by performing a filtering step before segmentation. Classic approaches such as thresholding using a single threshold or adaptive multiple thresholds (e.g., Sahoo *et al.* [11.1]) and deterministic region growing (e.g., Chen and Pavlidis [11.2]) simply will not give the necessary accuracy. A proper model for these images that captures the essence of object characteristics, such as continuity, deterministic boundaries, and meaningful topologies, will be the vehicle to carry out the segmentation needed.

11.2 Image modelling

The goal of image modeling is to describe the visual characteristics of the image. Stochastic approaches, particularly random field models, have been used with impressive success to model various types of images. These models have been incorporated in various image processing and image analysis tasks, including filtering, coding, and segmentation, in the past three decades (we refer the reader to the work of Besag [11.3], [11.4]; Geman and Geman [11.5]; Derin and Elliott [11.6]; Zhu *et al.* [11.7]; Zhang *et al.* [11.8]; and Farag *et al.* [11.9], for sample papers on this very rich literature). Objects of interest in an image are characterized by their geometric shapes and visual appearance, although it is very difficult to define these notions formally. *A priori* information about the objects in the image is crucial for robust performance of various tasks in image understanding.

As a simple illustration, Figure 11.2 shows a star-shaped object in which additive Gaussian noise would frustrate the segmentation process. The outline and inside of the star would be detected in the upper image (and could thus be made into a binary image), but this is not the case for the lower image. *A priori* information about the object's shape (i.e. star) can provide a clue for the segmentation process. Modeling the appearance (intensity information), spatial interdependence (spatial interaction), and *a priori* information is an active research area, and a number of issues related to incorporating these models into image understanding remain unresolved owing to the ill-posed nature of the specific problems, e.g., segmentation.

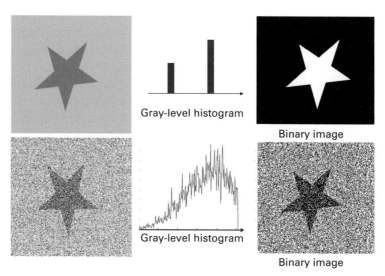

Figure 11.2 Simple objects in which degradation by white Gaussian noise would frustrate the segmentation process when using intensity information only. Proper modeling of the *a priori* information and incorporating it into the segmentation process will enhance the automatic segmentation.

This chapter will develop a general statistical approach for image segmentation using the MAP approach, focusing on three major issues:

(a) Proper estimation of the joint and marginal probability densities of objects in the image from the intensity information;

(b) Proper modeling of the spatial interdependence of pixel intensities with respect to neighboring pixels; and

(c) Formulating the segmentation process in terms of a sequential set of components that govern the objects characteristics in an image; e.g., intensity, texture, and shape, which may be implemented in an iterative yet cooperative fashion.

Figure 11.3 illustrates the framework of our modeling and segmentation approach for biomedical images. This has evolved over the past several years and has been shown to be particularly robust in a number of biomedical imaging applications.

11.2.1 Problem formulation and image models

The conventional approach for model-based image segmentation describes the input image and the desired map (labeled image) by a joint Markov–Gibbs random field (MGRF) model of independent image signals and interdependent region labels. Let $\mathbf{G} = \{0\ldots,Q-1\}$ and $L = \{1,\ldots,K\}$ denote sets of gray levels g and region labels l, respectively. Here, Q is the number of gray levels, and K is the number of image modes, i.e. peaks in the gray-level frequency distribution. We assume that each dominant image mode corresponds to a particular class of objects to be found in the image. Let P be the set

11.2 Image modelling

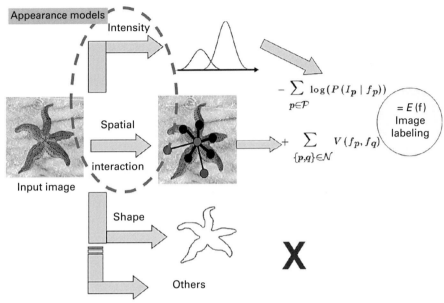

Figure 11.3 A model-based segmentation may incorporate an object's intensity, texture, and shape. (a) LDCT; (b) DCE-MRI; (c) MRA.

of image pixels; then we can define the gray-level image $I : P \to G$ and its desired map $f : P \to L$. A two-level probability model of the original image and its desired map is given by a joint distribution

$$P(I, f) = P(f)P(I|f) \tag{11.1}$$

where $P(I|f)$ is a conditional distribution of the original image given the map and $P(f)$ is an unconditional probability distribution of the map. The Bayesian MAP estimate of the map f, given the image I,

$$f^* = \arg\max_{f \in \mathcal{F}} L(I, f) \tag{11.2}$$

where $\mathcal{F}$ is the set of all region maps with labels $l \in \mathbf{L}$ on P, maximizes the log-likelihood function:

$$L(I, f) = \log P(I|f) + \log P(f). \tag{11.3}$$

To find this log-likelihood function, we need to estimate the conditional $P(I|f)$ and the unconditional $P(f)$ image models, and identify their parameters.

11.2.1.1 The conditional image model

To estimate the conditional distribution of the original image given the map, we assume that this model is an independent random field of gray levels with different distributions of the gray values:

$$P(I \mid f) = \Pi_{p \in \mathcal{P}} P(I_p \mid f_p), \quad (11.4)$$

where for each pixel $p \in \mathcal{P}$ $I_p = g$ is the pixel gray level, and $f_p = l$ is the pixel label. To accurately estimate this conditional distribution $P(I \mid f)$, we need to approximate the gray-level marginal density of each class P $(I_p \mid f_p)$. Although precise classification cannot be achieved by using only a mixed marginal probability distribution, many important applications (e.g. analysis of images obtained by computer tomography, magnetic resonance imaging, or magnetic resonance angiography) depend on this type of data classification. Since the borders between data classes are usually formed by intersecting tails of the class distributions, classification of the data using distributions created by approximating only the peaks (the modes of the data) of the probability density function is often not enough to give an accurate solution. For more accurate classification, the probability density function approximation should describe the function behavior between the peaks.

In this chapter, we use the LCG model (Farag et al. [11.9]) with $C_{p,l}$ positive and $C_{n,l}$ negative components, to approximate the gray-level marginal density of each class as follows:

$$P(I_p = g \mid f_p = l) = \sum_{r=1}^{C_{p,l}} w_{p,r,l} \emptyset(g \mid \theta_{n,s,l}) - \sum_{s=1}^{C_{n,l}} w_{n,s,l} \emptyset(g \mid \theta_{n,s,l}) \quad (11.5)$$

where $\emptyset(g \mid \theta)$ is a Gaussian density with parameter θ (mean μ and variance σ^2), $w_{p,r,l}$ means the rth positive weight in class l, and $w_{n,s,l}$ means the sth negative weight in class l. As both sides in Eq. (11.5) must integrate to 1, $\sum_{r=1}^{C_{p,l}} w_{p,r,l} - \sum_{s=1}^{C_{n,l}} w_{n,s,l} = 1$ is immediate since $\emptyset(g \mid \theta)$ is a Gaussian PDF; however, the integration should be conducted over the finite domain, $[0, Q-1]$.

In order to estimate the parameters of the LCG model, we used the modified EM algorithm (e.g. [11.9]) to deal with the positive and negative components. However, in the modified EM algorithm, the number of classes K and the initial parameters of its dominant modes were set manually. An automatic approach to estimate these parameters is given in Ali and Farag [11.10], which we briefly describe below.

11.2.1.2 Dominant mode estimation

Assume for any given multimodal image that its number of classes is equal to the number of dominant modes (peaks in the gray-level frequency distribution), and each dominant mode is roughly approximated with a single Gaussian distribution. The image is described by a mixture of Gaussian distributions, and the number of dominant modes is estimated by finding the minimum number of Gaussian distributions that maximizes the likelihood function of this model. Since this complete log-likelihood is actually unknown, we use a "partial" likelihood function that leads to a partial AIC (pAIC):

$$pAIC \propto \sum_{p,l} \hat{\Delta}_{pl} \log \emptyset(\theta_l, I_p) - (K+1)n = \sum_{p,l} \hat{\Delta}_{pl} \left(\log \emptyset(\theta_l, I_p) - (K+1)n/|P| \right) \equiv D(K),$$

$$(11.6)$$

where n is the model component penalty, and $\hat{\Delta}_{pl}$ is the posterior probability of the label l given the input image. Let the prior estimate of label $\hat{\pi}_l = \sum_p \hat{\Delta}_{pl}/|P|$. For given values of the parameter π, θ, and Δ we would like to increase the RHS of Eq. (11.6) by assigning $\min_l \hat{\pi}_l = 0$ and re-weighting the remaining $(K-1)$ $\hat{\pi}$ values so as to satisfy the constraint $\sum_l \hat{\pi}_l = 1$. This could then be used later in the iterative steps of the EM-type procedure.

Assume that we have re-labeled the mixtures so as to have $\min_l \hat{\pi}_l = \hat{\pi}_1$. Denote the modified $D(K)$ by $\tilde{D}(K-1)$, $\beta_{\min} = \min_{p,l|l\geq 2} \log \emptyset\,(\theta_l, I_p)$, and $\beta_{\max} = \max_p \log \emptyset(\theta_l, I_p)$.

It is easy to prove the following:

$$\tilde{D}(K-1) - D(K) - D(K) \geq |P|\hat{\pi}_1(\beta_{\min} - \beta_{\max}) + n \quad (11.7)$$

Thus if the condition

$$\hat{\pi}_1(\beta_{\min} - \beta_{\max}) + n/|P| \geq 0 \quad (11.8)$$

is satisfied then $\tilde{D}(K-1) - D(K) \geq 0$ and the pAIC is increased as a result of the adjustment. The *pAIC-EM algorithm* is summarized in Box 11.1 below.

The initial values of this algorithm are selected to be $K = 10$ Gaussians with $\hat{\theta}_l(\mu_l = l^*(Q-1)/(K+1)$ and $\sigma_l^2 = 5)$, $\hat{\pi}_l = 1/K$ and the model component penalty $n = 100$.

11.2.1.3 The unconditional region map model

In order to estimate the unconditional probability distribution for the region map $P(f)$, the region map $f = \{f_1, \ldots, f_P\}$ is presented as realizations of random variables, and the probability measure representing the joint distribution of all pixel labels on an image grid is presented as a Markov–Gibbs random field (MGRF) with respect to a neighborhood system $\mathcal{N}$. Fitting a Markov random field (MRF) model to an image requires estimating its parameters from a sample of the image. The literature is rich with proposals of different MGRF models, which are suitable for a specific system behavior. The maximum likelihood estimates (MLE) are most popular in finding unknown

---

Box 11.1 The pAIC-EM algorithm
1. Initialize the estimates of model parameters $\hat{\pi}$, $\hat{\theta}$, and $\hat{\Delta}$ by over-fitting the number of mixtures K (i.e. fitting a higher-order model than necessary).
2. Perform the expectation step of the EM algorithm.
3. For the smallest $\hat{\pi}$ check the condition Eq. (11.8). If it is satisfied, remove the corresponding component and adjust the remaining $\hat{\pi}$ values, otherwise do nothing.
4. Perform the maximization step of EM.
5. Repeat 2–4 until pAIC does not change by more than pre-specified error.

parameters of a distribution (e.g. Dubes and Jain [11.11], Gimel'farb [11.12], and Picard [11.13].) Let Θ be a vector of potential parameters (e.g. in a second-order neighborhood system) for a homogeneous anisotropic Potts model with pairwise cliques[1]: $\Theta = [\gamma_1, \gamma_2, \gamma_3, \gamma_4]$. The Gibbs probability distribution is represented as a function of Θ as follows:

$$P(f) = \frac{1}{Z} \exp\left(-\sum_{\{p,q\} \in \mathcal{N}} V(f, \Theta)\right) \qquad (11.9)$$

where Z is a normalizing factor, V is the potential function, and f is a realization of the MGRF. Thus, the MLE of Θ is defined by

$$\Theta^* = \arg\max_{\Theta} \frac{-1}{|P|} \left(\sum_{\{p,q\} \in \mathcal{N}} V(f, \Theta) + \log(Z(\Theta))\right) \qquad (11.10)$$

Equation (11.10) cannot be solved by the differentiation of the log-likelihood because the second term, $\log(Z(\Theta))$, is intractable. Thus, numerical techniques are usually used to find a solution for this problem. The coding method (CM) [11.3], and least square error (LSQR) method [11.6] are among the most popular MRF parameter estimators. However, CM performance varies widely for different data and its estimations sometimes need adjustment [11.13]. Also, to estimate the model parameters using LSQR, one needs to solve an overdetermined system of linear equations. This is not practical in the case of realizations with many colors, where the number of equations in the overdetermined system may be up to the number of colors to the power of 8. Farag et al. [11.9] proposed an analytical approach to estimate the parameter of the homogenous isotropic MGRF model. Ali and Farag [11.14] developed an approach for parameter estimation for asymmetric pairwise co-occurrences of the region labels. The asymmetric Potts model is chosen to guarantee more instances where the Gibbs energy function is submodular, so it can be globally minimized using a standard "graph cuts" approach in polynomial time. To identify the homogeneous isotropic Potts model that describes the image f, we need to estimate only one potential value $\gamma_1 = \gamma_2 = \gamma_3 = \gamma_4 = \gamma$. The Gibbs potential governing asymmetric pairwise co-occurrences of the region labels can be described as follows:

$$V(f_p, f_q) = \gamma \delta(f_p \neq f_q) \qquad (11.11)$$

where the indicator function $\delta(A)$ equals 1 when the condition A is true and zero otherwise. Notice that because γ is constant, we simplify the notation $V(f, \Theta)$, which is is in this case $V(f_p, f_q, \gamma)$, to $V(f_p, f_q)$. Then the MGRF model of region maps is specified by the following Gibbs probability distribution:

$$P(f) = \frac{1}{Z} \exp\left(-\sum_{\{p,q\} \in \mathcal{N}} V(f_p, f_q)\right) = \frac{1}{Z} \exp\left(-\gamma |T| F_{\text{neq}}(f)\right) \qquad (11.12)$$

Here, $T = \{\{p,q\} : p, q \in P; \{p,q\} \in \mathcal{N}\}$ is the family of the neighboring pixel pairs supporting the Gibbs potentials, $|T|$ is its cardinality, and $F_{\text{neq}}(f)$ denotes the relative frequency of the non-equal labels in the pixel pairs of that family:

---

[1] As in Chapter 6, a clique is defined as a set of sites (e.g. image pixels) such that all pairs of sites are mutual neighbors in accord with a given neighborhood system.

$$F_{neq}(f) = \frac{1}{|T|} \sum_{\{p,q\} \in T} \delta(f_p \neq f_q) \qquad (11.13)$$

To completely identify the Potts model that describes the image f, the potential value γ specifying the Gibbs potential has to be estimated. In doing so, the MGRF model is identified using a reasonably close first approximation of the maximum likelihood estimation of γ. Using (11.12), the model log likelihood can be written as follows:

$$L(f|\gamma) = -\gamma \frac{|T|}{|P|} F_{neq}(f) - \frac{1}{|P|} \log \sum_{\hat{f} \in \mathcal{F}} \exp\left(-\gamma |T| F_{neq}(\hat{f})\right) \qquad (11.14)$$

The model log-likelihood (11.14) can be approximated by truncating the Taylor's series expansion of $L(f|\gamma)$ to the first three terms in the close vicinity of the zero potential, $\gamma = 0$:

$$L(f|\gamma) \approx L(f|0) + \gamma \frac{dL(f|\gamma)}{d\gamma}\bigg|_{\gamma=0} + \frac{1}{2}\gamma^2 \frac{d^2L(f|\gamma)}{d\gamma^2}\bigg|_{\gamma=0} \qquad (11.15)$$

In the vicinity of the origin $\gamma = 0$, the approximate log-likelihood of Eq. (11.15) becomes (e.g [11.15]):

$$L(f|\gamma) \approx -|P|\log K + \frac{|T|}{|P|}\gamma\left(F_{neq}(f) - \frac{1}{K}\right) - \frac{1}{2}\gamma^2 \frac{|T|}{|P|} \frac{K-1}{K^2} \qquad (11.16)$$

For the approximate log-likelihood, let $\frac{dL(f|\gamma)}{d\gamma} = 0$. This results in the following approximate MLE of γ:

$$\gamma^* = \frac{K^2}{K-1}\left(\frac{K-1}{K} - F_{neq}(f)\right). \qquad (11.17)$$

11.2.1.4 Graph cuts optimal segmentation

After we have estimated the image models, the goal is now to find the desired map f by maximizing the likelihood in Eq. (11.2). Unfortunately, this problem has no analytical solution. However, using Eqs. (11.3), (11.4), and (11.9) (in the case of pairwise Gibbs potential), and simple algebra, one can easily prove that maximizing the likelihood in Eq. (11.2) is equivalent to minimizing the following energy function:

$$E(f) = \sum_{\{p,q\} \in \mathcal{N}} V(f_p, f_q) - \sum_{p \in P} \log\left(P(I_p|f_p)\right). \qquad (11.18)$$

As described in the flowchart in Figure 11.4, to minimize this energy we initially segment the input image based on its gray-level probabilistic model described in Section 11.3, and use the resultant labeled image as the best initialization to the α-expansion move algorithm (e.g. [11.16]). The α-expansion move algorithm repeatedly minimizes the energy function Eq. (11.18), which is defined over a finite set of labels by minimizing another version of this function with binary variables using the optimization algorithms Max-flow and Min-cut. In each iteration of the α-expansion move algorithm, we use the resultant labeled image to update the MGRF potentials γ as in Eq. (11.17).

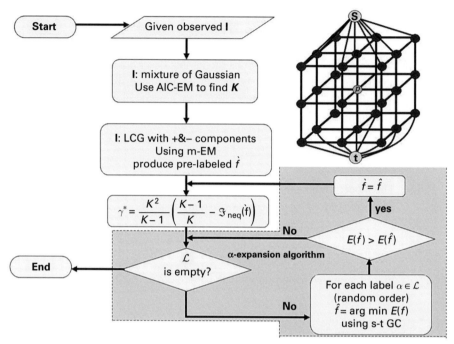

Figure 11.4 Flowchart of the proposed framework, and an example of a graph used in volume segmentation. Note: Terminals should be connected to all the voxels in the volume, but for the sake of illustration we have not done this.

We should point out that the shape information of the objects can be added to the formulation of the energy function in Eq. (11.18), but that will not be considered in this chapter.

In order to minimize this binary version of the energy function, we create a weighted undirected graph with vertices corresponding to the set of image pixels/voxels P and two special terminal vertices s (source, the new label "0"), and t (sink, the current label "1"). We use the neighborhood system N, the nearest 4-neighborhood in the 2D case (or 6-neighborhood in the 3D case). Each edge in the set of edges connecting the graph vertices is assigned a non-negative weight. Then we obtain the optimal segmentation (the boundary of each class) by finding the segmentation resulting from minimum cost (min-cut) on this graph. The minimum cost cut is computed in polynomial time for two terminal graph cuts with positive edges weighted via the s/t min-cut/max-flow algorithm (see e.g. Boykov and Kolmogorov [11.17]).

11.3 Experiments and discussion

To assess the performance of the proposed segmentation framework, we conducted several experiments for segmenting N-dimensional multimodal images. These experiments included ground-truth experiments, done on synthetic images to measure the performance

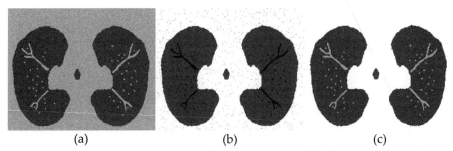

Figure 11.5 Effect of different terms of the energy function Eq. 11.18. (a) Original image; (b) the output using the first term only; and (c) the output using both terms.

of the proposed framework. We have also conducted many experiments to illustrate the performance of applicability of the proposed framework to biomedical images.

11.3.1 Ground-truth experiments

To illustrate the contribution of each term of the energy function Eq. (11.18), in the segmentation framework, Figure 11.5 shows (a) a synthetic image; (b) the output using the first term only; and (c) the output using both terms.

11.3.1.1 Spatial interaction parameter γ effect

First, we will highlight the advantage of the adaptive analytical approach (shown in Figure 11.4) that we propose to compute the spatial interaction parameter γ. As shown in Figure 11.6, for a small value of γ the resultant labeled image (panel (b)) will be noisy (it emphasizes the data, the second term in Eq. (11.18)). For a large value of γ the corresponding labeled image is smoothed, and some classes have disappeared (panel (c)). For this image, Figure 11.6(d) shows the change of the relative error with γ. Also, values of γ computed with our adaptive analytical approach are shown by the range between the two asterisks. These values, located at the range that gives the minimum error, emphasize the correctness of the proposed approach.

Example 11.1 Synthetic 2D multimodal images.
To assess the robustness of the proposed approach, we tested it on 600 synthetic 2D multimodal images and compared the results with ground-truth images. Figure 11.7 shows examples of these images and results of our approach in comparison to ground truth and computation times, τ. Relative errors are given by:

$$\varepsilon = 100 \frac{\text{Number of misclassified pixels}}{\text{Total number of object pixels}} \%$$

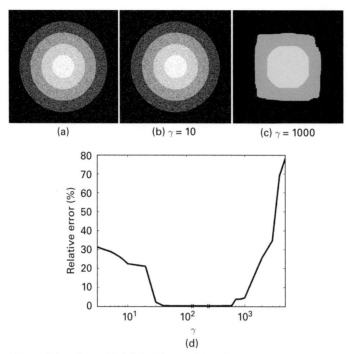

Figure 11.6 Effect of choosing γ. (a) Original image. (b) Noisy output. (c) Over-smoothed output. (d) Changes in the relative error, with proposed adaptive analytical approach values shown by asterisks.

11.3.1.2 Comparison with other approaches

We compare our approach with both the mean shift algorithm (e.g. [11.18]) and normalized cuts algorithm (e.g. [11.19]). Figure 11.7(e–h) shows the mean shift algorithm EDISON outputs ($h_s = 2$, $h_c = 1.5$, $M = 8000$) and NCUTS outputs (default parameters with $nsg = 3$ and 5). To obtain more statistics, we generated 10 three-modal data sets, each of which consists of 30 images, with different signal to noise ratios (SNR). We ran the proposed algorithm on the data sets and computed the average relative error for each data set. Figure 11.7(i) shows the SNR and the corresponding average relative segmentation error. The error at SNR -5 dB is very large, and the proposed algorithm missed one of the objects owing to the high noise. The same scenario is repeated for some five-modal images, and the corresponding error versus SNR is plotted in Figure 11.7(j). For comparison purposes, the segmentation errors of the ICM algorithm [11.4], EDISON, and NCUTS techniques are also illustrated.

11.3.2 Examples of applicability to biomedical images

Example 11.2 Lung segmentation in LDCT scans

Figure 11.8 shows the gray-level histogram of a typical slice from spiral-scan low-dose computer tomography (LDCT). The 8-mm-thick LDCT slices, taken from a scan of the chest, were reconstructed every 4 mm with a scanning pitch of 1.5 mm.. An obvious

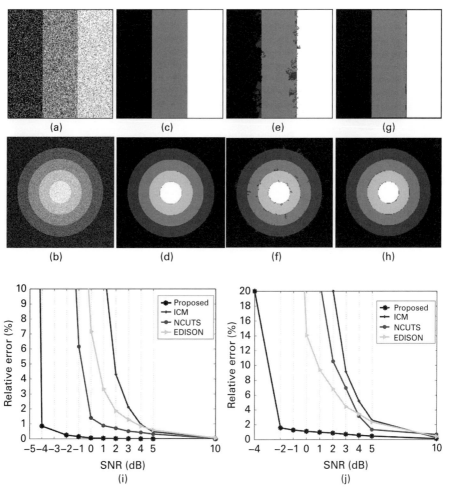

Figure 11.7 Segmentation results. (a) Gray-level image with SNR = 1 dB, (b) gray-level image with SNR = 5 dB. (c, d) Proposed approach segmentation, $\varepsilon = 0.04\%$, $\tau = 1$ sec and $\varepsilon = 0.41\%$, $\tau = 7$ sec, respectively. (e, f) EDISON output, $\varepsilon = 3.86\%$, $\tau = 26$ sec and $\varepsilon = 1.48\%$, $\tau = 13$ sec, respectively. (g, h) NCUTS output, $\varepsilon = 2.24\%$, $\tau = 2$ sec and $\varepsilon = 1.44\%$, $\tau = 18$ sec, respectively. (Error shown in dark portion.) (i, j) The change of the misclassification error with SNR for (i) three-modal and (j) five-modal images.

characteristic is the bimodal nature of the histogram and the clear distinction between the modes; therefore our proposed framework is a good fit in this case. The proposed algorithm is designed to segment the whole lung volume simultaneously. This helps to overcome the large gray-level inhomogeneities in lung data. The proposed approach has been applied to several human chest CT scans. Some of these results are presented in Figure 11.9.

For comparison, results from the statistical analysis of ICM technique [11.4], and the iterative threshold (IT) approach [11.20] are also shown in Figure 11.10. The unpaired *t*-test is used to

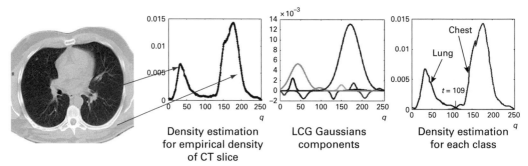

Figure 11.8 Modeling the gray-level distribution of a typical LDCT lung slice.

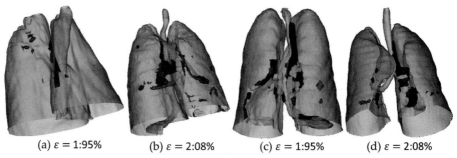

(a) $\varepsilon = 1{:}95\%$ (b) $\varepsilon = 2{:}08\%$ (c) $\varepsilon = 1{:}95\%$ (d) $\varepsilon = 2{:}08\%$

Figure 11.9 Examples of 3D lung segmentation results for different subjects.

show that the differences in the mean errors between the proposed segmentation, and that of ICM and IT, are statistically significant (the two-tailed value P is less than 0.0006). All misclassified pixels in our results are located at the boundary. Therefore, our segmentation did not miss any abnormal tissues, which are important if lung segmentation is a pre-step in a system for detection of lung nodules. Figure 11.10 illustrates this issue on a 2D segmented slice.

Modern approaches for lung tissue analysis may be found in Farag et al. [11.21] and in Farag [11.22], where segmentation of the lung tissue and analysis of lung nodules are conducted.

Example 11.3 Spinal segmentation from CT

Bone mineral density (BMD) measurements and fracture analysis of the spinal bones are restricted to the vertebral bodies (VBs). Accurate segmentation of VBs is therefore a key step in this analysis. We use our proposed framework to segment the VB from volumetric computed tomography (CT) images of the vertebral bones of spine column. Since it is a challenge to segment the VB directly from the CT slice (e.g. Figure 11.11(a)), we use a preprocessing step (e.g. [11.39]) to find the VB region (e.g. Figure 11.11(b)) in the CT slice; then we apply our segmentation framework to that region, as shown in Figure 11.11(c). Examples of segmented 3D VBs are shown in Figure 11.12. Aslan et al. [11.22] compared this method with other alternatives, using

11.3 Experiments and discussion

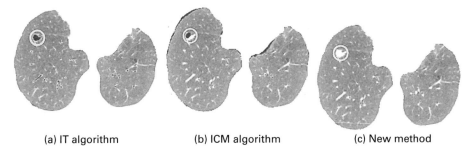

(a) IT algorithm   (b) ICM algorithm   (c) New method

Figure 11.10 Examples of segmented lung slices that have nodules (bounded by the circles). Panels (a) and (b) misclassified these parts (error is shown in dark portion contained in the circles). However, (c) correctly classified them as a lung nodule.

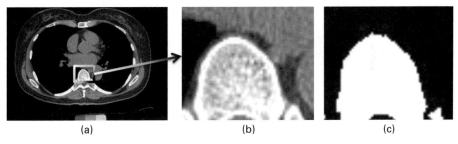

(a)   (b)   (c)

Figure 11.11 (a) The clinical CT data set; (b) the VB region; and (c) segmentation results.

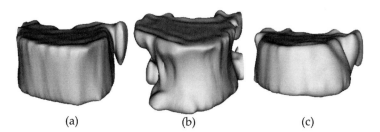

(a)   (b)   (c)

Figure 11.12 Examples of 3D segmented VBs using the proposed framework.

10 clinical 3D CT scans, and showed very impressive performance in terms of accuracy and speed.

Example 11.4 Kidney segmentation from DCE-MRI
Isolating the kidney from its surrounding anatomical structures is a crucial step in many unsupervised frameworks that assess the renal functions, such as frameworks proposed for automatic classification of normal kidneys and acute rejection transplants from Dynamic Contrast Enhanced Magnetic Resonance Imaging (DCE-MRI).

Gray-level modeling for a typical DCE-MRI slice is shown in Figure 11.13. Segmentation examples of a DCE-MRI of human kidneys are shown in Figure 11.14. Yuskel et al. [11.24] show algorithmic evaluation of kidney segmentation. The results in Figure 11.13 and 11.14 are based on the algorithm devised by Ali et al. [11.25].

Example 11.5 Extraction of the vascular tree in MRA
Blood vessel segmentation in the brain is not a simple task, owing to their intersection with brain tissues and their very low prior probability. Figure 11.15 shows a magnetic resonance angiography (MRA) slice and its gray-level distribution estimation with three dominant modes, which represent dark bones and fat, brain tissues, and bright blood vessels, respectively. Our segmentation result with respect to ground truth (i.e. what the radiologist would detect) is also illustrated. Details of two statistical approaches for extraction of the vascular tree are given in Hassouna et al. [11.26] and El-Baz et al. [11.27].

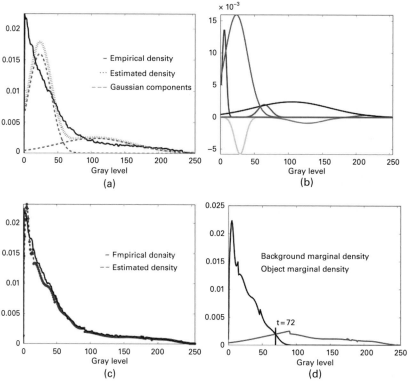

Figure 11.13 Gray-level probabilistic model for DCE-MRI kidney slice. (a) pAIC-EM algorithm result, (b) LCG components, (c) final density estimation, and (d) marginal densities.

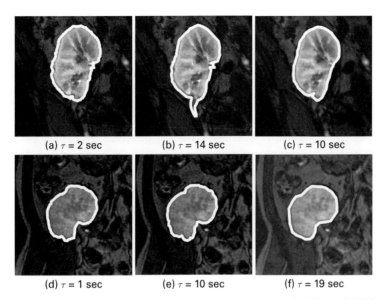

Figure 11.14 Kidney segmentation results of (a) proposed algorithm, $\varepsilon = 1.7\%$; (b) EDISON (hs = 5, hc = 6.1, $M = 9000$), $\varepsilon = 1.1\%$. (c) NCUT (nsg = 2, of = 0.01, th = 0.04, et = 0.01) $\varepsilon = 1.1\%$.. (d) Proposed algorithm $\varepsilon = 0.1\%$. (e) EDISON (hs = 7, hc = 6.6, $M = 9000$.), $\varepsilon = 0.01\%$. (f) NCUT (nsg = 2, and the default parameters), $\varepsilon = 0.6\%$.

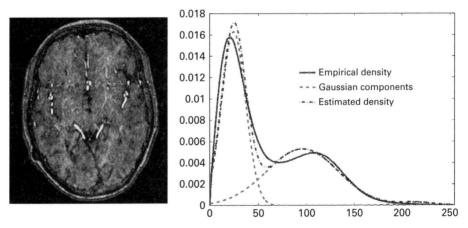

Figure 11.15 Blood vessel examples. (a) MRA slice; (b) empirical marginal gray-level distribution approximated with the dominant normal mixture.

11.4 Summary

In this chapter, we have presented a framework for modeling and segmentation of multimodal images. The classic approaches for modeling the intensity and the spatial interaction were studied with respect to this class of images. The focus of the chapter has been on model identification such that the front-end process of segmentation is entirely unsupervised; hence, important problems of object recognition and computer-assisted diagnosis systems in biomedical images, for example, can be enhanced and evaluated with respect to certain ground truth or standards. Modeling of the intensity or the spatial interaction of pixel (or voxel) information entails model selection and parameter estimation. Approaches to estimate the number of modes in the histogram (components of the LCG model) and the corresponding parameters of the Gaussian kernels were presented. An analytical approach to estimate spatial interaction potentials in the MGRF model is presented and evaluated. A MAP approach was presented which uses the LCG and the MGRF models, resulting in an energy function that can be minimized iteratively using the graph cuts approach. Experimental results on synthetic and biomedical images show the power of statistical models in image segmentation. Ali *et al.* [11.28] have extensive surveys and algorithmic evaluations of statistical image segmentation of bimodal imaging.

11.5 Exercises

11.1 Derive the general maximum-*a-posteriori* (MAP) image segmentation algorithm for generalized spatial appearance.
11.2 Create a statistical phantom to test various appearance models of segmentation. Study the effect of size and occlusion.
11.3 Derive the generalized energy functional in the statistical segmentation model, and explain how the graph cuts approach works.
11.4 Compare the graph cuts, simulated annealing, and dynamic programming approaches for segmenting synthetic multimodal images.

References

[11.1] P. K. Sahoo, A. A. Farag and Y. P. Yeap, Threshold selection based on histogram modeling. *IEEE Int. Conf. Systems, Man, and Cybernetics, Chicago, IL* (1992) 351–356.
[11.2] P. C. Chen and T. Pavlidis, Segmentation by texture using a cooccurrence matrix and a split-and-merge algorithm. *Comput. Graph. Image Proc.* **10** (1979) 172–182.
[11.3] J. E. Besag, Spatial interaction and the statistical analysis of lattice systems. *J. Roy. Stat. Soc. B* **36** (1974) 192–236.
[11.4] J. E. Besag, On the statistical analysis of dirty pictures. *J. Roy. Stat. Soc. B* **48** (1986) 259–302.
[11.5] S. Geman and D. Geman, Stochastic relaxation, Gibbs distributions, and the Bayesian restoration of images. *IEEE Trans. Pattern Anal. Mach. Intel.* **6** (1984) 721–741.
[11.6] H. Derin and H. Elliott, Modeling and segmentation of noisy and textured images using Gibbs random fields. *IEEE Trans. Pattern Anal. Mach. Intel.* **9** (1) (1987) 39–55.
[11.7] S. Zhu, Y. Wu and D. Mumford, Filters, random fields and maximum entropy (FRAME): Towards a unified theory of texture modeling. *Int. J. Comp. Vision* **27**(2) (1998) 107–126.
[11.8] Y. Zhang, M. Brady and S. Smith, Segmentation of brain MR images through a hidden Markov random field model and the expectation-maximization algorithm. *IEEE Trans. Med. Imaging* **20**(1) (2001) 45–57.
[11.9] A. A. Farag, A. El-Baz and G. L. Gimel'farb, Precise segmentation of multimodal images. *IEEE Trans. Image Processing* **15**(4) (2006) 952–968.

[11.10] A. M. Ali and A. A. Farag, Density estimation using a new AIC-type criterion and the EM algorithm for a linear combination of Gaussians. *Proc. IEEE Int. Conf. Image Processing (ICIP08)* (2008) 3024–3027.

[11.11] R. C. Dubes and A. K. Jain, Random field models in image analysis. *J. Appl. Stat.* **16** (1989) 131–164.

[11.12] G. L. Gimel'farb, Texture modeling with multiple pairwise pixel interactions. *IEEE Trans. Pattern Anal. Mach. Intel.* **18** (11) (1996) 1110–1114.

[11.13] R. W. Picard, Gibbs random field: Temperature and parameter analysis. *Proc. ICASSP* **III**, San Francisco, March (1992) 45–48.

[11.14] A. M. Ali, A. A. Farag and G. Gimel'farb, Analytical method for MGRF Potts model parameters estimation, in *Proc. Int. Conf. Pattern Recognition (ICPR-08)*, Tampa, Florida (2008) 1–4.

[11.15] Y. Y. Boykov and M. P. Jolly, Interactive graph cuts for optimal boundary & region segmentation of objects in N-D images. *Proc. ICCV* **1** (2001) 105–112.

[11.16] Y. Boykov, O. Veksler and R. Zabih, Fast approximation energy minimization via graph cuts. *IEEE Trans. Pattern Anal. Mach. Intel.* **23**(11) (2001) 1222–1239.

[11.17] Y. Boykov and V. Kolmogorov, An experimental comparison of min-cut/max-flow algorithms for energy minimization in vision. *IEEE Trans. Pattern Anal. Mach. Intel.* **26**(9) (2004) 1124–1137.

[11.18] D. Comaniciu and P. Meer, Mean shift: A robust approach toward feature space analysis. *IEEE Trans. Pattern Anal. Mach. Intel.* **24** (5) (2002) 603–619.

[11.19] J. Shi and J. Malik, Normalized cuts and image segmentation. *IEEE Trans. Pattern Anal. Mach. Intel.* **22**(8) (2000) 888–905.

[11.20] S. Hu, E. A. Hoffman and J. M. Reinhardt, Automatic lung segmentation for accurate quantitation of volumetric X-ray CT images. *IEEE Trans. Med. Imag.* **20**(6) (2001) 490–498.

[11.21] Amal Farag, J. H. Graham and A. A. Farag, Robust segmentation of lung tissue in chest CT scanning. *Proc. IEEE Int. Conf. Image Processing (ICIP)* (2010) 2249–2252.

[11.22] A. A. Farag, Modeling small objects under uncertainties: novel algorithms and applications. Unpublished Ph.D. thesis, University of Louisville, Department of Electrical and Computer Engineering, (2012).

[11.23] M. S. Aslan, A. Ali, A. A. Farag et al., 3D vertebral body segmentation using shape based graph cuts. *20th Int. Conf. Pattern Recognition, ICPR'10, Istanbul, Turkey* (2010) 3951–3954.

[11.24] S. E. Yuksel, A. El-Baz, A. A. Farag et al., Automatic detection of renal rejection after kidney transplantation, *Proc. Computer Assisted Radiology and Surgery (CARS)*, Berlin, Germany, June 22–25, (2005) 773–778.

[11.25] A. Ali, A. A. Farag and A. El-Baz, Graph cuts framework for kidney segmentation with prior shape constraints, *Proc. Int. Conf. Medical Image Computing and Computer-Assisted Intervention (MICCAI'07)*, Sydney, Australia, October 29 – November 2 (2007) 384–392.

[11.26] M. S. Hassouna, A. A. Farag, S. Hushek and T. Moriarty, Cerebrovascular segmentation from TOF using stochastic models, *Med. Image Anal.* **10** (1) (2006) 2–16.

[11.27] A. El-Baz, A. A. Farag, G. L. Gimel'farb, M. Abou El-Ghar and T. Eldiasty, A new adaptive probabilistic model of blood vessels for segmenting MRA images, *Proc. Int. Conf. Medical Image Computing and Computer-Assisted Intervention (MICCAI'06)*, Copenhagen, Denmark, October 1–6 (2006) 799–806.

[11.28] A. Ali, A. Farag, N. Al-Ajlan and A. A. Farag, Multimodal imaging-modeling and segmentation with biomedical applications. *Brit. Comp. Vision J.*, IET-CV **6** (2012) 524–539.

12 Segmentation: variational approach

12.1 Introduction

This chapter deals with image segmentation using the variational and level-set methods discussed in Chapter 10. Over three decades of work in the literature (1960–1990) has been devoted to gradient-based and statistical-based approaches for detection and linking of objects' boundaries. These approaches have a mixed record of success owing to the ill-posed nature of the problem, and they do not easily adapt to fusion of *a priori* information about the objects or the imaging sensors. Variational approaches provide an alternative view to purely gradient-based and statistical-based methods. These approaches extract the object boundaries through an energy minimization framework that controls the propagation of a parametric curve or surface (sometimes called a front, as indicated in Chapter 10) inside the objects of interest. Two techniques have been proposed for controlling the curve propagation: active contours (snakes), introduced by Kass, Witkin and Terzopoulos in 1987 [12.1] (see also 12.2],[12.3]), and the level-sets approach, introduced by Osher and Sethian in 1988 [12.4]. At the heart of the active contours and the level-set approaches is an energy formulation that implicitly describes the curve/surface propagation in terms of a set of partial differential equations that can be solved numerically to determine the steady state position of the front. The level-set methods (LSM) have proven to be more efficient and flexible than active contours; the image segmentation algorithms developed in this chapter will be mainly based on the LSM.

As stated in the previous chapter, image segmentation deals with separating objects using the intrinsic information in the image (its intensity statistics, edge information, and other salient characteristics) and whatever known (*a priori*) shape information is available about the objects in the image (e.g. the kidney shape in the medical images in Figure 12.1). Other than providing a comprehensive survey and comparison of methods, this chapter will augment the theoretical foundation of the curve/surface modeling and propagation covered in Chapter 10 as applied to the segmentation problem.

As a refresher, we overview a few basic formulations on the variational methods covered in Chapter 10.

Snakes [12.1]–[12.3], as a deformable model, are defined as a parametric contour embedded in the image plane (x, y). That contour is represented by $\mathbf{C}(p) = [x(p)\ y(p)]^T$ where $p \in [0,1]$ is defined as the curve parameter. The contour starts from an intial location inside the object and then is required to evolve, expanding to cover the object in the image $I(x, y)$ by minimizing a certain energy function defined as follows:

12.1 Introduction

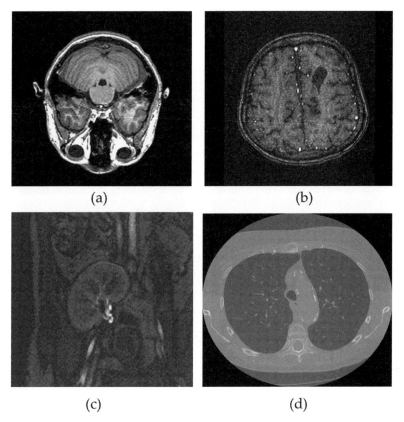

Figure 12.1 Biomedical images that can be segmented by variational methods, despite uncertainties in object definitions due to noise, blurring, low resolution, and size. (a) CT slice of the human brain; (b) MRI slice of the human brain; (c) a dynamic contrast-enhanced magnetic resonance imaging (DCE-MRI) slice of the kidney; and (d) low-dose CT (LDCT) slice of the human chest.

$$E(\mathbf{C}) = E_{\text{internal}}(\mathbf{C}) + E_{\text{external}}(\mathbf{C}). \tag{12.1}$$

The first term is the internal energy, which characterizes the deformation of the contour, and has the following form [12.1]:

$$E_{\text{internal}}(\mathbf{C}) = \int_0^1 \left(w_1(p)|\mathbf{C}_p|^2 + w_2(p)|\mathbf{C}_{pp}|^2 \right) dp. \tag{12.2}$$

The non-negative values w_1 and w_2 are important in controlling the stretching and bending of the contour. The length of the contour may be reduced by increasing w_1, which removes the ripples and loops. Large values of w_2 increase the bending rigidity and smoothness of the contour.

The external energy represents the image force which drives the contour towards the object boundaries. Traditionally, the edges of an object are used to designate the external energy term as follows:

$$E_{\text{external}}(\mathbf{C}) = -\lambda \int_0^1 |\nabla(G_\sigma * I(\mathbf{C}))| \, dp \qquad (12.3)$$

where λ is the magnitude of the external energy term and G_σ is a Gaussian smoothing filter with width σ. Using the calculus of variations, the contour evolution may be described by using the gradient descent vector-valued PDE. McInerney and Terzopoulos [12.2] provide a survey of active contours in medical image analysis. Xu and Prince [12.3] provide further extensions to active contour formulations and applications.

Level-set formulation was proposed by Osher and Sethian [12.4] (see also Sethian [12.5]) to handle topology changes by embedding the contour into a higher-dimensional function. An object is outlined through an energy formulation involving the object's boundaries (external energy) and its evolution (internal energy). These energies aim to minimize the arc-length and the area enclosed; the equation has the following form:

$$E(\phi) = \lambda \int_\Omega g(I) \delta(\phi) |\nabla \phi| \, d\Omega + \nu \int_\Omega g(I) H(\phi) \, d\Omega \qquad (12.4)$$

where H and δ are the Heaviside and the univariate Dirac delta functions, respectively. The indicator function g depends on the edge of the object and is defined as follows:

$$g(I) = \frac{1}{1 + |\nabla(G_\sigma * I)|.} \qquad (12.5)$$

This function approximately vanishes at the object edges where the contour evolution stops. The arc-length term aims to smooth the contour with a positive weight λ. The area terms speed up the evolution with a weight ν which can be positive or negative depending on the position of the contour relative to the object of interest (inside or outside).

12.2 Variational segmentation without edges

Below we discuss two energy formulations for the variational segmentation problem: those introduced by Mumford and Shah [12.6], and by Chan et al. [12.7][12.8].

12.2.1 The Mumford–Shah energy formulation

Mumford and Shah [12.6] assumed that the image can be divided into two smooth parts. A representation u of an image I is obtained by minimizing the following energy function:

$$E(u, \mathbf{C}) = \int_{\Omega} |u - I|^2 d\Omega + \lambda \int_{\Omega|C} |\nabla u| d\Omega + \gamma \oint_{C} ds \qquad (12.6)$$

where **C** represents a smooth closed segmenting curve. The first term is a mean square data term, the second term smoothes the rough "cartoon" model, and the third term minimizes the length of the contour **C**. The given weighting coefficients are positive real scalar values which control the competition between various terms.

12.2.2 Chan and Vese variational approach

Chan et al. [12.7][12.8] proposed the following energy function:

$$E(\mu_o, \mu_b) = \int_{\Omega} (I - \mu_o)^2 H(\phi) d\Omega + \int_{\Omega} (I - \mu_b)^2 H(-\phi) d\Omega + \lambda \int_{\Omega} |\nabla H(\phi)| d\Omega \qquad (12.7)$$

The contour evolves to minimize this energy function or to maximize the difference between the object (the level set positive side) mean μ_o and the background (the level set negative side) μ_b, which is represented by the sum of squared difference in the first two terms. The last term of the energy, weighted by λ, smoothes the contour evolution by minimizing the arc-length. The energy function is minimized with respect to the changing surface ϕ and also the regions means μ_o and μ_b. Using the calculus of variations, the following PDEs describe their change with time:

$$\mu_o = \frac{\int_{\Omega} I H(\phi) d\Omega}{\int_{\Omega} H(\phi) d\Omega} \qquad (12.8)$$

$$\mu_b = \frac{\int_{\Omega} I H(-\phi) d\Omega}{\int_{\Omega} H(-\phi) d\Omega} \qquad (12.9)$$

$$\phi_t = \delta(\phi) \left(\lambda \operatorname{div} \left(\frac{\nabla \phi}{|\nabla \phi|} \right) - (I - \mu_o)^2 + (I - \mu_b)^2 \right) \qquad (12.10)$$

where ϕ_t is the level set function (propagating front). A simple interpretation of the above equation is as follows: if a pixel (in the narrow band region) in the image has a color intensity more similar to that of the object, the function rate of change will be positive. Hence, at these points the contour (zero level) will expand, otherwise it will shrink. The above equation can be simplified by defining the following term:

$$v(x, y) = \begin{cases} +1 & \text{if } (I - \mu_b)^2 - (I - \mu_o)^2 \geq 0 \\ -1 & \text{if } (I - \mu_b)^2 - (I - \mu_o)^2 < 0 \end{cases} \qquad (12.11)$$

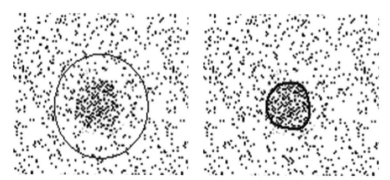

Figure 12.2 The noise effect on the segmentation problem.

which changes Eq. (12.10) into the following:

$$\phi_t = \delta(\phi)\left(\lambda\operatorname{div}\left(\frac{\nabla\phi}{|\nabla\phi|}\right) + v\right). \tag{12.12}$$

The above formulation has the regularization term $\kappa = \operatorname{div}\left(\frac{\nabla\phi}{|\nabla\phi|}\right)$, weighted by λ, which helps in segmenting objects under the effect of uncertainties. Figure 12.2 is an image containing two noisy regions with different noise densities. This makes segmentation using the edges impossible, yet a level-set approach still possible.

12.3 Image segmentation using multiple level-set functions

The Chan and Vese approach [12.8] divides the image into N regions or classes, with N a power of 2. Each level-set function represents two regions, one region located on the positive side and the other on the negative side. A number of algorithms have been reported on multimodality image segmentation in the past decade, in which regions are assumed to be homogeneous such that a Gaussian model would be suitable to describe the region statistics (e.g. Samson *et al.* [12.9] and Farag *et al.* [12.10]). The functional used has the following form:

$$E(\phi_1,\ldots,\phi_N) = \frac{\alpha}{2}\int_\Omega \left(\sum_{i=1}^N H(\phi_i) - 1\right)^2 d\Omega + \sum_{i=1}^N \beta_i \int_\Omega H(\phi_i)\frac{(I-\mu_i)^2}{\sigma^2} d\Omega$$
$$+ \sum_{i=1}^N \gamma_i \int_\Omega \delta(\phi_i)|\nabla\phi_i| d\Omega, \quad \text{with } \alpha \in R^+, \text{ and } \beta_i, \gamma_i \in R. \tag{12.13}$$

This energy function has three terms: the first term penalizes the overlap between regions, the second term (the data term) assumes a Gaussian model for each region, and the last term is a functional that minimizes the interface length between regions. This approach assumes that the Gaussian parameters of each region (the mean and variance) are known *a priori*. Smeared versions of the delta and Heaviside functions are used to replace the sharp functions which cannot be practically implemented. Each level-set function changes according to its calculus of variation.

Two issues are crucial for convergence of algorithms based on the functionals in Eq. (12.13): the initialization of the contours in each region, and the selection of the weighting functional coefficients α, β, and γ. Manual initialization can be used to set the position of the initial level-set contours as shown in Figure 12.3 (here we show a wildly random initialization). Selection of the weighting coefficients is crucial. In many cases, failing to obtain good weights leads to inaccurate results.

These methods are not robust for segmenting images with large inhomogeneities and occluded objects. For example, in Figure 12.4, the tooth region has large inhomogeneities such that a discrimination between the object and background average intensity cannot be achieved.

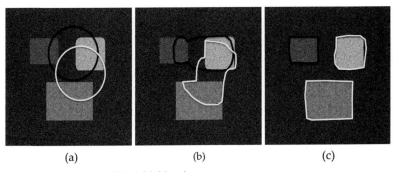

(a) (b) (c)

Figure 12.3 Manual initialization of the initial level-set contours.

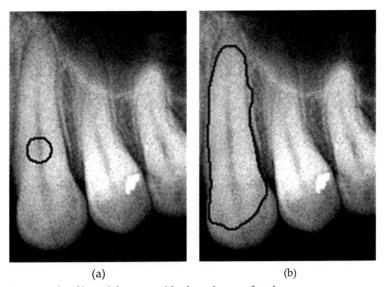

(a) (b)

Figure 12.4 An example of large inhomogeneities in an image of teeth.

12.4 Implicit shape representation

Shape modelling is an active research area (e.g. [12.11]–[12.17]). In this book, several chapters deal with shape representations and modelling. More detailed treatment of shape models will be provided in Chapter 14 in the context of shape registration. A shape representation (in vector form) was proposed by Faugeras and Gomes [12.13] (see also [12.14]) and has been popular in various image analysis applications. The method, called the *vector distance function* (VDF) method, uses a vector that connects any point in space to its closest point on the object of interest. Given a manifold $\mathcal{M}$ in $\mathbb{R}^n$, $(n = 2,3)$, let $\mathbb{d}(\mathbf{x}) = \text{dist}(\mathbf{x}, \mathcal{M})$ denote the distance from a point $\mathbf{x} \in \mathbb{R}^n$ to $\mathcal{M}$: that is, $\mathbb{d}(\mathbf{x}) = \|\mathbf{x}-\mathbf{x}_0\|$ with $\mathbf{x}_0$ being the closest point to $\mathbf{x}$ on $\mathcal{M}$. The function $\mathbb{d}(\mathbf{x})$ is Lipschitz continuous and hence differentiable, and so is the squared distance function defined by

$$\mathbb{D}(\mathbf{x}) = \frac{1}{2}\mathbb{D}^2(\mathbf{x}). \tag{12.14}$$

The vector distance function $V(\mathbf{x})$ is defined as the derivative of $\eta\;(\cdot)$. That is,

$$V(\mathbf{x}) = \nabla \mathbb{D}(\mathbf{x}) = \mathbb{D}(\mathbf{x})\nabla \mathbb{D}(\mathbf{x}). \tag{2.15}$$

The VDF, $V(\cdot)$, is an implicit representation of the manifold $\mathcal{M}$, with $\mathcal{M} = V^{-1}(0)$. For each $\mathbf{x} \in \mathbb{R}^n$, $V(\mathbf{x})$ is a vector of length $\mathbb{d}(\mathbf{x})$ since $\mathbb{d}(\cdot)$ satisfies the *Eikonal* equation:

$$\|\nabla \mathbb{d}(\mathbf{x})\| = 1$$

Let $\mathbf{x}$ be a point where $\mathbb{d}(\cdot)$ is differentiable, and let $\mathbf{x}_0 = P_{\mathcal{M}}(\mathbf{x})$ be the unique projection of $\mathbf{x}$ onto $\mathcal{M}$, i.e., $\mathbb{d}(\mathbf{x}) = \|\mathbf{x}-\mathbf{x}_0\|$. If $\mathcal{M}$ is smooth at $\mathbf{x}$, then the VDF to $\mathcal{M}$ at $\mathbf{x}$ is given by (e.g. [12.13][12.14]):

$$V(\mathbf{x}) = \mathbf{x} - \mathbf{x}_0 = \mathbf{x} - P_{\mathcal{M}}(\mathbf{x}). \tag{12.16}$$

Figure 12.5 shows a few examples of the *x*- and *y*-components of the VDFs corresponding to different 2D shapes.

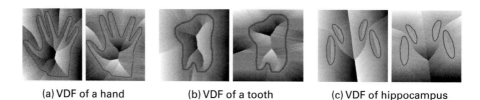

(a) VDF of a hand   (b) VDF of a tooth   (c) VDF of hippocampus

Figure 12.5   Shape representation using the VDF. Left: *x*-component; right: *y*-component.

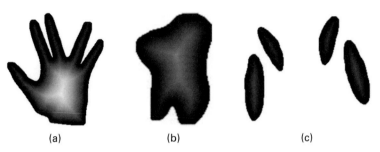

Figure 12.6 Examples of the distance map inside 2D shapes. (a) Hand. (b) Tooth. (c) Hippocampus.

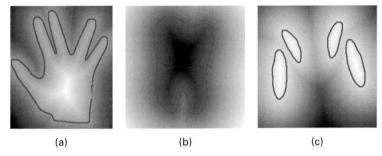

Figure 12.7 Examples of the signed distance representation of 2D shapes by negating the distance outside the shapes. (a) Hand. (b) Tooth. (c) Hippocampus.

The distance transform, or the distance map, of a given shape assigns to each point **x** in the image its minimal Euclidean distance, $D(\mathbf{x})$, from the shape boundary. Some 2D examples of such representations are shown in Figure 12.6.

The boundary is modelled as the zero-level set of the distance transform. In many applications, including the present work, a signed variant of the distance transform is considered. This variant negates the values of the distance transform either inside or outside the region enclosed by the shape. Let S denote an imaged shape in $\mathbb{R}^n$ which defines a partition of the image domain Ω into two regions: the region enclosed by S, Ω_S, and its complement in Ω, $\Omega \backslash \Omega_S$. The shape S can be implicitly defined by the following signed distance transform

$$\Phi_S(\mathbf{x}) = \begin{cases} 0, & \text{if } \mathbf{x} \in S, \\ +\text{dist}(\mathbf{x}, S) & \text{if } \mathbf{x} \in \Omega_S, \\ -\text{dist}(\mathbf{x}, S) & \text{if } \mathbf{x} \in \Omega \backslash \Omega_S, \end{cases} \qquad (12.17)$$

where dist($\mathbf{x}$, S) refers to the minimum Euclidean distance between an image point **x** and the shape S. Examples of such representation are presented in Figure 12.7 for the 2D shapes in Figure 12.6.

The signed variant has the advantage of eliminating the singularities at the shape outline, and leads to a linear transition as one crosses the object boundary. It is advantageous to use the signed distance transform rather than the distance transform for shape representation. First and foremost, this representation provides a feature space in which the registration energy functionals that can be optimized using gradient descent can be conveniently and efficiently used. Second, the signed distance representation is invariant to rotations and translations. Third, in the context of shape-based segmentation, since this representation is set in an Eulerian framework, it does not require point correspondences during the phase of building a shape model from a set of training samples. In addition, it has the ability to handle topological changes, such as merging and breaking. This ability is of great value for segmenting medical images where some organs or lesions can present as one confluent object or as a union of disconnected islands. In the context of shape registration, one can reduce the sample domain for registration to a narrow band around the input shape in the embedding space.

12.4.1 Shape registration

Shape registration involves a transformation that moves a point from a given shape (source) to another (target) according to some dissimilarity measure (e.g. Paragios *et al.* [12.18], and Abdelmunim and Farag [12.19]). The dissimilarity measure can be defined with respect to a boundary or a region enclosed by that boundary. Implicit functions are used as matching criteria, and an energy function may be formulated to obtain the summation of squared differences between the implicit functions of the source and target shapes.

The gradient descent is a commonly used optimization approach for solving the resulting PDEs in order to estimate the optimal transformation parameters that move the source to its target. The motion can be global or elastic. Global transformations always rotate, translate, and scale the source template. Elastic motion means that each point can handle its own transformation independently of the whole shape. The objective of this process is to generate point correspondences between the given two shapes. An example for elastic registration of two medical shapes is given in Figure 12.8, in which point correspondences are established for different anatomical points.

Shape models will be further detailed in Chapter 14 in the context of shape registration and in Chapter 15 in the context of object modeling.

12.5 Shape-based segmentation

Shape-based segmentation is a process of embedding a template into the image domain. Human anatomical structures such as the lungs, liver, kidney, eyes, and heart may have common shapes that do not differ greatly from one individual to another. An average

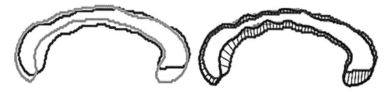

Figure 12.8 An example of elastic registration of two medical shapes.

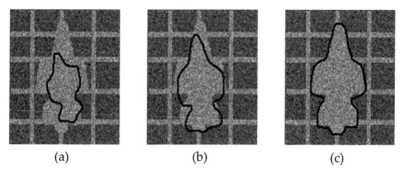

(a)   (b)   (c)

Figure 12.9 An example of shape-based segmentation.

shape or template may be generated for a certain structure given an ensemble of these shapes. For example, an active shape model provides interpolation of the variations in a certain shape within an ensemble (e.g. Cootes *et al.* [12.20]). The active shape model is sometimes considered as a weighted sum of the implicit representations of the training shapes. An example of shape-based segmentation is shown in Figure 12.9, in which a set of shapes for a fighter jet is used to form the active shape model. The shape model is transformed to the image domain in order to minimize an energy related to the image intensity. The objective is to maximize the distance between the average intensity of the internal and external regions of the active shape. The gradient descent method is used to estimate the parameters. The evolution occurs from left to right. Interpolation between the training shapes gives the final object as shown in Figure 12.9(c).

A general formulation for shape-based segmentation may be as follows: Take an n-dimensional image I with $n \in \mathcal{N}$, (typically, $n = 2$ or 3). The information in I may be grayscale, color (RGB), or multispectral information (e.g. in satellite imagery). At a location X in the spatial support of I, $I(X)$ may take a certain value depending on the image intensity; i.e., $I(X)$ is an element of q^m, where $q \in R$ and m is a small integer ($m = 1$ for grayscale images, $m = 3$ for RGB and $m = 7$ for seven-band satellite images, etc.). Typically, q has 2^8 levels for grayscale images, 2^{12} for DICOM format, 2^{24} for RGB color images, etc. The image information may be described as a mapping from R^n to R^m; i.e. $I : R^n \rightarrow R^m$.

As indicated in Chapter 10, an object O in I may be represented by its boundary, which can be achieved by evolving a hyper front (curve or surface in several dimensions) Γ from an initial location inside the object. The evolving front Γ is implicitly represented by a level set function $\Phi(\mathbf{X}, t)$ such that at any given instant t, the front of Γ is given by $\Phi(\mathbf{X}, t) = 0$. In other words, the object outline at an instant t is the intersection of $\Phi(X, t)$ with the zero-plane. This representation is applicable for multiple objects as well.

The front evolution process can be cast as an energy minimization formulation that depends on the properties of the image (e.g., edge information), the level set function Φ, its derivatives, and the *a priori* shape information about the object of interest, Φ_{prior}; i.e., $E = E(I, \nabla I, \Phi, \nabla\Phi, \Phi_{\text{prior}})$. The quantity Φ_{prior} may be represented by a shape model (e.g., an average model from an ensemble of objects), a transformation function $\mathbf{A}$ that aligns this shape model to the object of interest, and the weights $\mathbf{w}$ that represent the shape variations.

The variational approach for minimization of E leads to a set of partial differential equations that can be solved iteratively to generate the outlines of the desired objects.

The above description is generic for object description using variational methods and highlights the large number of issues involved which can be summarized as follows: (1) representation of the image information; (2) implicit representation of the front Γ and control of its initialization; (3) representation of the prior shape model; (4) selection of the shape alignment process that maps the prior shape to the object of interest; and (5) choice of the optimization criterion or approach that governs the energy minimization process. There is a tremendous literature on the subject of shape-based segmentation and registration, and various approaches are application-dependent (e.g. [12.15]–[12.19]).

12.6 Curve/surface modeling by level sets

Within the level-set framework (e.g. [12.4] [12.5]), the evolving curve/surface is a propagating front embedded as the zero level of a scalar function $\phi(\mathbf{X}, t)$. This function is usually defined as the signed distance function, which is positive inside, negative outside, and zero on the boundary of a region. The continuous change of ϕ can be described by the partial differential equation:

$$\frac{\partial \phi(\mathbf{X}, t)}{\partial t} + F|\nabla \phi(\mathbf{X}, t)| = 0, \qquad (12.18)$$

where F is a scalar velocity function depending on the local geometric properties (local curvature) of the front and on the external parameters related to the input data, e.g. image gradient. The hyper curve/surface ϕ deforms iteratively according to F, and the position of the front is given at each iteration step by the equation $\phi(\mathbf{X}, t) = 0$.

The design of the velocity function F plays a major role in the evolutionary process. Among several formulations, the following equation is chosen:

$$F = v + \varepsilon \kappa, \qquad (12.19)$$

where $v = 1$ or -1 for the contracting or expanding front, respectively, ε is a smoothing coefficient that is always small with respect to 1, and K is the local curvature of the front. The latter parameter acts as a regularization term.

With this representation, a single level set either contracts until vanishing, or expands to cover all the space. To stop the evolution at the edge, F can be multiplied by a value which is a function of the image gradient. However, if the edge is missed, the surface vanishes. So depending only on the edge is not sufficient for accurate segmentation, and other information from the image should be used. The segmentation partitions the image into regions, each belonging to a certain class. In Farag *et al.* [12.10] (see also [12.17]) a separate level-set function is defined for each class, and automatic seed initialization is used.

Given the parameters of each class, the volume is initially divided into equal non-overlapping subvolumes. For each subvolume, the average gray level is used to specify the most probable class with the initial parameters estimated by the Stochastic Expectation Maximization algorithm (SEM) (e.g. [12.21]). Such initialization differs from that used in Samson et al. [12.9], where only the distance to the class mean is used. A signed distance level set function for the associated class is then initialized. Therefore selection of the class parameters is very important for successful segmentation. The probability density functions of classes are embedded into the velocity term of each level set equation. The parameters of each of these density functions are re-estimated at each iteration. The automatic seed initialization produces initially non-overlapping level set functions. The competition between level sets based on the probability density functions stops the evolution of each level set at the boundary of its class region.

A segmented image I consists of homogeneous regions characterized by statistical properties related to a visual consistency. The inter-region transitions are assumed to be smooth. Let $\Omega \in R^p$ be an open (i.e. not solid) and bounded p-dimensional volume. Let $I : \Omega \to R$ be the observed p-dimensional image data. The number of classes K is assumed to be known. Let $p_i(I)$ be the Gaussian intensity probability density function of class i. Each density function must represent the region information that is needed to discriminate between two different regions. In this work, such density functions, mean μ_i, covariance Σ_i, and prior probability π_i are associated with each class i. The priors satisfy the obvious condition:

$$\sum_{i=1}^{K} \pi_i = 1. \qquad (12.20)$$

In accordance with the estimation method in Chan and Vese [12.8], the model parameters are updated at each iteration as follows:

$$\mu_i = \frac{\int_\Omega H_\alpha(\phi_i) I d\Omega}{\int_\Omega H(\phi_i) d\Omega} \qquad (12.21)$$

$$\Sigma_i = \frac{\int_\Omega H_\alpha(\phi_i)(\mu_i - I)(\mu_i - I)^T dx}{\int_\Omega H_\alpha(\phi_i) d\Omega}. \qquad (12.22)$$

The following equation is proposed to estimate the prior probability by counting the number of pixels in each region and dividing it by the total number of pixels:

$$\pi_i = \frac{\int_\Omega H_\alpha(\phi_i) d\Omega}{\sum_{i=1}^{K} \int_\Omega H_\alpha(\phi_i) d\Omega}. \qquad (12.23)$$

Here, $H_\alpha(z)$ is the Heaviside step function defined in Chan and Vese [12.8] as a smoothed differentiable version of the unit step function. The function $H_\alpha(z)$ changes smoothly at the boundary of the region. From the above equations, the model parameters are estimated based on the region information.

12.7 Variational model for evolution-based region statistics

The problem is now formulated as a minimization of an energy function. The energy depends on maximizing *a posteriori* probability of the regions represented by the positive side of each level set function. The length shortening term is very necessary to smooth the evolution of the fronts and to avoid creating islands in the curve/surface. The functional is written as:

$$E(\phi_1,\ldots,\phi_K) = -\sum_{i=1}^{K}\left[H_\alpha(\phi_i)\log(\pi_i p_i) + H_\alpha(-\phi_i)\log\left(\sum_{j=1, j\neq i}^{N}\pi_j p_j\right)\right]d\Omega$$
$$+ \varepsilon\sum_{i=1}^{K}\delta_\alpha(\phi_i)|\nabla\phi_i|d\Omega \qquad (12.24)$$

The use of the log function is just for numerical issues. The first term is designed to maximize the *posteriori* probability for each class inside the region and at the same time for the other classes outside. The evolution of each front is described in a straightforward manner as follows:

$$\frac{\partial}{\partial t}\phi_i = \delta_\alpha(\phi_i)\left(\log\left(\frac{\pi_i p_i}{\sum_{j=1, j\neq i}^{N}\pi_j p_j}\right) + \varepsilon\kappa_i\right) \qquad (12.25)$$

The above equation can be compared to Eq. (12.18). The magnitude of the level-set function gradient is 1 owing to the signed distance property. The term $\log\left(\frac{p_i}{\sum_{j=1,j\neq i}^{N}\pi_j p_j}\right)$ can be replaced by the directional function v. If a pixel belongs to the class i (the object in this case) that means its $\pi_i p_i > \pi_b p_b$, this relation guarantees that $\pi_i p_i > \pi_j p_j \ \forall j \neq i$, which coincides with the classification decision based on Bayes' rule, and the following relation holds:

$$i^*(\mathbf{X}) = \arg\max_{i=1,\ldots,K}(\pi_i p_i(I(x))). \qquad (12.26)$$

where

$$v_i(\mathbf{X}) = \begin{cases} -1 & \text{if } i = i^*(\mathbf{X}) \\ 1 & \text{otherwise} \end{cases} \qquad (12.27)$$

If the pixel x belongs to the front of the class $i = i^*(\mathbf{X})$ associated to the level set function, the front will expand; otherwise it will contract. The function selects the narrow band of points around the front. Solution of the $\delta_\alpha(z)$ requires numerical processing at each point of the image or volume, which is a time-consuming process. In practice, only the changes of the front are considered, so that the solution is important at the points near the front. The parameters here have a theoretical derivation, while Brox and Weickert [12.22] used an empirical approach to estimate the parameters.

12.8 Examples and evaluation

12.8.1 Performance on images and volumes

2D images Image and inhomogeneities represent a challenge for the segmentation process, so to obtain better segmentation results, images are pre-processed by an anisotropic diffusion filter, described for example in Perona and Malik [12.23] (see also treatments in Sapiro [12.24]). Results on synthetic images are shown in Figure 12.10, and results on biomedical images are shown in Figure 12.11 and Figure 12.12. All the initialization of the level-set functions is done using automatic seed initialization to specify the class of each seed.

Segmentation of 3D brain MR images Four classes are considered: (i) bones, (ii) gray matter (GM), (iii) white matter (WM), and (iv) cerebral spinal fluid (CSF). Applying the automatic seed initialization directly may result in misclassifying some pixels that share the gray-level range of the brain. That may lead to segmenting the eye as brain, for example. Therefore gray levels alone are not sufficient for accurate segmentation. To solve this problem, the level sets for the classes have automatic seed initialization, except that the WM class is initialized manually inside the volume as small balloons. However,

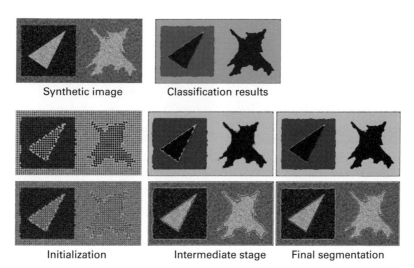

Figure 12.10 Multi-phase level-set segmentation results on synthetic images. First row: left, original image; right, ground-truth segmented image. Second row: left, initialization; middle, intermediate segmentation; right, final result. Third row: as for second row, except original synthetic image is more noisy.

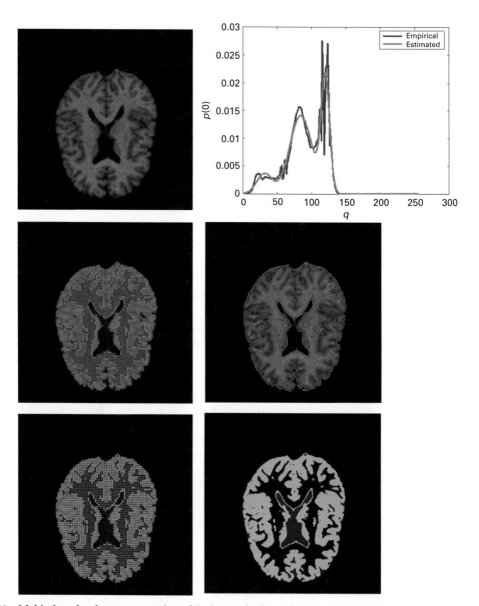

Figure 12.11 Multi-phase level-set segmentation of the human brain 1. First row: left, original image; right, histogram (dark is original and light is estimated using the kernel estimation of Chapter 7). Second row: left, initialization; right, segmented image. Third row: left, another initialization; right, final segmentation.

such initialization yields a lower prior probability of the WM region than it should have in Eq. (12.23) compared with the other two classes. To avoid this problem, the prior probabilities are computed for all the classes by Eq. (12.23), but for the WM prior we use the condition $\pi_3 = 1 - \pi_1 - \pi_2 - \pi_4$, and Eq. (12.23) is modified as follows:

12.8 Examples and evaluation

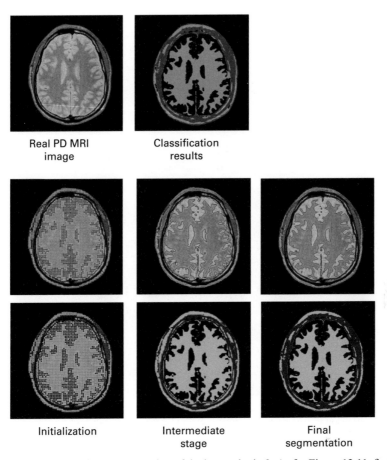

Figure 12.12 Multi-phase level-set segmentation of the human brain 2. As for Figure 12.11, first row: left, original image; right, histogram (dark is original and light is estimated using the kernel estimation of Chapter 7). Second row: left, initialization; right, segmented image. Third row: left, another initialization; right, final segmentation.

$$\pi_i = \frac{\int_\Omega H_\alpha(\phi_i)dx}{\int_\Omega dx}, \quad \forall i = 1, 2, 4. \tag{12.28}$$

After these modifications, the initial balloons will evolve to cover the WM region without overlapping other regions, as shown in Figure 12.13 for different brain scans. Results are visualized for WM regions that represent the object of interest.

12.8.2 Validation experiment on a real phantom

The above approach can be tested on a phantom as well as on real data of magnetic angiography. A real part of a tree (used to model blood vessel bifurcations) is scanned and

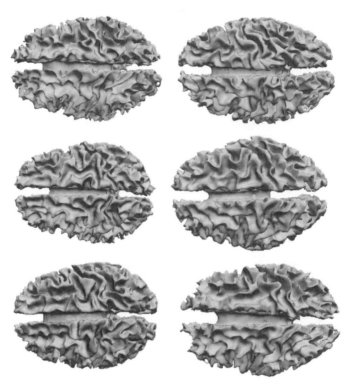

Figure 12.13 An example of segmentation of 3D brain MR images.

ground-truth data achieved by manual segmentation of the model. The ground truth is corrupted by three different types of noise as shown in Figure 12.14 to simulate different blood vessel imaging modalities (phase contrast, CT angiography, MR angiography). In each case the phantom is segmented and compared with the ground truth. Accuracy results are given in Figure 12.15 with average error per slice less than 1.1% in the three cases. This guarantees that the approach is suitable to segment blood vessels.

12.8.3 Blood vessel extraction

Magnetic resonance angiography (MRA) is based on amplification of signals from blood vessels and suppression of signals from other tissues. The blood vessels appear as lighter spots in the image. Traditional segmentation needs an extra post-processing to remove the non-blood-vessel areas from the final region maps. The data set has three classes, namely CSF with bones, GM with WM, and blood vessels (BV) combined with the fat around the brain which has practically the same range of gray levels as the blood vessels. Once again, the level set function for the BV class is initialized manually as balloons inside the vessels that have the largest cross-sectional area, as shown in Figure 12.16 (left image), and the prior probabilities are estimated as in the previous section (with the

12.8 Examples and evaluation 333

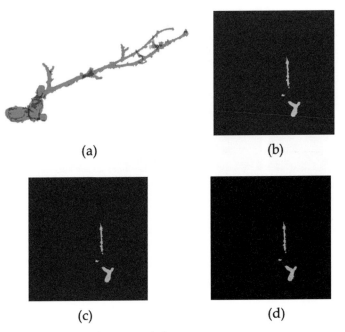

Figure 12.14 Level-set segmentation on a real phantom.

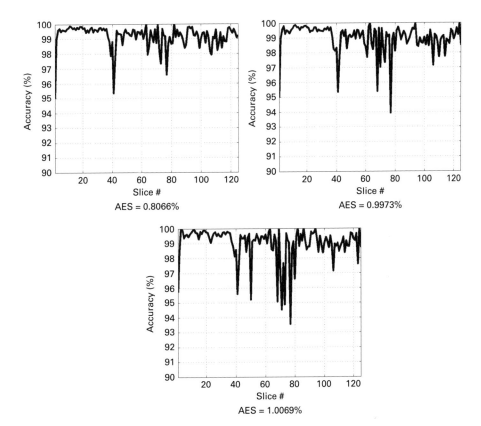

Figure 12.15 Accuracy results. AES, absolute error square.

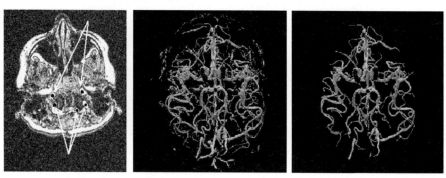

Figure 12.16 Extraction of blood vessels.

obvious changes of the class indices). As a result, the fat does not appear in the final segmentation results. Data sets were collected using a Picker 1.5T Edge MRI scanner. It consists of $512\times512\times93$ axial slices with slice thickness 1 mm, TR = 27 ms, TE = 6 ms. The proposed segmentation approach is shown to the right.

12.9 Clinical example: lung nodule segmentation

This section describes a variational approach for segmentation of small-size lung nodules which may be detected in low-dose CT (LDCT) scans. These nodules do not have distinct shape or appearance characteristics; hence, their segmentation is enormously difficult, especially at small size (≤ 1 cm). Variational methods hold promise in these scenarios despite the difficulties in estimation of the energy function parameters and the convergence. The proposed method is analytic and has a clear implementation strategy for LDCT scans.

Despite the wide range of nodule classifications among radiologists, the nodule classification of Kostis *et al.* [12.25] is found to be particularly useful in the algorithmic evaluation presented in this work, where nodules are grouped into four categories:

(i) Well-circumscribed, where the nodule is located centrally in the lung without being connected to vasculature;
(ii) Vascularized, where the nodule has significant connection(s) to the neighboring vessels while being located centrally in the lung;
(iii) Pleural tail, where the nodule is near the pleural surface, connected by a thin structure; and
(iv) Juxta-pleural, where a significant portion of the nodule is connected to the pleural surface.

Figure 12.17 shows examples of small nodules (≤ 1 cm in diameter) from the four categories. The upper and lower rows show zoomed images of these nodules. Notice the ambiguities associated with shape definition, location in the lung tissues, and lack of crisp discriminatory features.

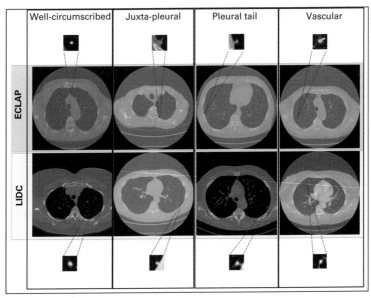

Figure 12.17 Examples of lung nodules of size below 10 mm from two clinical studies. The upper and lower rows show zoomed pictures of the nodules.

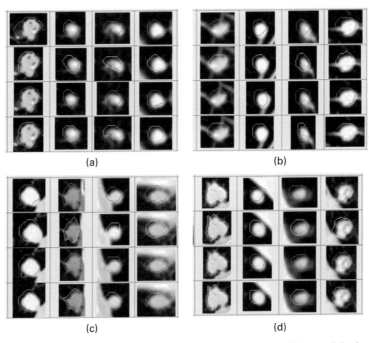

Figure 12.18 Manual annotation of the main portion of the spatial support of lung nodules by four radiologists. Note the difference in size and shape of the annotations. (a) Outlines of four well-circumscribed nodules; (b) outlines of four vascular nodules; (c) outlines of four juxta-pleural nodules; (d) outlines of four pleural-tail nodules.

A major difficulty with small-size nodules lies in the lack of exact boundary definition. For example, radiologists may differ in outlining the spatial support (the span or domain of independent variables) of the lung nodules, as shown in Figure 12.18. Difference in manual annotation is common for small objects that do not have a well-defined description. This adds another dimension of difficulty for automatic approaches, as they are supposed to provide outputs that mimic human experts. In other words, if human experts differ among themselves, how would they judge a computer output? Validation of automatic approaches for lung nodule detection, segmentation and classification – using only the visible information in an image – is an order of magnitude more difficult than that of automatic face recognition, for example.

The lungs are a complex organ which includes several structures, such as vessels, fissures, bronchi, or pleura, that can be located close to lung nodules. Also, the main "head" of the nodule is what radiologists consider when computing the size. In the case of detached nodules (i.e. well-circumscribed nodules), the whole segmented nodule is considered in size computations and growth analysis, while in detached nodules (i.e. juxta-pleural, vascularized and pleural-tail) the "head" is required to be extracted from the anatomical surrounds. Intensity-based segmentation [12.26, 12.27] has been applied to nodule segmentation using local density maximum and thresholding algorithms. These classes of algorithms are primarily effective for solitary nodules (well-circumscribed), but fail in separating nodules from juxtaposed surrounding structures, such as the pleural wall (i.e., juxta-pleural and pleural-tail nodules) and vessels (vascular nodules), owing to their similar intensities.

More sophisticated approaches have been proposed to incorporate nodule-specific geometrical and morphological constraints (e.g. [12.25, 12.28–12.30]). However, juxta-pleural, or wall-attached, nodules still remain a challenge because they can violate geometrical assumptions and appear frequently. Robust segmentation of the juxta-pleural cases can be addressed by two approaches: (i) global lung or rib segmentation (e.g. [12.31]), and (ii) local non-target removal or avoidance [12.32]. The first can be effective but also computationally complex and dependent on the accuracy of the whole-lung segmentation. The second is more efficient than the former, but it is more difficult to achieve high performance owing to the limited amount of information available for the non-target structures. Other approaches have been proposed in the literature (e.g. [12.33]) but require excessive user interaction. In addition, some approaches assume predefined lung walls before segmenting the juxta-pleural nodules (e.g. [12.34]).

12.9.1 Variational approach for nodule segmentation

The level-set function as a signed distance map is able to capture complicated topological deformations. A level-set function $\emptyset : \Omega \subset R^2 \to R$ can be defined as the minimum Euclidean distance between the point $X \in \Omega$ and the shape boundary points. A curve can be initialized inside an object, and then evolves to cover the region, guided by image information. The evolving curve within the level-set formulation is a propagating front embedded as the zero level of a 3D scalar function $\emptyset(X,t)$, where X represents a location in space. In order to formulate the intensity segmentation problem, it is necessary to involve contour representation. Given an image $I : \Omega \subset R^2 \to R$, the segmentation process aims to partition the image into two regions: object (inside the contour, denoted by **o**) and background (outside the contour, denoted by **b**). An error term can be computed by counting the number of correctly classified pixels and then measuring the difference with respect to the total number of pixels. This can be done by summing up the probabilities of the internal pixels to be classified as *object* and the external pixel probabilities to be classified as *background*. This is measured by the term:

$$\text{Error} = 1 - \pi_o \int_{\Omega_o} p_o\big(I(X)\big) d\Omega - \pi_b \int_{\Omega_b} p_b\big(I(X)\big) d\Omega \quad (12.29)$$

where p_o and p_b are the probabilities of the object and background according to the intensity values (Gaussian distributions are used to model these regions). Prior probabilities of regions (π_o and π_b) are involved in the formulation as well. Minimizing this error term is equivalent to minimizing the energy functional:

$$E(\varnothing) = -\pi_o \int_{\Omega_o} p_o H_\epsilon(\varnothing) d\Omega - \pi_b \int_{\Omega_b} p_b H_\epsilon(-\varnothing) d\Omega \quad (12.30)$$

where H is the Heaviside step function and $\epsilon \in R^+$ represents the narrow band region width. An extra term is added to the energy function to represent the contour arc-length (L) which also needs to be minimal to guarantee a smooth evolution. The new energy will be:

$$E(\varnothing) = -\pi_o \int_{\Omega_o} p_o H_\epsilon(\varnothing) d\Omega - \pi_b \int_{\Omega_b} p_b H_\epsilon(-\varnothing) d\Omega + \lambda L \quad (12.31)$$

where $\lambda \in R^+$. The level-set function evolves to minimize such a functional using the Euler–Lagrange formulation with the gradient descent optimization:

$$\frac{\partial \varnothing}{\partial t} = \delta_\epsilon(\varnothing)(\pi_o p_o - \pi_b p_b) + \lambda \kappa \quad (12.32)$$

where δ is the derivative of the Heaviside function and κ is the curvature. Thus, the evolution depends on the local geometric properties (local curvature) of the front and the external parameters related to the input data I. The function $\varnothing(\cdot,\cdot)$ deforms iteratively according to the above equation, while solving $\varnothing(X,t) = 0$ gives the position of the 2D front iteratively. Let $\varnothing_g$ denote the intensity segmented region function representation. The Gaussian distribution and prior probabilistic parameters are computed according to the method in Abdelmunim and Farag [12.17].

12.9.2 Shape alignment

This process aims to compute a transformation **A** that moves a source shape (α) to its target (β). The inhomogeneous scaling matching criterion from [12.17] is adopted, where the source and target shapes are represented by the signed distance functions $\varnothing_\alpha$ and $\varnothing_\beta$, respectively. The transformation function is assumed to have scaling components $\mathbf{S} = \text{diag}(s_x,s_y)$, rotation angle θ (associated with a rotation matrix $\mathbf{R}$), and translations $\mathbf{T} = [T_x,T_y]^T$. A dissimilarity measure to overcome the scale variance issue is formulated by assuming that the signed distance function can be expressed in terms of its projections in the coordinate directions as $\mathbf{d}_\alpha = [d_x, d_y]^T$ at any point in the domain of the shape α. Applying a global transformation $\mathbf{A}$ on $\emptyset_\alpha$ results in a change of the distance projections to $\mathbf{d}'_\alpha = \mathbf{RSd}_\alpha$ which allows the magnitude to be defined as: $\emptyset'_\alpha = \|\mathbf{Sd}_\alpha\|$ which implies that $\emptyset'_\alpha \leq \max(s_x, s_y)\emptyset$. Thus, a dissimilarity measure to compute the difference between the transformed shape and its target representation can be directly formulated as:

$$r(\mathbf{X}) = \|\mathbf{RSd}_\alpha(\mathbf{X})\| - \emptyset_\beta(\mathbf{A}). \tag{12.33}$$

By summing the squared difference between the two representations, an energy function can be formulated as:

$$E_1 = \int_\Omega \delta'_\epsilon(\emptyset_\alpha, \emptyset_\beta) r^2 d\Omega \tag{12.34}$$

where δ'_ϵ reduces the complexity of the problem and ε is the width parameter of the band around the shape contour. The given measure r, from the derivations shown, satisfies the relation $r \leq s\emptyset_\alpha(\mathbf{X}) - \emptyset_\beta(\mathbf{A})$, where $s = \max(s_x, s_y)$.

Thus, an energy function can be obtained where $E \leq E_1$:

$$E = \int_\Omega \delta'_\epsilon(\emptyset_\alpha, \emptyset_\beta) \left(s\emptyset_\alpha(\mathbf{X}) - \emptyset_\beta(\mathbf{A}) \right)^2 d\Omega \tag{12.35}$$

The above functional better describes the registration since it incorporates a scaled version of the source shape representation. In this work, the gradient descent optimization is used to solve the problem, which requires the involved functions to be differentiable. A smeared version of s $(s_x, s_y) = \max(s_x, s_y)$ is used at the line $(s_x = s_y)$ since the function is not differentiable there, which is based on its original definition:

$$s(s_x, s_y) = \max(s_x, s_y) = s_x H_\epsilon(s_x - s_y) + s_y \left(1 - H_\epsilon(s_x - s_y) \right) \tag{12.36}$$

which will return s_x if $s_x - s_y \geq 0$, otherwise s_y. The smeared Heaviside step function H is used to obtain a smooth transition around the line $s_x = s_y$ allowing the function to be differentiable everywhere. The function derivatives will be calculated as

$$\frac{\partial s}{\partial s_x} = H_\epsilon(s_x - s_y) + (s_x - s_y)\delta_\epsilon(s_x - s_y) \tag{12.37}$$

$$\frac{\partial s}{\partial s_y} = H_\epsilon(s_y - s_x) + (s_y - s_x)\delta_\epsilon(s_y - s_x) \tag{12.38}$$

The parameters $\{s_x, s_y, \theta, T_x, T_y\}$ are required to minimize the energy functional E.

12.9.3 Level-set segmentation algorithm with shape prior

The above steps have resulted in an algorithm whose input is LDCT scans and whose output is segmented lung nodules. The algorithm can be summarized as follows.

Lung nodule segmentation algorithm

1. **Lung tissue segmentation:** Segment the lungs from their surroundings (e.g. [12.35]).
2. **Lung nodule modeling:** Train the lung nodule modeling step on a portion of the data at hand.
3. **Nodule detection and ROI determination:** Apply the lung nodule detection approach to compute the positions of the candidate nodules and hence crop them for classification. Cropping here means setting a box around the nodule center and extracting its neighbor area from the surroundings; i.e., a region of interest, ROI, is cropped around the detected nodules.
4. Based on the input image size, construct the initial prior shape circle and its shape model representation ϕ_p.
5. Solve Eq. (12.31) to compute the intensity segmentation region representation ϕ_g. Solution is iterative until the function converges (reaches a certain state). Note that the function keeps the sign distance property by following the approach in [12.35].
6. Initialize the transformation parameters to $s_x = 1$, $s_y = 1$ and $\theta = 0$. At this moment the nodule center location is manually selected, which initializes the translation parameters t_x and t_y.
7. Solve the gradient descent approach to minimize the energy in Eq. (12.34). Parameters converge to their steady state values, and hence the final boundaries of the ellipse are computed.
8. Threshold the region inside the ellipse to accurately mark the nodule pixels. The resulting region may undergo a median filter smoothing step to remove noisy pixels.

12.9.4 Some results

This work is validated using four different databases. The first is the ELCAP [12.37] public database, DB1. This database has nodules of diameter ranging from 2 mm to 5 mm. The second (DB2) contains 108 nodules from LDCT scans of slice thickness 2.5 mm and a pixel-spacing of 0.72461 mm× 0.72461 mm (diameter from 2.9 to 6 mm). The third (DB3) has 28 nodules, 1.25 and 2.5 mm slice thickness, and nodules diameter ranging from 7 to 20 mm. The fourth database (DB4) is from the Lung Image Database Consortium (LIDC) which contains nodules of a range of sizes. The slices are both low-dose and high-dose CT images [12.38].

Figure 12.17 demonstrates the performance of a number of model-based methods for nodule segmentation. Nodules have been cropped by four different radiologists, and the approaches are applied to these cropped nodules. Overall, the variational shape-based level-set method provided the best segmentation results for obtaining the "head" of the nodule region. Intensity-based approaches may be used as an initial estimate in conjunction with shaped-based level-set methods. Also, approaches where a shape model can

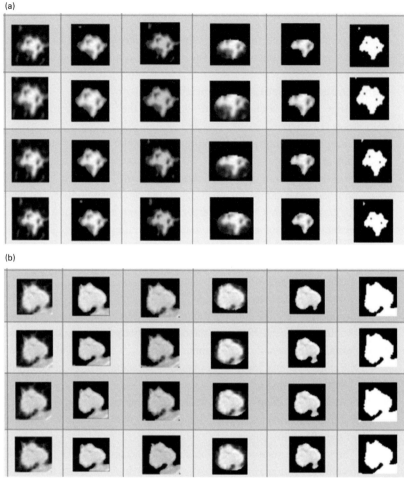

Figure 12.19 Nodule segmentation, by a number of approaches. (a), Nodules within lung tissue; (b), nodules bulging outward from the lung surface. In each case, columns 5 and 6 show results of the variational approach with and without shape alignments. The first column is a nodule segmented by four radiologists. The second column is the EM segmentation. The third column is the level-set method. The fourth column is level sets plus shape priors. The fifth column is EM plus shape priors. Last column is graph cuts.

be embedded into the formulation of the segmentation method are necessary for such cases as nodule segmentation.

The developed approach uses a region of interest (ROI) image that contains the lung nodule as input. Image intensity segmentation using level sets (as described above) is used to extract the non-lung regions from the lung tissue regions and represents the slices by a level set function (ϕ_g). Different scales, rotation, and translation parameters are computed in each case to obtain an ellipse exactly around the nodule head (see Figure 12.18). Changes of the shape model can be noted until a steady state around the nodule boundaries is reached. Also, the axis of the ellipse rotates and varies in size to

12.9 Clinical example: lung nodule segmentation

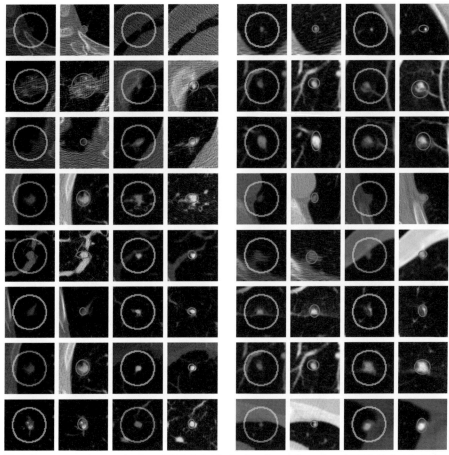

Figure 12.20 Nodule segmentation results from DB1 (left block: first four columns) and DB2 (right block: last four columns). Initialization is larger circles, while final nodule boundaries are shown in smaller circles/ellipses.

include the maximum boundary information of the nodule. Similar results are obtained from other databases (e.g. [12.36][12.39]).

12.9.5 Extensions

Among the possible extensions of the above algorithm are the following:

(i) Proper modeling of the shape priors in the statistical segmentation approach.
(ii) Generalizing the transformation parameters that embed the shape model into the image domain, thus avoiding the post EM step.
(iii) Incorporation of the shape priors into the energy function of general topological cliques in the MGRF models, and evaluation of the segmentation algorithm with respect to variational shape-based techniques such as level sets.

Nodule segmentation is a component of the CAD system for analysis of lung nodules; it requires exhaustive validation by large-scale clinical studies and various radiologists.

12.10 Summary

Variational methods are very powerful for image segmentation. They provide a continuous boundary and handle various uncertainties such as noise, blurring artifacts, occlusion and degradations. The approaches lend themselves to incorporating priors about objects, especially shape. The resulting formulations involve energy functionals which can be optimized by various numerical approaches. The material in the chapter has been tested on various types of images. As the literature on variational methods is rich, the chapter only presents a few of the basic foundations. The reader is encouraged to examine the modern literature on the subject.

12.11 Exercises

12.1 Define the segmentation problem, specifying the challenges with different examples of medical imaging and natural images.
12.2 Why do we consider registration in the shape-based segmentation process?
12.3 Derive the relation between the distance function and the vector distance representation of the corresponding shape.
12.4 Using the vector distance representation of a shape, prove that the magnitude of the gradient of its distance transform equals unity.
12.5 Derive the energy function for an adaptive segmentation using level sets without re-initialization. Give the gradient descent formulation for your resulting energy. Your energy will be very similar to that described in this chapter except that it will have an extra term for re-initialization.

12.12 Computer laboratory

Task 1 Implement the bimodal image segmentation for the object and background problem using the Chan and Vese model. Give results for manual and automatic initializations.

Task 2 Implement the image segmentation for the four-regions problem using the Chan and Vese model. Give results for manual initializations.

Task 3 Implement the image segmentation using Gaussian probability density functions, rather than the Chan and Vese model, to describe regions.

References

[12.1] M. Kass, A. Witkin and D. Terzopoulos, Snakes: active contour models. *Int. J. Comp. Vis.* **1** (1987) 321–331.

[12.2] T. McInerney and D. Terzopoulos, Deformable models in medical image analysis: a survey. *Med. Image Anal.* **1**(2) (1996) 91–108.

[12.3] C. Xu and J. L. Prince, Snakes, shapes, and gradient vector flow. *IEEE Trans. Image Processing* **7**(3) (1998) 359–361.

[12.4] S. Osher and J. Sethian, Fronts propagating with curvature-dependent speed: algorithms based on the Hamilton–Jacobi formulation. *J. Comp. Phys.* **79** (1988) 12–412.

[12.5] J. A. Sethian, *Level Set Methods and Fast Marching Methods*, Cambridge: Cambridge University Press. (1999).

[12.6] D. Mumford and J. Shah, Boundary detection by minimizing functionals. In *Proc. Int. Conf. Computer Vision and Pattern Recognition (CVPR)*, San Francisco, CA (1985) 22–26.

[12.7] T. Chan, B. Sandberg and L. Vese, Active contours without edges for vector valued images. *J. Vis. Commun. Image Represent.* **2** (2000) 130–141.

[12.8] T. Chan and L. Vese, A multiphase level set framework for image segmentation using the Mumford and Shah model. *Int. J. Comp. Vis.* **50**(3) (2002) 271–293.

[12.9] C. Samson, L. Blanc-Féraud, G. Aubert and J. Zerubia, *Multiphase Evolution and Variational Image Classification*. Technical Report 3662, INRIA, France (1999).

[12.10] A. A. Farag, H. Hassan, R. Falk and S. G Hushek, 3D volume segmentation of MRA data sets using level sets. *Acad. J. Radiol.* **5** (2004) 419–435.

[12.11] R. Malladi, J. Sethian and B. Vemuri, Shape modeling with front propagation: A level set approach. *IEEE Trans. Pattern Anal. Mach. Intel.* **17**(2) (1995) 158–175.

[12.12] M. Leventon, E. Grimson and O. Faugeras, Statistical shape influence in geodesic active contours'. *Proc. IEEE Conf. Computer Vision and Pattern Recognition* **1** (2000) 316–323.

[12.13] O. Faugeras and J. Gomes, Dynamic shapes of arbitrary dimension: The vector distance functions. In *Proc 9th IMA Conference on the Mathematics of Surfaces*, London: Springer (2000) 227–262.

[12.14] J. Gomes and O. Faugeras, The vector distance functions. *Int. J. Comp. Vis.* **52**(2–3) (2003) 161–187.

[12.15] M. Rousson, N. Paragios and R. Deriche, Implicit active shape models for 3D segmentation in MRI imaging. *Proc. Conf. Medical Image Computing and Computer Assisted Intervention (MICCAI)*, Part 1, Saint Malo, France (2004) 209–216.

[12.16] H. E. Abd El Munim and A. A. Farag, A shape-based segmentation approach: an improved technique using level sets. *Proc. IEEE Int. Conf. Computer Vision (ICCV)*, Beijing, China (2005) 930–935.

[12.17] H. E. Abd El Munim and A. A. Farag, Curve/surface representation and evolution using vector level sets with application to the shape-based segmentation problem. *IEEE Trans. Pattern Anal. Machine Intel.* **29**(6) (2007) 945–958.

[12.18] N. Paragios, M. Rousson and V. Ramesh, Matching distance functions: a shape-to-area variational approach for global-to-local registration. *Eur. Conf. Computer Vision*, Copenhagen, Denmark (2002), Vol. **2**, 775–790.

[12.19] H. E. Abd El Munim and A. A. Farag, A new global registration approach of medical imaging using vector maps. *Proc. Int. Symp. Biomedical Imaging*, Metro Washington, DC (2007) 584–587.

[12.20] T. Cootes, C. Taylor, D. Cooper and J. Graham, Active shape models-their training and application. *Comp. Vis. Image Understanding*, **61**(1) (1995) 38–59.

[12.21] C. Baillard, C. Barillot and P. Bouthemy, *Robust adaptive segmentation of 3D medical images with level sets*. Technical Report, INRIA, France (2000).

[12.22] T. Brox and J. Weickert, Level set based image segmentation with multiple regions. *Pattern Recog.*, **3175** (2004) 415–423.

[12.23] P. Perona and J. Malik, Scale-space and edge detection using anisotropic diffusion. *IEEE Trans. Pattern Anal. Machine Intel.*, **12**(7) (1990) 629–631.

[12.24] G. Sapiro, *Geometric Partial Differential Equations and Image Analysis*. Cambridge University Press (2001).

[12.25] W. J. Kostis, D. F. Yankelevitz, A. P. Reeves et al., Small pulmonary nodules: reproducibility of three-dimensional volumetric measurement and estimation of time to follow-up. *Radiology* **231** (2004) 446–452.

[12.26] B. Zhao, D. Yankelevitz, A. Reeves and C. Henschke, Two-dimensional multi-criterion segmentation of pulmonary nodules on helical CT images. *Med. Phys.* **26**(6) 1999 889–895.

[12.27] J. P. Ko, H. Rusinek, E. L. Jacobs et al., Small pulmonary nodules: volume measurement at chest CT-phantom study. *Radiology* **228**(3) (2003) 864–870.

[12.28] J. M. Kuhnigk, V. Dicken, L. Bornemann et al., Morphological segmentation and partial volume analysis for volumetry of solid pulmonary lesions in thoracic CT scans. *IEEE Trans. Med. Imaging* **25**(4) (2006) 417–434.

[12.29] T. Kubota, A. K. Jerebko, M. Dewan, M. Salganicoff and A. Krishnan, Segmentation of pulmonary nodules of various densities with morphological approaches and convexity models. *Med. Image Anal.* **15**(1) (2011) 133–154.

[12.30] D. Wu, L. Lu, J. Bi et al., Stratified learning of local anatomical context for lung nodules in CT images. *Proc. Computer Vision and Pattern Recognition (CVPR)*, San Francisco, California, USA, June, (2010).

[12.31] S. G. Armato III, M. L. Giger, C. J. Moran et al., Computerized detection of pulmonary nodules on CT scans. *J. Radio Graphics* **19** (1999) 1303–1311.

[12.32] N. Petrick, H. J. Kim, D. Clunie et al., Comparison of 1D, 2D and 3D nodule sizing methods by radiologists for spherical and complex nodules on thoracic CT phantom images. *Acad. Radiol.* **21** (2014) 30–40.

[12.33] S. Diciotti, S. Lombardo, M. Falchini, G. Picozzi and M. Mascalchi, Automated segmentation refinement of small lung nodules in CT scans by local shape analysis. *IEEE Trans. Biomed. Eng.* **58**(12) (2011) 3418–3428.

[12.34] S. Diciotti, G. Picozzi, M. Falchini et al., 3-D segmentation algorithm of small lung nodules in spiral CT images. *IEEE Trans. Information Technol. Biomed.* **12**(1) (2008) 7–19.

[12.35] A. Farag, J. Graham and A. Farag, Robust segmentation of lung tissue in chest CT Scanning. *Proc. 2010 IEEE Int. Conf. Image Processing (ICIP)* (2010) 2249–2252.

[12.36] A. A. Farag, Modeling small objects under uncertainties: novel algorithms and applications. Unpublished PhD Dissertation, University of Louisville, CVIP Lab, 2012.

[12.37] ELCAP public lung image database. www.via.cornell.edu/databases/lungdb.html.

[12.38] G. Armato, G. McLennan, M. F. McNitt-Gray, et al., Lung image database consortium: developing a resource for the medical imaging research community, *Radiology* **232**(3) (2004) 739–748.

[12.39] A. A. Farag, A variational approach for small-size lung nodule segmentation, *Proc. ISBI'13*, San Francisco, CA (2013) 81–84.

13 Basics of registration

Registration is the process of relating source data to a target or model. It is a fundamental process in image analysis and machine learning. When the source and target are rigid, the process of registration involves obtaining a coordinate translation, rotation, and scaling to align the two entities. The alignment is performed according to a similarity (or dissimilarity) measure, usually involving minimization of square distance or maximizing common attributes (e.g. information content). Registration is performed for object recognition, for tracking changes and in image-guided interventions. When elasticity, or motion, is also present, the registration process takes on an extra layer of complexity. Elastic registration is used for tracking tumors, image-guided surgeries, and assessment of therapy. Some anatomical structures (e.g. heart and lungs) naturally move; hence, registration in such cases is inherently elastic. As it is common to use linearization over small spatial areas to analyze non-linear systems, elastic registration may be analyzed by successive and incremental applications of rigid registration over small regions of interest. Elastic registration may be conducted in two steps: global (rigid) registration followed by a local registration step to handle changes/deformations that the first step cannot handle. This chapter introduces the basic principles and terminology used in classic approaches for image registration.

13.1 Introduction

In general, the process of registration depends on: (1) the representation of the objects' shapes or intensities; (2) the nature of the transformation to move the points from the experimental data (source) toward the model (target), or from model to data; and (3) a similarity/dissimilarity measure. The latter can be defined according to either the shape boundary or its entire region. This chapter addresses the basic fundamentals of registration. The following chapter is devoted to shape registration using variational models. Numerical examples will be provided for two common approaches: distance-based rigid registration using the iterated closest point (ICP) approach, and intensity-based image registration using the mutual information (MI) approach.

This chapter will cover the ICP and MI approaches from their historical prospective, as were introduced for free form registration (e.g. Besl and McKay [13.1] and Zhang [13.2], and used in various applications, e.g. Yamany *et al*. [13.3]–[13.5]) and for multimodality image registration (e.g. Viola *et al* [13.6], Wells *et al*. [13.7], Collingnon *et al*. [13.8],

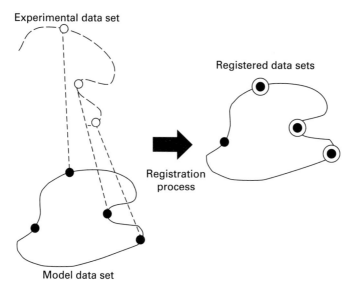

Figure 13.1 A pictorial explanation of registration, where the experimental data is registered, or aligned, to the model data set using local point set matching. Note that the registration process needs to account for translational offset, rotational misalignment, and partial data sets.

Maes *et al.* [13.9] [13.10]). We should point out that the ICP and MI approaches, on their own, are optimization/search criterion which may be deployed with rigid or elastic registrations, in general.

13.2 Basic concepts and definitions

DEFINITION 13.1 *Registration (also known as alignment) refers to the process of transforming an experimental (source) data set to the coordinate system of a model data (target) set for the purposes of establishing point correspondences between the two sets, such that a dissimilarity measure between them is optimized.* ∎

Figure 13.1 illustrates the process of aligning incomplete experimental data about an object to a model (target) which is complete.

Image registration

Given two images referred to as model (template) T, and source (reference) R, of the same object, image registration is thus to find homologous (corresponding) points in both images.

Assume that in continuous variables, the two images can be represented in a D-dimensional space by two compactly supported functions (i.e. functions with finite domain), $R: \Omega \subseteq \mathbb{R}^D \to \mathbb{R}^C$ and $T: \Omega \subseteq \mathbb{R}^D \to \mathbb{R}^C$, where $D = 2$ or 3, and C represents the dimension of the image data, e.g. $C = 1$ for gray-level images while $C = 3$ for color images. As such the functions R and T assign to each image point $\mathbf{x}$ in the compact domain Ω the intensities $T(\mathbf{x}) \in \mathbb{R}^C$ and $R(\mathbf{x}) \in \mathbb{R}^C$, respectively. Note that by intensities we mean any image-representing feature such as grayscale values, the edge map, a distance transform with respect to a locus of points, etc. The image domain Ω is assumed to be a bounded region of $\mathbb{R}^D$ whose boundary, $\partial\Omega$, fulfils some regularity constraints.

The goal of matching the images, T and R, is to find a displacement field $\mathbf{u} = (u_1, u_2, \ldots, u_D)^T : \Omega \to \mathbb{R}^D$ such that the transformed template $T(\mathbf{x} + \mathbf{u}(\mathbf{x}))$ matches the reference $R(\mathbf{x})$. Generally, the displacement field $\mathbf{u}$ is searched for in a space of admissible functions, χ, whose definition depends on how much is known about the relation between the two images and what regularity constraints can be imposed on the unknown $\mathbf{u}$. For instance, for some camera calibration problems, it is known that corresponding points should belong to epipolar lines, and hence the mapping transformation is a homography.

Shape registration

Shape represents objects in a way invariant to scale, translation, and rotation. Shape models may be in terms of object contours or a unique transform such that no two shapes have the same model coefficients. The registration between a source/reference shape S and model/template/target shape T requires encoding the shape landmarks/control points such that a possible correspondence may be found.

Let the source/reference shape be represented by a set of points $X_R = \{\mathbf{x}_R^i\}$ where $i = 1, 2, \ldots, N_R$ and N_R is the number of points in the reference shape, such that $\mathbf{x}_R^i \in \mathbb{R}^D$. Similarly, let the model/template/target shape be represented by a set of points $X_T = \{\mathbf{x}_T^i\}$ where $i = 1, 2, \ldots, N_T$ and N_T is the number of points in the template shape, such that $\mathbf{x}_T^i \in \mathbb{R}^D$. Such points can be extracted from the same or different imaging modalities. The task of registration hence can be defined as finding a mapping between the coordinate systems of the model/reference shape and the data/template shape. In particular, we are after a mapping/warping function $W : \mathbb{R}^D \to \mathbb{R}^D$ which warps the corresponding anatomical points in the template frame to the reference frame such that: $\mathbf{x}_R^i = W(\mathbf{x}_T^i)$. Hence the resulting mapping would align pairs of corresponding anatomical features to share the same coordinate frame.

Registration process/workflow

The registration workflow is illustrated in Figure 13.2. Starting from an initial estimate of the transformation parameters (also referred to as the deformation field), the template image is transformed and the similarity/dissimilarity between the transformed template and the reference/source is iteratively measured while the transformation parameters are updated through an optimization procedure. The process stops when the difference between the transformed template and the reference is below a certain threshold, or when a maximum number of iterations is attained.

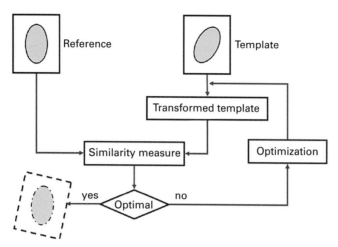

Figure 13.2 Registration work flow. Only the main components of the registration process are shown.

The above workflow of registration applies for image, volume, and shape registration. We will provide some basic definitions in the rest of this section. Again, we will devote the next chapter to shape registration.

DEFINITION 13.2 *In a D-dimensional space, a **transform** on $\mathbb{R}^D$ is a mapping $W : \mathbb{R}^D \to \mathbb{R}^D$ which maps each point $\mathbf{x} \in \mathbb{R}^D$ to exactly one point $W(\mathbf{x})$ also in $\mathbb{R}^D$.* ∎

DEFINITION 13.3 *Let $W : \mathbb{R}^D \to \mathbb{R}^D$ be a transform. W is said to be a **linear** transform/warp if and only if:*

(a) $\forall \alpha \in \mathbb{R}$ and $\mathbf{x} \in \mathbb{R}^D$ we have $W(\alpha \mathbf{x}) = \alpha W(\mathbf{x})$.
(b) $\forall\, \mathbf{x}, \mathbf{y} \in \mathbb{R}^D$ we have $W(\mathbf{x} + \mathbf{y}) = W(\mathbf{x}) + W(\mathbf{y})$. ∎

An example of a linear transform/warp is the identity transform given by $W(\mathbf{x}) = \mathbf{x}$.

DEFINITION 13.4 *Let $W : \mathbb{R}^D \to \mathbb{R}^D$ be a transform. W is said to be a **translation** if there exists $\mathbf{t} \in \mathbb{R}^D$ such that $\forall\, \mathbf{x} \in \mathbb{R}^D$ we have $W(\mathbf{x}) = \mathbf{x} + \mathbf{t}$. A translation moves all vectors or points by a fixed distance in a fixed direction.* ∎

DEFINITION 13.5 *An **affine** transform is a transform that can be written as $W(\mathbf{x}) = L(\mathbf{x}) + \mathbf{t}$ where $L(.)$ is a linear transform.* ∎

Any linear transform in $\mathbb{R}^3$ can be represented by a 3×3 matrix of the following form:

$$\mathbf{L} = \begin{pmatrix} \ell_{11} & \ell_{12} & \ell_{13} \\ \ell_{21} & \ell_{22} & \ell_{23} \\ \ell_{31} & \ell_{32} & \ell_{33} \end{pmatrix} \tag{13.1}$$

To transform a point we apply the matrix $\mathbf{L}$ to the point $\mathbf{x} \in \mathbb{R}^3$ where $\mathbf{x} = \{x, y, z\}$ to obtain:

$$x' = L(x) \equiv \mathbf{L}x = \begin{pmatrix} \ell_{11} & \ell_{12} & \ell_{13} \\ \ell_{21} & \ell_{22} & \ell_{23} \\ \ell_{31} & \ell_{32} & \ell_{33} \end{pmatrix} \begin{pmatrix} x \\ y \\ z \end{pmatrix} \quad (13.2)$$

Linear transforms can also be represented as transforms on homogeneous coordinate systems as follows:

$$\mathbf{L} = \begin{pmatrix} \ell_{11} & \ell_{12} & \ell_{13} & 0 \\ \ell_{21} & \ell_{22} & \ell_{23} & 0 \\ \ell_{31} & \ell_{32} & \ell_{33} & 0 \\ 0 & 0 & 0 & 1 \end{pmatrix} \quad (13.3)$$

This allows affine transforms to be represented as a matrix product of a linear transform and a translation.

13.2.1 Components of the registration transformation

Scaling

Assuming that the object of interest is centered at the origin, scaling amounts for changing the size of that object in $\mathbb{R}^3$. If the size changes by the same proportion in all directions, this is called uniform scaling, which can be given by:

$$L \equiv \mathbf{S} = \begin{pmatrix} s & 0 & 0 \\ 0 & s & 0 \\ 0 & 0 & s \end{pmatrix} \quad (13.4)$$

where $s \in \mathbb{R}$. Uneven scaling would define the *non-uniform scaling* matrix,

$$L \equiv \mathbf{S} = \begin{pmatrix} s_x & 0 & 0 \\ 0 & s_y & 0 \\ 0 & 0 & s_z \end{pmatrix} \quad (13.5)$$

where $s_x, s_y, s_z \in \mathbb{R}$. Similarly, scaling matrices can be defined in the 2D space where $\mathbf{S} = \begin{pmatrix} s & 0 \\ 0 & s \end{pmatrix}$ in the case of uniform scaling and $\mathbf{S} = \begin{pmatrix} s_x & 0 \\ 0 & s_y \end{pmatrix}$ in the case of non-uniform scaling. See Figure 13.3 for an illustration.

Translation

To allow a unified representation for affine transforms, we can use the homogeneous coordinate system to write translations in a matrix form (see Figure 13.4 for illustration). A translation by $t = (t_x, t_y, t_z)^T$ is given by a 4×4 matrix defined as:

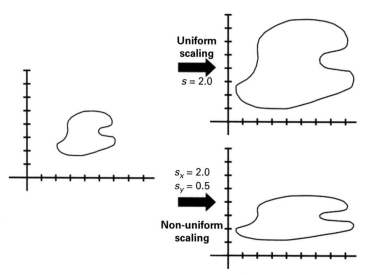

Figure 13.3 Scaling a coordinate means multiplying each of its components by a scalar to change the size of the object of interest. Uniform scaling means that this scalar is the same for all components, whereas in non-uniform scaling, a different scalar is used for each component.

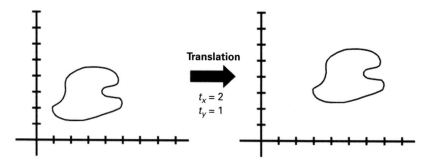

Figure 13.4 Translation moves all the points of the object of interest by a fixed distance in a fixed direction.

$$L \equiv \mathbf{T} = \begin{pmatrix} 1 & 0 & 0 & t_x \\ 0 & 1 & 0 & t_y \\ 0 & 0 & 1 & t_z \\ 0 & 0 & 0 & 1 \end{pmatrix}. \quad (13.6)$$

In the same manner, translation matrices can be defined in the 2D space as:

$$\mathbf{T} = \begin{pmatrix} 1 & 0 & t_x \\ 0 & 1 & t_y \\ 0 & 0 & 1 \end{pmatrix}.$$

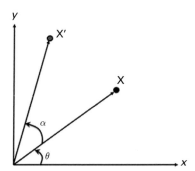

Figure 13.5 Rotation in the 2D Cartesian plane.

Rotation

In the 2D space, rotation can be derived as follows. In Figure 13.5, we have a point $\mathbf{x} = (x, y)^T$ which is rotated anticlockwise by an angle α to obtain $\mathbf{x}' = (x', y')^T$. It can be seen that $x = \|\mathbf{x}\| \cos \theta$ and $y = \|\mathbf{x}\| \sin \theta$, where the norm $\|\mathbf{x}\|$ is the distance between the origin (0,0) and the point $\mathbf{x}$. Since this distance will not be changed by rotation, we will have:

$$x' = \|\mathbf{x}\| \cos(\theta + \alpha) = \|\mathbf{x}\| \cos \theta \cos \alpha - \|\mathbf{x}\| \sin \theta \sin \alpha = x \cos \alpha - y \sin \alpha. \quad (13.7)$$

Likewise we can compute y' as follows;

$$y' = \|\mathbf{x}\| \sin(\theta + \alpha) = \|\mathbf{x}\| \cos \theta \sin \alpha + \|\mathbf{x}\| \sin \theta \cos \alpha = x \sin \alpha + y \cos \alpha. \quad (13.8)$$

As such, the transform can be written as the orthogonal matrix;

$$\mathbf{R}_{z,\alpha} = \begin{pmatrix} \cos \alpha & -\sin \alpha \\ \sin \alpha & \cos \alpha \end{pmatrix}. \quad (13.9)$$

$\mathbf{R}_{z,\alpha}$ rotates in the Cartesian plane, i.e. rotation around the z-axis.
In $\mathbb{R}^3$, the rotation matrix about the z-axis can be written as:

$$\mathbf{R}_{z,\alpha} = \begin{pmatrix} \cos \alpha & -\sin \alpha & 0 \\ \sin \alpha & \cos \alpha & 0 \\ 0 & 0 & 1 \end{pmatrix} \quad (13.10)$$

In the same manner, the rotation matrices about the x and y axes are defined as follows:

$$\mathbf{R}_{x,\alpha} = \begin{pmatrix} 1 & 0 & 0 \\ 0 & \cos \alpha & -\sin \alpha \\ 0 & \sin \alpha & \cos \alpha \end{pmatrix} \quad (13.11)$$

and

$$\mathbf{R}_{y,\alpha} = \begin{pmatrix} \cos\alpha & 0 & -\sin\alpha \\ 0 & 1 & 0 \\ \sin\alpha & 0 & \cos\alpha \end{pmatrix} \qquad (13.12)$$

Usually, the *Euler transform* is used to represent the orientation of an object. It is defined as $E(\alpha, \beta, \gamma) = \mathbf{R}_{z,\gamma}\mathbf{R}_{x,\alpha}\mathbf{R}_{y,\beta}$, where the angles α, β, and γ define yaw, pitch, and roll angles. Since a degree of freedom can be lost in some cases, the Euler transform suffers from *gimbal lock*. Instead of using the Euler transform, we use a general rotation matrix and use concatenated transforms to specify rotations. Quaternions (presented later in this chapter) also form an efficient way to represent rotations in 3D space.

13.2.2 Choice of transformation

Whether we are aligning images or shapes, it is important to formalize the type of mapping we are looking for. Most registration problems deal with finding a mapping either between images at different times or images using different modalities. While global transformation resolves for translational offset, scale difference, and rotational misalignment, local (non-rigid/elastic) transformation aims to find the local deformations sustained by the imaged anatomy.

Global transformation

Global transformation models are usually defined by a small set of parameters. These models include, among others, the rigid transformation (translations and rotations), the similarity transformation (translations, rotations, and isotropic scaling), and the affine transformation, which in addition to translations and rotations accounts for anisotropic scaling and/or shearing. Such a transformation can be used alone to align two shapes efficiently, or it can be used as a pre-step for a local matching algorithm.

Several techniques have been proposed to achieve global alignment between shapes. Some of these are feature-based and proceed by extracting salient features and using them to match a set of corresponding points. Finally, the matched points are used to recover the transformation parameters. Other methods, in contrast, recover these parameters by directly optimizing a similarity/dissimilarity criterion between the two shape representations.

For a D-dimensional space, there are $2D + 1$ degrees of freedom: D *rotational* degrees of freedom about each axis and D *translational* degrees of freedom in the direction of each axis, and one degree of freedom for *scaling*. Thus it is necessary for the registration process to correct for misalignments in all the degrees of freedom and then calculate an error measure, which is a calculation of the dissimilarity between the scene/template and model/reference data sets. The result of the registration process is a direct transformation from the template data set to the reference data set and an error measure between the rotated, translated, and scaled experimental data set and the model data set.

The registration process must compensate for translational offset, rotational misalignment, and partial data sets. Translational offset occurs when the coordinate origins of the template and reference data are different. This can be demonstrated by calculating the point-by-point error of two identical objects located at different locations in the D-dimensional space. Even though the objects are identical, the average error measure will be equal to the distance of the offset between the two objects.

Rotational misalignment can be visualized by viewing a non-symmetrical object from two different angles. The views may appear very different even though they come from the same object. Once the views are rotated into correct alignment, an accurate value for the error measure can be obtained. Assume that the template shape is a rigid deformed version of the reference shape. According to *rigid transformation*, such deformation can be expressed as a combination of translation **t** and rotation **R** as follows:

$$\mathbf{x}_R^i = \mathbf{R}\mathbf{x}_T^i + \mathbf{t} \tag{13.13}$$

Consequently, rigid registration seeks the values of the rotation matrix **R** and the translation vector **t** that minimize a similarity criterion which entails how a transformed template shape is aligned to the reference shape.

If isotropic scaling factor s is incorporated in the transformation model such that $\mathbf{x}_R^i = s\mathbf{R}\mathbf{x}_T^i + \mathbf{t}$, this is referred to as a *similarity transformation*. Considering a more general global transformation, *affine transformation* takes into account an anisotropic scaling matrix **S** where different scaling factors are considered for each dimension.

Local transformation

In many applications, the global matching has to be completed by dense one-to-one displacement field in the presence of local deformations. Explicitly determining the displacement field plays a key role in various medical applications. For instance, the statistics of such a field over a set of subjects can help in classifying typical versus atypical subjects, as was done in research work dedicated to classifying the brains of autistic individuals versus typically developing brains [13.14]. Complementary to the global registration field, the local coordinate transformation between the two globally aligned shapes is explicitly estimated by minimizing an energy functional which encodes a discrepancy measure between the two shape representations while penalizing the deviation of the representation of the globally warped template shape from the reference shape. Typically, a regularization term is added which enforces the smoothness of the recovered deformations.

While global transformations do not capture deformation of anatomical structures, local transformations seek to find a local warping function which maps any point in the template domain to its corresponding point in the reference domain. As such, the warping function $W(.)$ acts as a correspondence operator which keep track of local deformations.

13.2.3 Similarity measures

The similarity measure or matching score is usually measured by a disparity functional $\mathcal{D}(R, T, \mathbf{u})$ which is defined in terms of statistical measures on the intensities of the

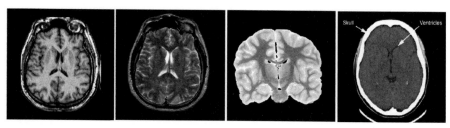

Figure 13.6 Examples of different medical imaging modalities of the human brain. From left to right: T1-weighted MR image, T2-weighted MR image, proton-density MR image and CT image.

images R and $T(\mathbf{x}+\mathbf{u}(\mathbf{x}))$. Different measures, depending on the nature of the data, have been proposed to map corresponding points to each other. For example, if the intensities of the given images are comparable (i.e., the images have been acquired by the same sensors or modality), then a reasonable way of matching the two images is by finding a geometric transformation which minimizes the sum of squared differences (SSD):

$$\mathcal{D}^{\text{SSD}}(R,T,\mathbf{u}) = \int_\Omega \left(T\big(\mathbf{x}+\mathbf{u}(\mathbf{x})\big) - R(\mathbf{x})\right)^2 d\mathbf{x}. \quad (13.14)$$

However, if the two images have different intensity maps, so-called *multimodal registration*, this simple way of measuring their similarity is no longer used. Consider, for example, the tracking problem under different illumination conditions, or the problem of registering different medical image modalities (see Figure 13.6). In such a case, more general measures have to be considered. This is the role of statistical and information-theoretic-based similarity measures, such as the *maximization of mutual information* (MI) [13.6–13.10].

The similarity measure for the mutual information (MI) is defined as follows:

$$\mathcal{D}^{\text{MI}}(R,T,\mathbf{u}) = H(R) + H\big(T\big(\mathbf{x}+\mathbf{u}(\mathbf{x})\big)\big) - H\big(R,T\big(\mathbf{x}+\mathbf{u}(\mathbf{x})\big)\big) \quad (13.15)$$

where $H(I)$ is the Shannon entropy of the image I, computed on the probability distribution of the gray values, $p^I(\cdot)$, and $H(I_1,I_2)$ is the joint entropy between I_1 and I_2. Maximizing $\mathcal{D}^{\text{MI}}(.)$ with respect to $\mathbf{u}$ is equivalent to maximizing the *Kulback–Leibler* distance between the joint distribution $p^{R,T(\mathbf{x}+\mathbf{u}(\mathbf{x}))}(\cdot,\cdot)$ and the product distribution $p^R(\cdot)\cdot p^T(\mathbf{x}+\mathbf{u}(\mathbf{x}))(\cdot)$, given by:

$$\mathcal{D}^{\text{MI}}(R,T,\mathbf{u}) = \int_\Omega p^{R,T(\mathbf{x}+\mathbf{u}(\mathbf{x}))}(l_1,l_2) \log\left(\frac{p^{R,T\big(\mathbf{x}+\mathbf{u}(\mathbf{x})\big)}(l_1,l_2)}{p^R(l_1)\cdot p^{T(\mathbf{x}+\mathbf{u}(\mathbf{x}))}(l_2)}\right) dl_1 dl_2. \quad (13.16)$$

Other measures, including the *correlation ratio* (CR) [13.11], have also been used to cope with the difficulty of registering images with different modalities. The correlation ratio measures the functional dependence between R and T, taking on values between 0 (no functional dependence) and 1 (purely deterministic dependence):

$$\mathcal{D}^{CR}(R, T, \mathbf{u}) = \frac{\text{Var}\left[E\left(T\left(\mathbf{x} + \mathbf{u}(\mathbf{x})\right)|R\right)\right]}{\text{Var}\left[T(\mathbf{x} + \mathbf{u}(\mathbf{x}))\right]} \tag{13.17}$$

where Var denotes variance and E denotes expectation.

13.3 Surface registration by the ICP algorithm

The problem of surface-based registration can be stated as aligning two partially overlapping meshes given an initial guess for relative transformation. If correct point correspondences are known in advance, it is possible to find a correct relative transformation which maps one surface to the other. Yet it is not possible to be certain that point correspondences are correct. As an alternative, if we assume that closest points correspond to each other, we can compute the *best* transformation and iterate to find the required alignment. The convergence of such a paradigm depends on how far the starting position is from the final stage.

Besl and McKay [13.1] presented a general purpose, representation-independent, surface-based registration algorithm which is known as the ICP algorithm (already defined above). It matches points in the experimental data set after applying the previously recovered transformation (scale, translation, and rotation). Least-squares estimation is then used to reduce the average distance between the matched points in the two data sets. However, since a point in one data set and its closest point in the other set do not necessarily correspond to a single point in space, several iterations are indispensable.

Different shape and free-form object registration methods based on this technique are provided in the literature (e.g. [13.2–13.5]). Below, we highlight the mathematics for the ICP algorithm following the developments in Besl and McKay [13.1].

13.3.1 Mathematical preliminaries

In this subsection, we present preliminary concepts which help in understanding the ICP algorithm.

Eigenvalue problem
Consider scaling a vector $\mathbf{v} \in \mathbb{R}^D$: this changes only its length, not its direction. This observation comes to play in the transformation of matrices which leads to the formation of eigenvectors and eigenvalues.

Example 13.1 Consider the following:

$$\underbrace{\begin{bmatrix} 2 & 3 \\ 2 & 1 \end{bmatrix}}_{A} \times \underbrace{\begin{bmatrix} 3 \\ 2 \end{bmatrix}}_{v} = \begin{bmatrix} 12 \\ 8 \end{bmatrix} = 4 \times \begin{bmatrix} 3 \\ 2 \end{bmatrix} \tag{13.18}$$

Basics of registration

The square (transformation) matrix **A** scales **v** by a scalar 4. Now assume we take a multiple of **v**:

$$2 \times \underbrace{\begin{bmatrix} 3 \\ 2 \end{bmatrix}}_{\mathbf{v}} = \begin{bmatrix} 6 \\ 4 \end{bmatrix} \tag{13.19}$$

After applying the same transformation matrix we have:

$$\underbrace{\begin{bmatrix} 2 & 3 \\ 2 & 1 \end{bmatrix}}_{\mathbf{A}} \times \underbrace{\begin{bmatrix} 6 \\ 4 \end{bmatrix}}_{2\mathbf{v}} = \begin{bmatrix} 24 \\ 16 \end{bmatrix} = 4 \times \begin{bmatrix} 6 \\ 4 \end{bmatrix} \tag{13.20}$$

Hence, regardless of how much we scale **v** by, the solution (under the transformation matrix **A**) is always a multiple of 4.

DEFINITION 13.6 *The eigenvalue problem is any problem having the form:*

$$\mathbf{Av} = \lambda \mathbf{v} \tag{13.21}$$

*where $\mathbf{A} \in \mathbb{R}^{D \times D}$, $\mathbf{v} \in \mathbb{R}^D$ is a non-zero vector and $\lambda \in \mathbb{R}$. Any value for λ for which Eq. (13.16) has a solution is called the eigenvalue of **A** and the vector **v** which corresponds to this value is called the eigenvector of **A**.*

Therefore, in the previous example, $[3\ 2]^T$ is an eigenvector of the square matrix **A** and 4 is the corresponding eigenvalue of **A**.

Using simple linear algebra, we can see that,

$$\mathbf{Av} = \lambda \mathbf{v} \Leftrightarrow \mathbf{Av} - \lambda \mathbf{Iv} = 0 \Leftrightarrow (\mathbf{A} - \lambda \mathbf{I})\mathbf{v} = 0 \tag{13.22}$$

where **I** is the identity matrix with dimension D. Finding the roots of $|\mathbf{A} - \lambda \mathbf{I}|$ results in the eigenvalues, where for each of these eigenvalues there will be an eigenvector.

Example 13.2

Let $\mathbf{A} = \begin{bmatrix} 0 & -2 \\ 1 & -3 \end{bmatrix}$, then we have:

$$|\mathbf{A} - \lambda \mathbf{I}| = \left| \begin{bmatrix} 0 & -2 \\ 1 & -3 \end{bmatrix} - \lambda \begin{bmatrix} 1 & 0 \\ 0 & 1 \end{bmatrix} \right| = \left| \begin{bmatrix} -\lambda & -2 \\ 1 & -3-\lambda \end{bmatrix} \right| = \lambda^2 + 3\lambda + 2$$

Setting the determinant to be zero, we obtain the two eigenvalues as:

$$\lambda^2 + 3\lambda + 2 = 0 \rightarrow \lambda_1 = -1, \lambda_2 = -2$$

In the case of λ_1, the corresponding eigenvector will be:

$$(\mathbf{A} - \lambda_1 \mathbf{I})\mathbf{v}_1 = 0 \rightarrow \begin{bmatrix} 1 & -2 \\ 1 & -2 \end{bmatrix} \begin{bmatrix} v_{11} \\ v_{12} \end{bmatrix} = 0 \rightarrow v_{11} = 2v_{12}$$

Hence we are looking for a column vector whose second element is twice its first element. Therefore the first eigenvector can be written as $\mathbf{v}_1 = k_1 \begin{bmatrix} 1 \\ 2 \end{bmatrix}$ where k_1 is some constant.

Similarly, the second eigenvector is obtained for some constant k_2 as $\mathbf{v}_2 = k_2 \begin{bmatrix} 1 \\ 1 \end{bmatrix}$. Note that eigenvectors can only be obtained for square matrices where all eigenvectors of a symmetric matrix are perpendicular to each other regardless of the data dimension.

Quaternions

In 2D space, rotation is always performed anticlockwise in the *xy*-plane. In 3D space, things get more complicated when one needs to specify the plane of rotation, e.g. the *xz*-plane, *yz*-plane, or even an arbitrary plane. We could also indicate a vector perpendicular to the require plane of rotation, e.g. the *z*-axis, *y*-axis, or an arbitrary axis. Hence instead of using Euler angles, we can use quaternions to specify this normal vector. In this subsection, we present the definition of quaternions along with some of its operators which enable us to represent 3D rotations. Most of the definitions are adopted from [13.6].

DEFINITION 13.7 *A quaternion* **q** *can be defined as:*

(a) A vector with four components: $\mathbf{q} = [q_0, q_1, q_2, q_3]^T$
(b) A composite of a scalar and an ordinary vector: $\mathbf{q} = [q_0, \mathbf{v_q}]$
(c) A complex number with three different imaginary parts: $\mathbf{q} = q_0 + iq_x + jq_y + kq_z$ ∎

The *multiplication* of quaternions can be expressed in terms of the product of their individual components. Suppose we have, by definition, the following:

$$i^2 \equiv j^2 \equiv k^2 \equiv -1$$
$$ij \equiv k, \quad jk \equiv i, \quad ki \equiv j \quad (13.23)$$
$$ji \equiv -k, \quad kj \equiv -i, \quad ik \equiv -j$$

DEFINITION 13.8 *Let* **r**,**q** *be two arbitrary quaternions. Their multiplication can be defined as:*

(a) The product of their individual components:

$$\begin{aligned}\mathbf{rq} = &(r_0 q_0 - r_x q_x - r_y q_y - r_z q_z) + i(r_0 q_x + r_x q_0 + r_y q_z - r_z q_y) \\ &+ j(r_0 q_y - r_x q_z + r_y q_0 + r_z q_x) \\ &+ k(r_0 q_z + r_x q_y - r_y q_x + r_z q_0)\end{aligned} \quad (13.24)$$

(b) The product of an orthogonal 4 × 4 matrix and a vector with four components:

$$\mathbf{rq} = \begin{bmatrix} r_0 & -r_x & -r_y & -r_z \\ r_x & r_0 & -r_z & r_y \\ r_y & r_z & r_0 & -r_x \\ r_z & -r_y & r_x & r_0 \end{bmatrix} \mathbf{q} = \mathbf{Rq} \quad (13.25)$$

∎

Note that we can expand either quaternion in the product into an orthogonal 4×4 matrix.

$$\mathbf{qr} = \begin{bmatrix} r_0 & -r_x & -r_y & -r_z \\ r_x & r_0 & r_z & -r_y \\ r_y & -r_z & r_0 & r_x \\ r_z & r_y & -r_x & r_0 \end{bmatrix} \mathbf{q} = \overline{\mathbf{R}}\mathbf{q} \qquad (13.26)$$

where $\overline{\mathbf{R}}$ is the same as $\mathbf{R}$ except that the lower right-hand 3×3 sub-matrix is transposed.

DEFINITION 13.9 *Let $\mathbf{r},\mathbf{q}$ be two arbitrary quaternions. Their dot product can be defined as:*

$$\mathbf{r} \cdot \mathbf{q} = r_0 q_0 + r_x q_x + r_y q_y + r_z q_z \qquad (13.27)$$

■

DEFINITION 13.10 *Let $\mathbf{q}$ be an arbitrary quaternion. $\mathbf{q}$ is said to be a unit quaternion if and only if:*

$$\mathbf{q} \cdot \mathbf{q} = \|\mathbf{q}\|^2 = 1 \qquad (13.28)$$

■

DEFINITION 13.11 *Let $\mathbf{q}$ be an arbitrary quaternion. The conjugate of $\mathbf{q}$ is defined as:*

$$\mathbf{q}* = q_0 - iq_x - jq_y - kq_z \qquad (13.29)$$

Its 4×4 orthogonal matrix is $\mathbf{Q}^T$ where $\mathbf{Q}$ is the transpose of the matrix associated with the quaternion itself:

$$\mathbf{Q} = \begin{bmatrix} q_0 & -q_x & -q_y & -q_z \\ q_x & q_0 & -q_z & q_y \\ q_y & q_z & q_0 & -q_x \\ q_z & -q_y & q_x & q_0 \end{bmatrix} \qquad (13.30)$$

■

THEOREM 13.1 *Let $\mathbf{q}$ be a non-zero quaternion. Its inverse can be defined as:*

$$\mathbf{q}^{-1} = \frac{\mathbf{q}*}{\mathbf{q} \cdot \mathbf{q}} \qquad (13.31)$$

PROOF *Since $\mathbf{Q}$ is an orthogonal matrix, the product with its transpose is a diagonal matrix where:*

$$\mathbf{Q}\mathbf{Q}^T = \mathbf{Q}^T\mathbf{Q} = (\mathbf{q} \cdot \mathbf{q})\mathbf{I} \qquad (13.32)$$

where $\mathbf{I}$ is the 4×4 identity matrix. As such the product of $\mathbf{q}$ and its conjugate $\mathbf{q}\mathbf{q}^* = \mathbf{q} \cdot \mathbf{q}$ which is real. This completes the proof. ■

COROLLARY 13.1 *The inverse of a unit quaternion is just its conjugate.* ∎

THEOREM 13.2 *Quaternion dot products are preserved: i.e. for three arbitrary quaternions* **q**, **v** *and* **r**, *we have:*

$$(\mathbf{qv}) \cdot (\mathbf{qr}) = (\mathbf{q} \cdot \mathbf{q})(\mathbf{v} \cdot \mathbf{r}) \qquad (13.33)$$

PROOF *Using* Def. 13.8 and Eq. (13.27) we have:

$$(\mathbf{qv}) \cdot (\mathbf{qr}) = (\mathbf{Qv}) \cdot (\mathbf{Qr}) = (\mathbf{Qv})^T(\mathbf{Qr}) = \mathbf{v}^T\mathbf{Q}^T\mathbf{Qr} = \mathbf{v}^T(\mathbf{q} \cdot \mathbf{q})\mathbf{Ir} = (\mathbf{q} \cdot \mathbf{q})(\mathbf{v} \cdot \mathbf{r}) \qquad (13.34)$$

∎

COROLLARY 13.2 *The magnitude of a dot product is the product of the magnitudes, i.e.*

$$(\mathbf{qr}) \cdot (\mathbf{qr}) = (\mathbf{q} \cdot \mathbf{q})(\mathbf{r} \cdot \mathbf{r}) \qquad (13.35)$$

∎

Given an arbitrary vector, it can be represented using a pure imaginary quaternion such that if $\mathbf{x} = [x, y, z]^T$, we can write it as $\mathbf{x} = 0 + ix + jy + kz$. It is important to note that since vectors have zero real part, their associated matrices are skew-symmetric, that is,

$$\mathbf{X}^T = -\mathbf{X} \text{ and } \overline{\mathbf{X}}^T = -\overline{\mathbf{X}} \qquad (13.36)$$

DEFINITION 13.12 *Let* **x** *be a pure imaginary quaternion representing a 3D point or vector where* $\mathbf{x} = 0 + ix + jy + kz$. *Let* **q** *be a unit quaternion such that* $\mathbf{q} = q_0 + iq_x + jq_y + kq_z$. *Rotating the point or vector* **x** *by a unit quaternion* **q** *is achieved by the composite product which is defined as:*

$$\mathbf{x}' = \mathbf{qxq}* \qquad (13.37)$$

where **x**′ is a pure imaginary quaternion representing **x** after being rotated by **q**. ∎

13.3.2 The ICP algorithm

The problem statement of the ICP algorithm can be stated as follows. A model shape may be represented as a point cloud, set of line segments, implicit curves, parametric curves, triangular mesh, implicit surfaces or parametric surfaces. Given a target or scene shape which is represented as a point cloud, the target shape may correspond to the model shape. It is required to estimate the optimal rotation, translation, and scaling that aligns or registers the target shape to the model shape.

The ICP algorithm registers the scene to the model shapes by minimizing, iteratively, the Euclidian distance between them. The basic steps in obtaining the translation, rotation, and scaling using the ICIP algorithm are as follows (Figure 13.7).

360 Basics of registration

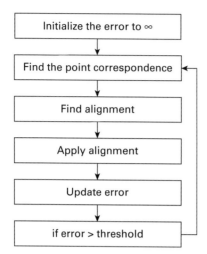

Figure 13.7 Block diagram outlining the basic steps of the ICP algorithm.

Basic steps in the ICP algorithm

(1) Begin with initial rotation, translation, and scaling (initial value for registration parameters).
(2) Fix the model shape and start moving the scene shape by applying the initial registration parameters, i.e. scale, rotate, and then translate.
(3) Compute the error metric that reflects the dissimilarity of the scene shape from the model shape.
(4) If the error is minimum, we have correctly aligned the scene shape to the model shape. Return the aligned scene shape.
(5) Else, calculate the new values for the registration parameters and go back to step 2 with the new parameter values.

Notations

Let the model shape be represented by a set of points $M = \{m_i\}$ where $i = 1, 2, \ldots, N_m$ and N_m is the number of points in the model shape, such that $m_i = [m_{xi}, m_{yi}, m_{zi}]^T \in \mathbb{R}^3$. Similarly, let the scene shape be represented by a set of points $P = \{p_i\}$ where $i = 1, 2, \ldots, N_p$ and N_p is the number of points in the scene shape, such that $p_i = [p_{xi}, p_{yi}, p_{zi}]^T \in \mathbb{R}^3$.

The registration parameters can be defined as follows. Let $s \in \mathbb{R}$ be a scalar representing the scaling parameter, $t \in \mathbb{R}^3$ be a vector representing the translation parameters, and $R(.)$ be an operator which applied rotation to its argument. Note that $R(.)$ will have a different definition according to the way we represent rotations. It can be Euler angles, a rotation matrix or a quaternion defining the rotation angle and axis of rotation.

Finding correspondences

A correct relative rotation and translation can be found if point correspondences are available. Yet finding such correspondences is the bottleneck of many registration

13.3 Surface registration by the ICP algorithm

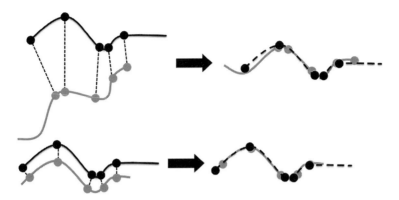

Figure 13.8 Illustration of the effect of the starting position on the registration process.

algorithms. ICP assumes closest points to correspond (hence the name). It is worth noting that such an assumption usually converges if the initial position is close enough to the true one (see Figure 13.8).

Finding correspondence can be estimated by searching the closest model point in the model shape to every scene point in the scene shape using the Euclidean distance.

DEFINITION 13.13 *Let $\mathbf{p}, \mathbf{m} \in \mathbb{R}^3$ be two given points. Their Euclidean distance is defined as:*

$$d(\mathbf{p}, \mathbf{m}) = \|\mathbf{p} - \mathbf{m}\| = \sqrt{(p_x - m_x)^2 + (p_y - m_y)^2 + (p_z - m_z)^2}. \tag{13.38}$$

∎

The Euclidean distance between a scene point (that is, a data point) $\mathbf{p}_i$ and the model point set M is the solution of the following minimization.

$$d(\mathbf{p}_i, M) = \min_k d(\mathbf{p}_i, \mathbf{m}_k) \tag{13.39}$$

Hence, the closest point $\mathbf{m}_j \in M$ satisfies:

$$d(\mathbf{p}_i, \mathbf{m}_j) = d(\mathbf{p}_i, M) \quad \Rightarrow \quad j = \operatorname*{argmin}_k d(\mathbf{p}_i, \mathbf{m}_k) \tag{13.40}$$

We denote the closest point in the model set which yields the minimum distance by $\mathbf{y}_i$. Hence $\mathbf{p}_i$ corresponds to $\mathbf{y}_i$. We also denote $Y = \{\mathbf{y}_i\}$ where $i = 1,2,\ldots,N_p$ as the set of closest points and C as the closest point operator such that $Y = C(P, M)$. Code 13.1 in Appendix 13.1 shows a sample implementation of the closest point operator.

Alignment calculation
The problem of alignment calculation can be stated as follows. Given a set of point correspondences Y between the scene shape P and the model shape M such that $Y \subseteq M$, it is required to find the optimal registration parameters, i.e. the scaling, rotation, and translation which bring the scene points $\{p_i\}$ to the closest model point $\{y_i\}$. Formally, we

are looking for a transformation of the form in Eq. (13.36) which registers/aligns the scene points P to the corresponding points Y.

$$Y = sR(P) + \mathbf{t} \quad (13.41)$$

where s denotes the scaling factor, $\mathbf{t}$ denotes the translational offset and $R(P)$ denotes the rotated version of the scene points P. Note that at the moment we are not referring to any particular notation for rotation.

Since point correspondences are not guaranteed to be perfect, in particular in the case of registration with partial information, we will not be able to find the exact registration parameters such that Eq. (13.36) is satisfied for each point in the scene shape. As such there will be a residual error for each point pair defined as:

$$\mathbf{e}_i = \mathbf{y}_i - \left(sR(\mathbf{p}_i) + \mathbf{t}\right) \quad (13.42)$$

where $sR(\mathbf{p}_i) + \mathbf{t}$ is the transformed version of the scene point $\mathbf{p}_i$. Hence the objective now is to find the registration parameters that minimize the total error, defined as the sum of squares of these residuals.

$$E = \sum_{i=1}^{N_p} \|\mathbf{e}_i\|^2 \quad (13.43)$$

In the following, we will consider the variation of the total error first with translation, then with scale and finally with respect to rotation.

Computing the translation

In order to remove the effect of the shape origin, it is useful to refer all points to their centroid, defined as:

$$\boldsymbol{\mu}_P = \frac{1}{N_P} \sum_{i=1}^{N_p} \mathbf{p}_i \quad \text{and} \quad \boldsymbol{\mu}_Y = \frac{1}{N_P} \sum_{i=1}^{N_p} \mathbf{y}_i \quad (13.44)$$

where each $\mathbf{p}_i$ is a point in the scene (data) and $\mathbf{y}_i$ is the closest point to it on the model. Hence the centered (zero-mean) points are given by:

$$\mathbf{p}'_i = \mathbf{p}_i - \boldsymbol{\mu}_P \quad \text{and} \quad \mathbf{y}'_i = \mathbf{y}_i - \boldsymbol{\mu}_Y \quad (13.45)$$

Now, the error term can be re-written as:

$$\mathbf{e}_i = \mathbf{y}'_i - \left(sR(\mathbf{p}'_i) + \mathbf{t}'\right) \quad (13.46)$$

where

$$\mathbf{t}' = \mathbf{t} - \boldsymbol{\mu}_Y + sR(\boldsymbol{\mu}_P) \quad (13.47)$$

Hence the sum of squares of errors becomes:

$$E = \sum_{i=1}^{N_p} \|\mathbf{e}_i\|^2 = \sum_{i=1}^{N_p} \|\mathbf{y}_i' - \left(sR(\mathbf{p}_i') + \mathbf{t}'\right)\|^2$$

$$= \sum_{i=1}^{N_p} [\|\mathbf{y}_i' - sR(\mathbf{p}_i')\|^2 - 2\mathbf{t}'\|\mathbf{y}_i' - sR(\mathbf{p}_i')\| + \|\mathbf{t}'\|^2] \quad (13.48)$$

$$= \sum_{i=1}^{N_p} \|\mathbf{y}_i' - sR(\mathbf{p}_i')\|^2 - 2\mathbf{t}' \sum_{i=1}^{N_p} \|\mathbf{y}_i' - sR(\mathbf{p}_i')\| + N_p \|\mathbf{t}'\|^2$$

Now the sum in the middle of the expression in Eq. (13.43) is zero since the points are referred to the centroid (i.e. zero-mean, and rotation and scaling do not affect the mean). Hence, the first and third terms are left:

$$E = \sum_{i=1}^{N_p} \|\mathbf{y}_i' - sR(\mathbf{p}_i')\|^2 + N_p \|\mathbf{t}'\|^2 \quad (13.49)$$

Remember that we are looking for the optimal translational offset $\mathbf{t}'$ which will minimize the total error E. The first term in Eq. (13.44) does not depend on the translation while the second term cannot be negative since

$$\|\mathbf{t}'\|^2 \geq 0 \text{ and } N_p > 0 \quad (13.50)$$

Thus the total error is obviously minimized with $\mathbf{t}' = 0$. Therefore the translational offset can be found as follows:

$$\mathbf{t}' = \mathbf{t} - \boldsymbol{\mu}_Y + sR(\boldsymbol{\mu}_P) = 0 \Rightarrow \mathbf{t} = \boldsymbol{\mu}_Y + sR(\boldsymbol{\mu}_P) \quad (13.51)$$

That is, the translation is just the difference of the centroid of the model points and the centroid of the scaled and rotated scene points. We return to this equation to find the translational offset once we have found the scale and rotation. At this point, we note that the error term can be written as:

$$\mathbf{e}_i = \mathbf{y}_i' - sR(\mathbf{p}_i') \quad (13.52)$$

Since $\mathbf{t}' = 0$, the total error to be minimized can be re-written as follows:

$$E = \sum_{i=1}^{N_p} \|\mathbf{y}_i' - sR(\mathbf{p}_i')\|^2 \quad (13.53)$$

Computing the scale
Expanding the total error in Eq. (13.48), we will get:

$$E = \sum_{i=1}^{N_p} \|\mathbf{y}'\|_i^2 - 2s \sum_{i=1}^{N_p} \mathbf{y}_i' R(\mathbf{p}_i') + s^2 \sum_{i=1}^{N_p} \|R(\mathbf{p}_i')\|^2 \quad (13.54)$$

Rotation preserves length, i.e.

$$\|R(\mathbf{p}'_i)\|^2 = \|\mathbf{p}'_i\|^2 \tag{13.55}$$

Therefore we obtain:

$$E = \underbrace{\sum_{i=1}^{N_p} \|\mathbf{y}'_i\|^2}_{S_y} - 2s \underbrace{\sum_{i=1}^{N_p} \mathbf{y}'_i R(\mathbf{p}'_i)}_{D} + s^2 \underbrace{\sum_{i=1}^{N_p} \|\mathbf{p}'_i\|^2}_{S_p} \tag{13.56}$$

Hence we have:

$$E = S_y - 2sD + s^2 S_p \tag{13.57}$$

where S_y and S_p are the sums of the squares of the points' lengths relative to their centroids, while D is the sum of the dot products of the corresponding points in the model with the rotated points in the scene.

Since we are looking for the scaling factor s, completing the square in Eq. (13.52) with respect to s will give us:

$$E = \left(s\sqrt{S_p} - \frac{D}{\sqrt{S_p}}\right)^2 + \frac{S_y S_p - D^2}{S_p} \tag{13.58}$$

The total error can be minimized with respect to the scaling factor s when the first term in Eq. (13.53) is set to zero, since the second term does not depend on s. Hence the scaling factor is obtained as:

$$s = \frac{D}{S_p} = \frac{\sum_{i=1}^{N_p} \mathbf{y}'_i R(\mathbf{p}'_i)}{\sum_{i=1}^{N_p} \|\mathbf{p}'_i\|^2} \tag{13.59}$$

If we exchange the roles of the scene and the model points as recommended by Horn [13.6], we will find the best fit instead of the transformation. As such we will find the inverse transformation defined as:

$$\mathbf{p}_i = sR^T(\mathbf{y}_i) + \bar{\mathbf{t}} \tag{13.60}$$

where the scale factor equation in this case becomes:

$$s = \sqrt{\frac{\sum_{i=1}^{N_p} \|\mathbf{y}'_i\|^2}{\sum_{i=1}^{N_p} \|\mathbf{p}'_i\|^2}} \tag{13.61}$$

Computing the rotation

To minimize the error with respect to scaling, we set the first term in Eq. (13.53) to zero, since the second term does not depend on scaling. Now after finding the scale factor which causes the first term to be zero, the error terms can be re-written as:

13.3 Surface registration by the ICP algorithm

$$E = \frac{S_y S_p - D^2}{S_p} \tag{13.62}$$

By their definition, $S_y \geq 0$ and $S_p \geq 0$, therefore $S_y S_p \geq 0$ and does not depend on the rotation, i.e. is constant with respect to $R(.)$, and $D^2 \geq 0$ (self evident) is the only part in the error expression that depends on $R(.)$, Thus $E = S_y S_p - D^2$ must be minimized, which is satisfied if we maximize D.

Recall that D is the sum of the dot products of the model points and the rotated scene points. Hence this maximization can be interpreted geometrically as follows:

$$\mathbf{y}'_i R(\mathbf{p}'_i) = \|\mathbf{y}'_i\| \|R(\mathbf{p}'_i)\| \cos \theta \tag{13.63}$$

where θ is the angle between the model points and the rotated scene points. To obtain the optimal rotation, θ should be zero, therefore $\cos \theta = 1$ which is the maximum value obtained by the cosine function. Since by definition $|.|\geq 0$, having $\theta = 0$ will lead to the maximum value of $\mathbf{y}'_i R(\mathbf{p}'_i)$. Therefore, maximizing D implicitly means minimizing the angle between the model points and the rotated scene points.

There are many ways to represent rotation, including Euler angles, axis and angle, orthonormal matrices and quaternions. Usually, orthonormal matrices are deployed in photogrammetry and robotics. However, there are a number of advantages to the unit-quaternion notation. Further, unit quaternions lend themselves directly to the geometrical intuition of axis and angle notation. Here we need to find the unit quaternion $\mathbf{q}$ which maximizes

$$D = \sum_{i=1}^{N_p} \mathbf{y}'_i R(\mathbf{p}'_i) = \sum_{i=1}^{N_p} \mathbf{y}'_i (\mathbf{q} \mathbf{p}'_i \mathbf{q}^*) = \sum_{i=1}^{N_p} (\mathbf{q} \mathbf{p}'_i \mathbf{q}^*) \mathbf{y}'_i = \sum_{i=1}^{N_p} (\mathbf{q} \mathbf{p}'_i) \cdot (\mathbf{y}'_i \mathbf{q}) \tag{13.64}$$

Suppose that $\mathbf{p}'_i = [p'_{xi}, p'_{yi}, p'_{zi}]^T$ and $\mathbf{y}'_i = [y'_{xi}, y'_{yi}, y'_{zi}]^T$, then:

$$\mathbf{q}\mathbf{p}'_i = \begin{bmatrix} 0 & -p'_{xi} & -p'_{yi} & -p'_{zi} \\ p'_{xi} & 0 & p'_{zi} & -p'_{yi} \\ p'_{yi} & -p'_{zi} & 0 & p'_{xi} \\ p'_{zi} & p'_{yi} & -p'_{xi} & 0 \end{bmatrix} \mathbf{q} = \overline{\mathbf{P}}_i \mathbf{q}$$

and

$$\mathbf{y}'_i \mathbf{q} = \begin{bmatrix} 0 & -y'_{xi} & -y'_{yi} & -y'_{zi} \\ y'_{xi} & 0 & -y'_{zi} & y'_{yi} \\ y'_{yi} & y'_{zi} & 0 & -y'_{xi} \\ y'_{zi} & -y'_{yi} & y'_{xi} & 0 \end{bmatrix} \mathbf{q} = \mathbf{Y}_i \mathbf{q} \tag{13.65}$$

Note that $\overline{\mathbf{P}}_i$ and $\mathbf{Y}_i$ are skew-symmetric and orthogonal since they are associated to purely imaginary quaternions. The sum that we need to maximize can now be written as:

$$D = \sum_{i=1}^{N_p}(\mathbf{q}\mathbf{p}'_i)\cdot(\mathbf{y}'_i\mathbf{q}) = \sum_{i=1}^{N_p}(\overline{\mathbf{P}}_i\mathbf{q})\cdot(\mathbf{Y}_i\mathbf{q}) = \sum_{i=1}^{N_p}(\overline{\mathbf{P}}_i\mathbf{q})^T(\mathbf{Y}_i\mathbf{q})$$
$$= \mathbf{q}^T\left(\sum_{i=1}^{N_p}\underbrace{\overline{\mathbf{P}}_i^T\mathbf{Y}_i}_{\mathbf{N}_i}\right)\mathbf{q} = \mathbf{q}^T\mathbf{N}\mathbf{q} \tag{13.66}$$

where

$$\mathbf{N} = \sum_{i=1}^{N_p}\mathbf{N}_i$$

$$\begin{bmatrix} S_{xx}+S_{yy}+S_{zz} & S_{yz}-S_{zy} & -S_{xz}+S_{zx} & S_{xx}-S_{yz} \\ S_{yz}-S_{zy} & S_{xx}-S_{yy}-S_{zz} & S_{xy}+S_{yx} & S_{xz}+S_{zx} \\ S_{zx}-S_{xz} & S_{yx}+S_{xy} & S_{yy}-S_{zz}-S_{xx} & S_{yz}+S_{zy} \\ S_{xy}-S_{yx} & S_{zx}+S_{xz} & S_{zy}+S_{yz} & S_{zz}-S_{yy}-S_{xx} \end{bmatrix} \tag{13.67}$$

with $S_{xx} = \sum_{i=1}^{N_p} p'_{xi}y'_{xi}$, $S_{xy} = \sum_{i=1}^{N_p} p'_{xi}y'_{yi}$ ... etc.

Hence we can define the S-matrix whose elements are sums of products of coordinates measured in the scene shape with coordinates measured in the model shape, such that:

$$S = \begin{bmatrix} S_{xx} & S_{xy} & S_{xz} \\ S_{yx} & S_{yy} & S_{yz} \\ S_{zx} & S_{zy} & S_{zz} \end{bmatrix} \tag{13.68}$$

Note that the scene (data) and model points were brought to the origin by subtracting their centroids; this basically resolves the translation issue, and what remains is scale and rotation.

THEOREM 13.3 *The unit quaternion that maximizes* $\mathbf{q}^T\mathbf{N}\mathbf{q}$ *is the eigenvector corresponding to the most positive eigenvalue of the matrix* **N**.

PROOF *Left* for exercise.

Code 13.2 shows a code snippet which presents the implementation of finding the rotation, the scaling factor, and the translational offset given pairs of point correspondences

13.4 Global image registration via mutual information

Medical imaging technologies provide different imaging modalities to allow for non-invasive imaging of patient anatomy. For instance, magnetic resonance imaging (MRI) has been found to be a sensitive marker of changes in disease progression. Despite this, evaluation of the disease cannot be completely based upon MRI findings. For example, multiple sclerosis[1] (MS) lesion activity observed in MRI studies of the brain does not always correspond to clinically observed deficits (see [13.11] for algorithmic evaluation

---

[1] Multiple sclerosis (MS) is a debilitating disease of the human nervous system (see [13.11]).

of registration methods to quantify MS deficits from MRI). Hence, using multiple imaging modalities usually aids disease diagnosis.

It is desirable to apply computer vision techniques to the study of diseases using different imaging modalities. Allowing a computer to identify normal and abnormal anatomical structures automatically would free an expert from the arduous task of manually examining each slice of a study, while generally increasing the reproducibility of the identification by removing the subjectivity of the human observer. The fields of segmentation and classification address this task. Computer vision tools would also be useful for automatic, retrospective *alignment* of patient studies, taken at different points in time, to allow for qualitative comparison of different studies of a patient over the course of treatment. This type of analysis would aid the expert in deciding if the disease is responding well to the present treatment, or if a change in treatment is warranted.

When different scans are taken of a patient (at different times and/or using different imaging modalities), two factors must be considered. First, scan parameters are likely to differ between scans, including voxel dimensions, and perhaps scan weightings[2]. Second, and most important, the patient will not be positioned in the same location in the scanning volume. Thus, anatomy in two different studies, taken with exactly the same scan parameters, will not be geometrically aligned in the scanning volume, disallowing the possibility of comparing earlier and later scans on a slice-by-slice basis. To allow for a comparison of multiple scans, a geometric alignment of the anatomy imaged must be found; this function is known as *volume registration*. The goal of registration, therefore, is to align the anatomy from one scan to the anatomy from a second. When this function is performed, the resulting volumes are said to be registered; without this function, the volumes are said to be misregistered.

Figure 13.9 illustrates the problem of misregistration in two dimensions. Here, the box represents a scanning area. Comparing the positioning of the anatomy in the left and right

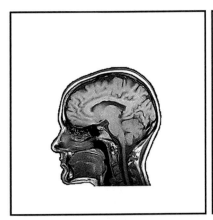 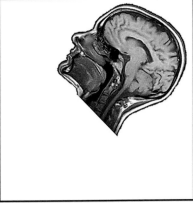

Figure 13.9 Illustration of the registration problem in two dimensions. The squares in the left and right figures represent the respective scanning areas. The anatomy is located at a different position between the two volumes, and has been rotated.

---

[2] By controlling the acquisition parameters of the scan, different image weightings may be obtained, allowing for different and/or improved image contrast between different types of tissue.

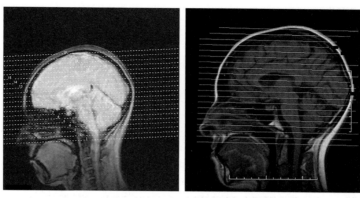

Figure 13.10 Scout scans for the same patient, at different time points. Note that the lines that indicate the slice planes do not correspond in the two different studies.

scanning areas, the volumes are out of alignment by three factors: two translation quantities (a horizontal and vertical), and a rotation angle. Registration is the function by which these quantities are discovered or calculated, thereby supplying the information necessary to relate one volume to another.

Figure 13.10 below provides further evidence of this problem. Shown are two different images, known as scout images[3], for the same patient, for MRI studies done at different points in time. The scout images show the positions of the imaging planes in a study, and are recorded by the technologist controlling the MRI machine at the time of data acquisition. As can be observed from the two scout images shown, the positions of these lines (dotted in the right image, solid in the left) do not correspond with one another, indicating that a slice-by-slice comparison of the studies will not allow comparison between the same physical locations in the patient's brain.

Finally, Figure 13.11 shows several slices from two brain studies. The sample slices shown in the first row are from a single study. The sample slices shown in the second row are the slices from a later study, which have the same slice number as the slices shown in the first row. As can be observed, the anatomy imaged is not geometrically aligned.

It is desirable to be able to perform registration using computer vision approaches, rather than imposing limitations in the scanning procedure, or affixing artificial fiducial markers on the patient which would be inconvenient and potentially painful for the patient. Additionally, this procedure would also introduce a risk of infection. Furthermore, using computer vision techniques, it is also desirable to be able to apply registration retroactively, allowing current data sets to be aligned with sets taken previously in a patient's history, or perhaps with an imaging modality that prevents the use of artificial markers.

Registration can also be used to assist in *segmentation*. For example, if a model of patient anatomy is known, then a study can be registered to that model, allowing segmentation of certain classes of problems to be made trivial, as the segmentation of the data set is then known *a priori* from the model. In this context, a well-known and

---

[3] The CT scout scan serves as an anatomic reference for the PET/CT scan.

13.4 Global image registration via mutual information

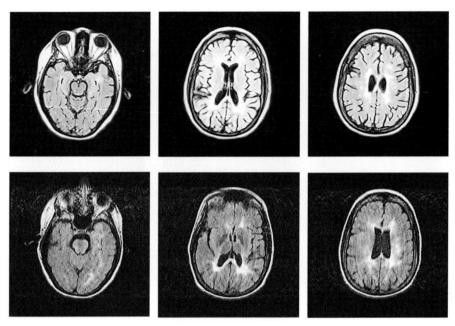

Figure 13.11 Sample slice comparison between two scans of the same patient, taken at different points in time. Each row contains sample slices from one study. The columns contain the same slice number from each study. As apparent, the anatomy is not geometrically aligned between the two scanning volumes.

useful volume registration technique, known as registration by maximization of mutual information (MI) [13.8–13.10], is presented in this section. This technique has generally been found to perform well, and is useful in clinical settings.

It relies on the evaluation of a metric function to quantify the quality of alignment of the source and target dataset, given a registration parameter vector. The metric function is based on information theoretical measure of the statistical dependencies between images [13.12]. An affine transformation is used to handle the global registration problem through a gradient descent optimization technique. It has been proven to be robust in multi-model image registration. Below, the implementation of this technique along with some mathematical preliminaries will be discussed.

13.4.1 Imaging model

Of preliminary concern is the construction of a volume from an imaging study, and modeling the relationship of this volume to 3D space. Data obtained from an imaging study such as an MRI-based modality or CT consists of a set of ordered slices, representing consecutive slices in parallel, along a direction normal to each slice; see Figure 13.12 for schematic illustration. Imaging studies are typically taken along one of three customary sets of planes: parasagittal, coronal, or axial planes. Parasagittal planes are those parallel to the sagittal plane, which itself divides the body of interest into two symmetrical parts; coronal planes are parallel to the long axis of the body, and normal to parasagittal planes;

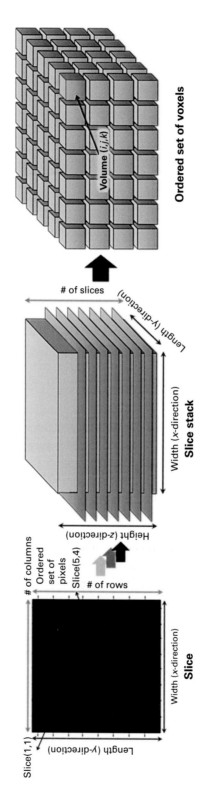

Figure 13.12 Schematic illustration of how an imaging study is formed. Image slices are stacked into a volume to construct a set of ordered voxels.

13.4 Global image registration via mutual information

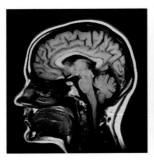 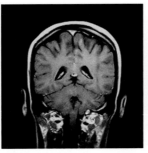 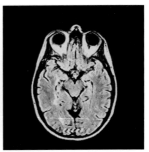

Figure 13.13 Examples of MRI sagittal scans (left), coronal scans (middle), and axial scans (right).

axial planes are normal to parasagittal and coronal planes. Given a choice of imaging planes, slices are then ordered in a particular direction, such as "patient left to right," and so forth. Examples of slices from each of the three imaging directions are shown below in Figure 13.13. Given a set of ordered image slices, a volume is formed by placing slices consecutively in the volume, ascending in a direction normal to each image plane by a fixed amount (determined by slice thickness and slice gap). Each slice is placed "squarely" upon the slice lower in the volume, such that the faces of the 3D volume formed have right angles between their edges.

13.4.2 Basics of information theory

Suppose we performed an experiment with N possible outcomes $x_1, x_2, \ldots, x_N$ and the outcome was x_k with probability $p(x_k)$. The question now becomes: what is the *information* that we have gained? There are several equivalent formulations of this question, among which is: what is the *uncertainty* that is removed? What is the amount of *surprise*? For example, the amount of surprise will be zero if $p(x_k) = 1$, that is, we are sure that we will obtain the outcome x_k whenever we perform the same experiment.

Our intuition implies the following. When $p(x_k) = 1$ we can say that surprise = uncertainty = information = 0. Zero uncertainty comes from our certainty that this outcome will occur, while zero information means that we do not gain any more information when this outcome occurs. Likewise if $p(x_k) = 0$, surprise = uncertainty = information = 1. Hence, according to this intuition, there is an *inverse relationship* between outcome probability and the information gained when that outcome occurs. This leads us to the proposal made by the father of information theory, Claude Elwood Shannon (April 30, 1916 – February 24, 2001) who was an American electronic engineer and mathematician.

DEFINITION 13.14 *The amount of information gained from an outcome x_k is quantified as:*

$$I(x_k) = \log \frac{1}{p(x_k)} = -\log p(x_k) \qquad (13.69)$$

where $I(x_k)$ is the information measure of outcome x_k which satisfies the following properties:

$$I(x_k) \begin{cases} = 0 & p(x_k) = 0 \\ \geq 0 & 0 < p(x_k) \leq 1 \end{cases} \quad (13.70)$$

The units are bits for base 2 logarithms and nats for natural logarithms. ∎

Since x_k is a random variable with probability $p(x_k)$ and the information measure $I(x_k)$ is defined as a function of a random variable, we can consider $I(x_k)$ as a random variable with probability $p(x_k)$. As such we can define the average amount of information gained from x_k as follows.

DEFINITION 13.15 *The entropy of the random variable X is defined as the mean value of $I(x_k)$, referring to the average amount of information gained from the occurrence of each outcome x_k where:*

$$H(X) = E[I(x_k)] = \sum_{k=1}^{N} p(x_k) I(x_k) = -\sum_{k=1}^{N} p(x_k) \log p(x_k) \quad (13.71)$$

∎

Entropy is a common measurement of information content. Information content is increased as entropy is increased, and decreased as entropy is decreased. The less concentrated a probability density or mass function is, the more information content that is encoded in the random variable. For example, consider a continuous random variable X. If X is distributed as a uniform random variable, the information content of X is greatest, because over the range of X, the probability of X taking on a value x_1 is equal in all cases to X taking on a value of x_2. For X distributed as a Gaussian random variable, with a mean μ and variance σ^2, X encodes less information, as the values of X around μ are more likely than values far from μ, with the spread or concentration of probability around μ quantified by the variance σ^2.

The entropy is bounded by:

$$0 \leq H(X) \leq \log N \quad (13.72)$$

such that

- $H(X) = 0$ iff $p(x_k) = 1$ for some k while the probabilities of all other outcomes are set to zero. This *lower bound* corresponds to the case where there is no uncertainty or no information gained.
- $H(X) = \log N$ iff $p(x_k) = \frac{1}{N}$ $\forall k$, i.e. uniform distribution. This *upper bound* corresponds to maximum uncertainty, i.e. new information gained for each outcome occurrence.

13.4 Global image registration via mutual information

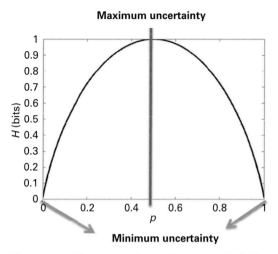

Figure 13.14 The entropy of tossing a coin as a function of XXX. Note that the maximum uncertainty occurs when both head and tail are equally likely to occur, while if one of them has a unit probability (and the other has zero probability) we are sure of the experiment outcome, hence minimum uncertainty occurs.

Example 13.3 Consider tossing a coin where the probability of getting a head is p while the probability of getting a tail is $1-p$. The entropy can be derived as follows:

$$H(X) = -\sum_{k=1}^{N} p(x_k) \log p(x_k) = -[p_1 \log p_1 + p_2 \log p_2] \quad (13.73)$$
$$= -p \log p - (1-p) \log(1-p)$$

When there are two random variables, the term used is joint or mutual entropy, which is defined as follows (see Figure 13.14).

DEFINITION 13.16 *Consider a random variable X taking values from the set* $\{x_1,\ldots,x_N\}$ *such that* $\sum_{k=1}^{N} p(x_k) = 1$ *and* $0 \le p(x_k) \le 1$. *Consider another random variable Y taking values from the set* $\{y_1,\ldots,y_M\}$ *such that* $\sum_{k=1}^{M} p(y_k) = 1$ *and* $0 \le p(y_k) \le 1$. *The joint entropy of X and Y is defined as:*

$$H(X,Y) = \sum_{i=1}^{N}\sum_{j=1}^{M} p(x_i,y_j) \log \frac{1}{p(x_i,y_j)} = -\sum_{k=1}^{N}\sum_{j=1}^{M} p(x_i,y_j) \log p(x_i,y_j) \quad (13.74)$$

where $p(x_i,y_j)$ is the joint probability density function of the two random variables, and refers to the probability of having both outcomes x_i and y_j occur together. ∎

Example 13.4 Let X be a random variable of rolling a fair die while Y is another random variable of flipping a coin. Assume they are independent[4]; as such their joint density function can be derived as follows:

$$p(x_i, y_j) = p(x_i)p(y_j) = \left(\frac{1}{6}\right)\left(\frac{1}{2}\right) = \frac{1}{12} \qquad (13.75)$$

Hence the joint entropy can be computed as:

$$H(X,Y) = -\sum_{k=1}^{N} p(x_i, y_j) \log p(x_i, y_j) = 2\left(6\left(\frac{1}{12}\log\frac{1}{12}\right)\right) = \log 12 \qquad (13.76)$$

DEFINITION 13.17 *Consider a random variable X taking values from the set $\{x_1,\ldots,x_N\}$ such that $\sum_{k=1}^{N} p(x_k) = 1$ and $0 \le p(x_k) \le 1$. Consider another random variable Y taking values from the $\{y_1, \ldots, y_M\}$ set such that $\sum_{k=1}^{M} p(y_k) = 1$ and $p(x_k) \le 1$. The conditional entropy describes the average uncertainty on Y that remains after a measurement of X. The conditional entropy of X given $Y = y_j$ is*

$$H(X|Y = y_j) = -\sum_{i=1}^{N} p(X = x_i|Y = y_j)\log p(X = x_i|Y = y_j) \qquad (13.77)$$

where $p(X = x_i|Y = y_j)$ is the conditional probability. The conditional entropy of X given Y can be given by:

$$H(X|Y) = -\sum_{i=1}^{N}\sum_{j=1}^{M} \underbrace{p(X=x_i|Y=y_j)p(Y=y_j)}_{p(X=x_i, Y=y_j)}\log p(X=x_i|Y=y_j) \qquad (13.78)$$

where $p(X = x_i, Y = y_j)$ is the joint probability density function. ∎

By simple algebraic manipulation, and using the definition of conditional probabilities, the joint entropy $H(X,Y)$ can be related to the entropy quantities as shown in Theorem 13.4.

THEOREM 13.4 *The joint entropy is related to conditional entropy according to the following relation:*

$$H(X,Y) = H(X) + H(Y|X) \qquad (13.79)$$

PROOF *Left for exercise.* ∎

Consider the average uncertainty on Y, i.e. $H(Y)$, and the average uncertainty on Y after measuring X, i.e. $H(Y|X)$. Hence $H(Y) - H(Y|X)$ can be interpreted as:

---

[4] Two events A and B are independent of each other if P(A) = P(A|B), i.e. knowing B does not add any information when measuring the probability of A, hence P(A,B) = P(A)P(B). Two events A and B are conditionally independent of each other given an event C if P(A|C) = P(A|B,C).

- The reduction in the uncertainty of Y by the knowledge of X.
- The information on Y resolved after measuring X.
- The amount of information that X contains about Y.

DEFINITION 13.18 *The mutual information between X and Y is defined as:*

$$I(X,Y) = H(Y) - H(Y|X) = H(X) - H(X|Y)$$
$$= H(X) + H(Y) - H(X,Y) \qquad (13.80)$$

where $I(X, Y) = I(Y, X)$. ∎

For two discrete random variables X and Y, with marginal probability mass functions $p_X(x)$ and $p_Y(y)$, and a joint distribution $p(x, y)$, the mutual information function $I(x, y)$ is the relative entropy between the joint distribution $p(x, y)$, and the distribution $p_X(x) p_Y(y)$, the joint distribution when X and Y are independent random variables. Thus, the mutual information of X and Y is given in Theorem 13.5 below.

THEOREM 13.5 *The mutual information is related to the entropy according to the following relation:*

$$I(X,Y) = \sum_{i=1}^{N} \sum_{j=1}^{M} p(x_i, y_j) \log \frac{p(x_i, y_j)}{p_X(x_i) p_Y(y_j)} \qquad (13.81)$$

PROOF Left for exercise. ∎

If X and Y are independent random variables, then p(x, y) is given by the product of the marginals p_X(x) and p_Y(y), and therefore, the quantity that is the argument of the logarithm function in Eq. (13.78) is 1. As the logarithm of 1 is 0, the mutual information $I(X, Y)$, when X and Y are statistically independent, is zero.

If the random variables X and Y are the image intensity values, x and y, of a pair of corresponding voxels in the two images that are to be registered, then estimations of the joint distribution $p_{XY}(x, y)$ and marginal distributions $p_X(x)$ and $p_Y(y)$ can be obtained by simple normalization of the joint and marginal histograms of the overlapping parts of both images.

Appendix 13.1 gives MATLAB realizations (Codes 13.3, 13.4, and 13.5) of the mutual information.

13.4.3 Registration metric

For volumetric registration, there will be two volumes, a floating volume, and a reference volume. The floating volume will be transformed by a transformation T_Θ, with registration parameters Θ. Using the intensities of the volumes as the features for registration, the random variable R will denote the intensities observed in the reference volume, the random variable F will denote the intensities observed in the floating volume, and the random variable $T_\Theta F$ will denote the intensities observed in the transformed floating volume, given the registration parameters Θ. The mutual information function $I(X,Y)$ will be used as a measure of alignment, by consideration of $I(R, T_\Theta F)$. Therefore, the registration problem is to maximize $I(R, T_\Theta F)$ by manipulation of the registration parameters Θ. The metric $I(R, T_\Theta F)$, from the definition of mutual information in Eq. (13.78), and the relationships of mutual information to entropy in Eq. (13.77_, can be written as below.

$$I(R, T_\Theta F) = \sum_{r \in R} \sum_{f \in F} p(r, T_\Theta f) \log\left(\frac{p(r, T_\Theta f)}{p_R(r) p_{T_\Theta F}(T_\Theta f)}\right) \quad (13.82)$$

$$I(R, T_\Theta F) = H(R) - H(R|T_\Theta F) \quad (13.83)$$

$$I(R, T_\Theta F) = H(R) + H(T_\Theta F) - H(R, T_\Theta F) \quad (13.84)$$

In the process of registration, only the overlapping portions of the reference and transformed floating volumes will be considered in computation of the mutual information metric, as will be discussed below. Therefore, the quantities $H(R)$ and $H(T_\Theta F)$ change little over the range of registration parameters considered.

Considering the relationship between the mutual information metric and entropy given in Eq. (13.83), it can be observed that maximization of $I(R, T_\Theta F)$ is equivalent to minimization of $H(R|T_\Theta F)$. Thus, by minimization of $H(R|T_\Theta F)$, given $T_\Theta F$, the information content of R is to be minimized. Qualitatively, if $T_\Theta F$ is known, then the information measure $H(R|T_\Theta F)$ is low, as minimization of $I(R, T_\Theta F)$ has established a relationship between the observations of R and the observations of $T_\Theta F$, regardless of the mathematical nature of the relationship. This property allows the mutual information metric to be useful for multimodal registration, where other similarity metrics perform poorly.

From Eq. (13.84), maximization of $I(R, T_\Theta F)$ is equivalent to minimizing $H(R, T_\Theta f)$. Thus, by minimization of $H(R, T_\Theta f)$, the information content of $(R, T_\Theta F)$ is minimized. In terms of the joint probability mass function $p(r, T_\Theta f)$, this corresponds to building concentrations of probability, as observed in a comparison of the information content of a random variable distributed as a Gaussian to that of a random variable distributed uniformly. This process allows for registration by favoring registration parameters that establish a relationship between the reference and floating volumes, with this relationship being the spatial alignment of anatomy, implicitly.

Computation of mutual information metric

Computation of the mutual information metric is based upon direct evaluation of Eq. (13.82). The codes in the Appendix show how to generate the marginal and joint densities, as well as the mutual information function. Three quantities are necessary: $p(r, T_\Theta f)$, $p_R(r)$, and $p_{T_\Theta F}(T_\Theta f)$. The marginals $p_R(r)$ and $p_{T_\Theta} F(T_\Theta f)$ may be obtained directly from the joint probability function $p(r, T_\Theta f)$, which can be approximated by the normalized joint histogram $h(r, T_\Theta f)$. Here, normalization refers to scaling of the histogram, such that the sum of approximated probabilities equals 1.0. The marginals are then approximated from $h(r, T_\Theta f)$ by summation over the rows of $h(r, T_\Theta f)$, and then the columns.

Computation of $h(r, T_\Theta f)$ involves a complete iteration over each sample in the floating volume. For each sample, the transformation T_Θ is applied, to arrive at a coordinate set in the image coordinate system of the reference volume. If the transformed coordinate is outside the measured reference volume, then the remaining operations are not executed, and the process starts again with the next sample in the floating volume. Otherwise, a sample in the reference volume at the transformed coordinates is approximated using trilinear interpolation (discussed below), and discretized. The two samples, one from the floating volume, and one from the reference volume, are then binned in the joint histogram.

Volume interpolation

With the application of T_Θ to convert between image coordinates in the floating volume to the reference volume, it is highly unlikely that the coordinate $x_R \in R^3$ will fall on a sampled point, and therefore, volume interpolation will be necessary to approximate the value of the volume at the coordinate x_R.

Trilinear interpolation is usually used as an extension of linear interpolation in one dimension, and bilinear interpolation in two dimensions, to the three-dimensional structure of a volume. An approximation of the value of the volume at the coordinate x_R is given by a linear weighting of the surrounding eight voxels that form the smallest bounding cube around x_R in the lattice. Trilinear interpolation uses the quantities given in Table 13.1 (in Appendix 13.1). The sample closest to the origin in the image coordinate system in the surrounding cube of eight voxels is selected as a reference. The image coordinates of this voxel are denoted by (*lower_left_N1, lower_left_N2, lower_left_N3*). The value of the volume at a coordinate $sample_i$ is denoted by V($sample_i$). The interpolated value in the volume V, denoted by *interpolated_value*, is given by the sum of the product of $weight_i$ and V($sample_i$), for i from 0 to 7, indexing the eight surrounding voxels.

13.4.4 Mutual information registration

The mutual information metric provides a quantitative measure of spatial alignment between two images/volumes, given a choice of registration parameters. To obtain the best alignment, it is necessary to maximize the metric. Maximization of the metric, which is parameterized in terms of the registration parameters, is numerically accomplished with the use of a search or maximization algorithm.

In the formulation of registration by maximization of mutual information in [13.9], Powell's multidimensional optimization method with Brent line minimizations was used for maximization of the mutual information metric (e.g. [13.12]). Subsequently, Maes *et al.* [13.10] compared different classical optimization methods maximizing the mutual information metric. One such method included in the study was the use of the classic Nelder and Mead or simplex algorithm for maximization. This method solely uses the objective function directly for optimization, and therefore does not require the expensive computation of derivatives; it is a geometry-based method, using the geometric operations of contraction, expansion, and reflection to manipulate a simplex to a maximum of the objective function. This method was found to perform well in [13.10], and is used here for maximization of the mutual information metric. The MATLAB function *fminsearch* minimizes a scalar function (mutual information in our case) of several variables

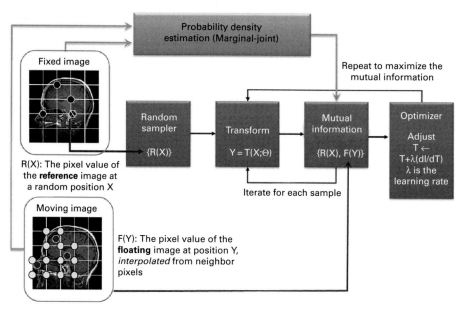

Figure 13.15 Mutual information registration framework.

(i.e. registration parameters) using the Nelder–Mead algorithm (e.g. implementations in Press *et al.* [13.13]).

13.5 Applications

The literature is rich in applications of image registration. Our applications (e.g. [13.3]–[13.5] and [13.12]) are a small sample of those in which registration plays a major role in reaching a decision. The reader should be able to follow the biomedical imaging literature on examples based on their interests and on the specifics of the problem at hand.

13.6 Summary

This chapter has introduced the basic concepts of image registration which serves as an integral part of image analysis in systems which are aimed at object recognition, visual navigation, and inspection/validation. We focused on two widely used algorithms. The first (the iterative closed point or ICP algorithm) deals with shapes explicitly represented as a point cloud. The other (mutual information or MI) makes use of a stochastic measure that is more appropriate for registering images with different modalities. Further, we presented examples of elastic shape registration algorithms based on thin-plate splines and implicit representation.

13.7 Exercises

13.1 Discuss the gimbal lock problem that affects Euler angles.

13.2 Imagine you are in a room with a cuboidal shape. You are on the floor in one corner looking along the base of one wall, and you want to turn to look at the top corner of your other neighboring wall. What angle do you have to turn through?

13.3 For each of the following matrices, determine the eigenvectors corresponding to each eigenvalue and determine a basis for the eigenspace of the matrix corresponding to each eigenvalue. Show intermediate steps.

a. $A = \begin{bmatrix} 6 & -1 \\ 16 & -4 \end{bmatrix}$

b. $A = \begin{bmatrix} 7 & 4 \\ -1 & 3 \end{bmatrix}$

c. $A = \begin{bmatrix} -4 & 3 \\ 2 & -5 \end{bmatrix}$

13.4 Two transformations are said to commute if and only if $AB = BA$. Show that the following sequence of transformations are commutative:
a. Two rotations about the x-axis;
b. Two translations;
c. A rotation and a uniform scaling.

13.5 Prove that the inverse of a unit quaternion is just its conjugate.

13.6 Prove that the composite product leads to a purely imaginary quaternion; hence it can be used to represent rotation.

13.7 Find the quaternions for $90°$ rotations about the x-axis and y-axis. Determine their product. What rotation is this?

13.8 Prove that, in the ICP algorithm, the translational offset between zero-mean points becomes $t' = t - \mu_Y + sR(\mu_P)$ where t is the translation offset between the original points, and μ_P and μ_Y are the centroids of the scene and the corresponding model point respectively.

13.9 Prove Eq. (13.53)

$$E = \left(s\sqrt{S_p} - \frac{D}{\sqrt{S_p}}\right)^2 + \frac{S_y S_p - D^2}{S_p}$$

13.10 Prove Theorem 13.3.

13.11 Computing the entropy $H(X)$ for the following cases, commenting on the result:
a. Tossing a fair die with $p(x_k) = \frac{1}{N}$ with $N = 6$ for $k = 1, 2, \ldots, 6$.
b. Tossing an unfair die with $p(x_1) = \frac{1}{2}$ and $p(x_2) = \ldots = p(x_6) = \frac{1}{10}$.

13.12 Prove Theorem 13.4.

13.13 Prove Theorem 13.5.

13.8 Computer laboratory

Task 1 Write your own matrix multiplication routines and use them to rotate, translate, and scale a rectangle. All transforms should be about the rectangle's local coordinate frame.

Task 2 Build your own graphical user interface (GUI) to allow the user to pick points from the space (2D and 3D) to form shapes of their own choice (e.g. lines, triangles, rectangle, polygons with arbitrary number of points). Allow the user to select the type of transformation to be performed on the drawn shape associated with its parameters and draw the shape after the transformation is applied. Note that you are required to draw the Cartesian coordinate system (2D and 3D) to understand the transformation effect. Provide a keyboard interface that allows the user to control the rotation angle, and to control separately the x- and y-components of translation and scale.

Task 3 Illustrate the coordinate system rotation in 3D space using a sequence of intrinsic rotations (Euler angles) using different conventions, e.g. ZXZ, ZYZ ...

Task 4 Use Codes 13.1 and 13.2 in a unified framework (shown in Figure 13.5) to allow the user to register two sets of points using the ICP algorithm.

Task 5 Use Codes 13.3, 13.4 and 13.5 in a unified framework (shown in Figure 13.15) to allow the user to register two volumes/images using the mutual information algorithm. Hint: you can use *fminsearch* as an optimizer.

References

[13.1] P. J. Besl and H. D. McKay, A method for registration of 3-D shapes. *IEEE Trans. Pattern Anal. Machine Intel.* **14**(2) (1992) 239–256.

[13.2] Z. Zhang, Iterative point matching for registration of free-form curves and surfaces. *Int. J. Comp. Vis.* **13**(2) (1994) 119–152.

[13.3] S. M. Yamany, M. N. Ahmed and A. A. Farag, A new genetic-based technique for matching 3D curves and surfaces. *Pattern Recog.* **32** (10) (1999) 1817–1820.

[13.4] S. M. Yamany and A. A. Farag, Free-form surface registration using surface signatures. *IEEE Int. Conf. Computer Vision (ICCV'99)*, Kerkyra, Greece (September 1999) 1098–1104.

[13.5] S. M. Yamany and A. A. Farag, Surface signatures: an orientation independent free-form surface representation scheme for the purpose of objects registration and matching. *IEEE Trans. Pattern Anal. Machine Intel.* **24**(8) (2002) 1105–1120.

[13.6] P. Viola and W. Wells, Alignment by maximization of mutual information. *IEEE Int. Conf. Computer Vision, MIT, June 20–23* (1995) 16–23.

[13.7] W. M. Wells, P. Viola, H. Atsumi, S. Nakajima and R. Kikinis, Multi-modal volume registration by maximization of mutual information. *Med. Image Anal.* **1** (1996) 35–54.

[13.8] A. Collignon, F. Maes, D. Vandermeulen, P. Suetens and G. Marchal, Automated multimodality image registration using information theory. *Proc. 14th Int. Conf. Information Processing in Medical Images*. Boston: Kluwer (1995) 263–274.

[13.9] F. Maes, A. Collignon, D. Vandermeulen, G. Marchal and P. Suetens, Multimodality image registration by maximization of mutual information. *IEEE Trans. Med. Imaging* **16**(2) (1997) 187–198.

[13.10] F. Maes, D. Vandermeulen and P. Suetens, Comparative evaluation of multiresolution optimization strategies for multimodality image registration by maximization of mutual information. *Med. Image Anal.* **3**(4) (1999) 373–386.

[13.11] A. Roche, G. Malandain, X. Pennec and N. Ayache, The correlation ratio as new similarity metric for multimodal image registration. In *Proc. Int. Conf. Medical Image Computing and Computer-Assisted Intervention (MICCAI'98)* (1998) 1115–1124.

[13.12] J. Nett, Image analysis for quantification of multiple sclerosis, Unpublished M. Eng. thesis, Computer Vision and Image Processing Laboratory, December 2001.

[13.13] W. H. Press, S. A. Teukolsky, W. T. Vetterling and B. P. Flannery, Section 10.5. Downhill simplex method in multidimensions. In *Numerical Recipes in C: The Art of Scientific Computing* 2nd Edition. Cambridge: Cambridge University Press (1992).

[13.14] M. F. Casanova, A. Farag, A. El-Baz *et al.*, Abnormalities of the gyral window in autism: a macroscopic correlate to a putative minicolumnopathy. *J. Spec. Ed. Rehabil.* **1** (2007) 85–101.

Appendix 13.1

MATLAB code implementations

Table 13.1 Samples and sample weightings for trilinear interpolation

$delta_X = x - lower\_left\_N1$
$delta_Y = y - lower\_left\_N2$
$delta_Z = z - lower\_left\_N3$
$weight_0 = (1-delta_X) * (1-delta_Y) * (1-delta_Z)$
$weight_1 = delta_X * (1-delta_Y) * (1-delta_Z)$
$weight_2 = (1-delta_X) * delta_Y * (1-delta_Z)$
$weight_3 = delta_X * delta_Y * (1-delta_Z)$
$weight_4 = (1-delta_X) * (1-delta_Y) * delta_Z$
$weight_5 = delta_X * (1-delta_Y) * delta_Z$
$weight_6 = (1-delta_X) * delta_Y * delta_Z$
$weight_7 = delta_X * delta_Y * delta_Z$
$sample_0 = (lower\_left\_N1, lower\_left\_N2, lower\_left\_N3)$
$sample_1 = (lower\_left\_N1+1, lower\_left\_N2, lower\_left\_N3)$
$sample_2 = (lower\_left\_N1, lower\_left\_N2+1, lower\_left\_N3)$
$sample_3 = (lower\_left\_N1+1, lower\_left\_N2+1, lower\_left\_N3)$
$sample_4 = (lower\_left\_N1, lower\_left\_N2, lower\_left\_N3+1)$
$sample_5 = (lower\_left\_N1+1, lower\_left\_N2, lower\_left\_N3+1)$
$sample_6 = (lower\_left\_N1, lower\_left\_N2+1, lower\_left\_N3+1)$
$sample_7 = (lower\_left\_N1+1, lower\_left\_N2+1, lower\_left\_N3+1)$

$$interpolated\_value = \sum_{i=0}^{7} weight_i * V(sample_i)$$

Code 13.1 Closest point operator

```
% finding correspondences
% for each point in the scene points set P we want to get the closest
% model point in the model points set M
Y = zeros(dim,Np); % set of closest points
for i = 1 : Np
  % current point
  pi = newP(:,i);
  % get the distance to all model points
  d = zeros(1,Nm);
  for k = 1 : Nm
    mk = M(:,k);
    d(k) = sqrt(sum((pi - mk).^2)); % euclidean distance
  end
  % the closest point will be ...
  [minD,j] = min(d);
  Y(:,i) = M(:,j);
end
```

Code 13.2 Finding alignment parameters (rotation, scale and translation)

```
function [s, R, t, err] = find_alignment(P,Y)
% Computes the scaling factor, rotation, and translational offset factor)
% for the transformation between two corresponding 3D point sets Pi
% and Yi such as they are related by:
%
%    Yi = sR*Pi + t
%
% Parameters:  P    3xN matrix representing the N scene 3D points
%              Y    3xN matrix representing the N model 3D points
% which correspond to the scene points P
%
% Return:  s    The scaling factor (uniform scaling)
% R   The 3x3 rotation matrix
% t   The 3x1 translation vector
% err   Residual error defined as err = sum(Yi-(sR*Pi+t))
%
% Notes: Minimum 3D point number is N > 4

%% Test the size of point sets
[dim_p Np] = size(P);
[dim_y Ny] = size(Y);

%Number of points
N = Np;
%% Compute the centroid of each point set
Mu_p = mean(P,2);
Mu_y = mean(Y,2);
```

```
% Remove the centroid: points measured relative to their centroids
Pprime = P - repmat(Mu_p,1,N);
Yprime = Y - repmat(Mu_y,1,N);
%%% Compute the optimal quaternion
% matrix of sums of products of the points,
Px = Pprime(1,:);      Yx = Yprime(1,:);
Py = Pprime(2,:);      Yy = Yprime(2,:);
Pz = Pprime(3,:);      Yz = Yprime(3,:);

Sxx = sum(Px.*Yx);
Sxy = sum(Px.*Yy);
Sxz = sum(Px.*Yz);

Syx = sum(Py.*Yx);
Syy = sum(Py.*Yy);
Syz = sum(Py.*Yz);

Szx = sum(Pz.*Yx);
Szy = sum(Pz.*Yy);
Szz = sum(Pz.*Yz);
Nmatrix = [ Sxx + Syy + Szz    Syz-Szy    -Sxz + Szx    Sxy – Syx;
   -Szy + Syz    Sxx – Szz – Syy    Sxy + Syx    Sxz + Szx;
   Szx – Sxz    Syx + Sxy    Syy – Szz – Sxx    Syz + Szy;
   -Syx + Sxy    Szx + Sxz    Szy + Syz    Szz – Syy – Sxx];

% Compute eigenvalues
[V,D] = eig(Nmatrix);

% the optimal quaternion is the one corresponding to the largest positive
% eigenvalue which is D(4,4).
q = V(:,4);

%%% Compute the rotation matrix
% individual components
q0 = q(1); q1 = q(2); q2 = q(3); q3 = q(4);

% matrices associated to the found quaternion
Qbar = [q0 -q1 -q2 -q3 ;
q1 q0 q3 -q2 ;
q2 -q3 q0 q1 ;
q3 q2 -q1 q0];

Q = [q0 -q1 -q2 -q3 ;
q1 q0 -q3 q2 ;
q2 q3 q0 -q1 ;
q3 -q2 q1 q0];

% The rotation matrix will be:
R = Qbar'*Q;
% Retrieve the 3x3 rotation matrix
R = R(2:4,2:4);
```

```
%% Compute the scaling factor
Sp = 0;
D = 0;
for i=1:N
    D = D + Yprime(:,i)' * Yprime(:,i) ;
    Sp = Sp + Pprime(:,i)' * Pprime(:,i);
end

s = sqrt(D/Sp);
s = s(:);
%% Compute the translational offset
t = Mu_y - s.*(R*Mu_p);

%% Compute the residual error
err = 0;
for i = 1:N
    d = (Y(:,i) - (s.*(R*P(:,i)) + t));
    err = err + d'*d;
end
err = err/N;
```

Code 13.3 Marginal density estimation

```
%% marginal density estimation
hist_bins = 0:255;

% histogram of the first image
a_hist = hist(A(:), hist_bins);

% normalized histogram - marginal density (unit area under curve)
prob_X = a_hist/sum(a_hist);

% histogram of the second image
b_hist = hist(B(:), hist_bins);

% normalized histogram - marginal density (unit area under curve)
prob_Y = b_hist/sum(b_hist);
```

Code 13.4 Joint density estimation

```
%% joint density estimation
sizeA = size(A,1) * size(A,2);
sizeB = size(B,1) * size(B,2);

if sizeA > sizeB
   % swap
   tempA = A ;
   A = B;
   B = tempA;
   clear tempA
end

min_val_A = min(A(:));
max_val_A = max(A(:));
min_val_B = min(B(:));
max_val_B = max(B(:));

% gray level normalization (both images will span the range from 0 to 255)
A = round((A-min_val_A)*(max_val_A)/(max_val_A-min_val_A ));
B = round((B-min_val_B)*(max_val_B)/(max_val_B-min_val_B));

L = 256;
for i = 0 : L-1 % for all gray levels
     % find pixels in A which have the current gray level
     j = find(A == i);
     ab_hist(i+1,:) = hist(B(j),0:L-1);
end

% normalized histogram - joint density (unit area under curve)
     prob_XY = ab_hist/sum(ab_hist(:));
```

Code 13.5 Mutual information computation

```
%% compute the mutual information
I_XY = 0;

L = 256;
for i = 1 : L
     for j = 1 : L
         curI = prob_XY(i,j) * ...
             log ((prob_XY(i,j)/(prob_X(i)*prob_Y(j)+eps)+eps));
         I_XY = I_XY + curI;
     end
end

I_XY = -I_XY;
```

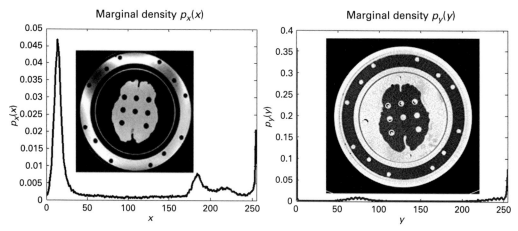

Figure 13.16 Marginal densities of sample images used in the presented implementation – Code (3). Note that the images do not need to be the same size, and objects within the images do not need to share the same color palette.

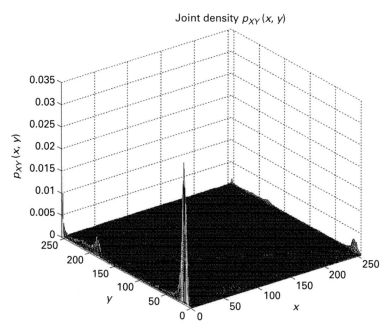

Figure 13.17 Joint density of sample images used in the presented implementation – Code (4).

14 Variational methods for shape registration

Variational methods are based on continuous modelling of input data through the use of partial differential equations (PDE), which benefits from the well-developed theory and numerical methods on PDEs. A novel variational framework for global-to-local shape registration is presented. A new sum-of-squared-differences (SSD) criterion, which measures the disparity between the "implicit" representations of the input shapes, is introduced to recover the global alignment parameters. This new criterion has some advantages over existing ones in accurately handling scale variations. Complementary to the global registration field, the local deformation field is explicitly established between two globally aligned shapes, by minimizing an energy functional which incrementally updates the displacement field while keeping the corresponding implicit representation of the globally warped source shape as close as possible to a "signed distance" function. The optimization is performed under regularization constraints that enforce the smoothness of the recovered deformations. The overall process leads to a coupled set of equations that are simultaneously solved through a gradient descent scheme. The finite element (FE) approach for solving PDEs may be used to validate the performance of the shape registration technique. This chapter provides a holistic approach for shape registration.

14.1 Introduction

The process of registering shapes is based on three main components, namely (1) the way to represent the shapes, (2) the transformation model, and (3) the mathematical framework selected to recover the registration parameters. The following section briefly reviews each of these components.

Shape representation is handled differently in each application. For instance, Paragios et al. [14.1] and Huang et al. [14.2] represent the shapes to be registered as the zero-level sets of distance functions in a higher-dimensional space. This implicit representation is known to be invariant to translation and rotation, and can efficiently handle the isotropic scaling case. Abdelmunim and Farag [14.3] used volumetric representation of shapes through vector level sets. Abdelmunim, Farag and Farag [14.4] used a vector distance function to represent shapes. Belongie et al. [14.5] represented shapes as clouds of points, where each sample point has a "shape context," which is then used to match shapes for object recognition purposes. Other shape descriptors include the medial axis [14.6] and Fourier descriptors [14.7].

Transformation models can be divided into two classes: global and local. The global transformation models are usually defined by a small set of parameters. These models include, among others, the rigid transformations (translations and rotations), the similarity transformations (translations, rotations, and isotropic scalings), and the affine transformations, which in addition to translations and rotations account for anisotropic scaling and/or shearing. In some cases, such transformations can be used alone to efficiently align two shapes. However, in the case of non-rigid deformations, more complex transformations are required in order to establish dense correspondences between the two given shapes. Figure 14.1 illustrates the elastic registration of multiple shapes.

Different techniques have been developed to solve the problem of non-rigid registration of shapes. Huang *et al.* [14.2] introduced a hierarchical shape registration algorithm using a B-spline-based incremental free-form deformation (IFFD) model to recover the local registration field between two globally aligned shapes. Li, Shen and Hunag [14.8] studied the optimization process in shape alignment, while Abdelmunim *et al.* [14.4] devised a closed-form solution to the optimization process involved in registering shapes. Registering shapes for biomedical applications has been studied by various groups (e.g., [14.9], [14.10]); Fahmi and Farag [14.11] used elastic registration of shapes in 3D space for analysis of facial expression.

Broadly speaking, given the transformation model and the selected shape representation model, most existing techniques that have been developed to recover the registration parameters are based on the optimization of a disparity measure between the two shapes. For instance, the SSD is a popular criterion that is mostly appropriate when the two data sets have comparable values (e.g., monomodal images), or when matching shapes with no scale variations, while the mutual information (MI) is a stochastic measure that is more appropriate for registering images with different modalities or matching shapes under scale variations (e.g. [14.2]). Smoothness constraints, using physically based functionals relying on elasticity or fluid theory are often introduced to guarantee that the problem is well posed, and to retain some smoothness properties of the recovered displacement field (e.g. [14.12]).

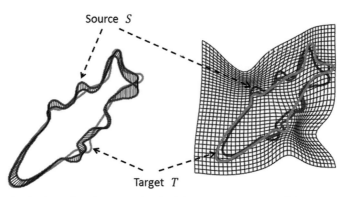

Figure 14.1 An elastic registration example of a fish shape using the implicit vector representation, showing correspondences and final grid deformation.

14.2 Shape modeling

Generally speaking, the shape of a geometrical figure (or object) is understood to refer to those geometrical attributes that are invariant to Euclidean similarity transformations – that is, attributes that remain unchanged when the object is rotated, translated, and scaled (e.g. [14.13]). Two objects are said to have the same shape if one is a transformed version of the other under a similarity transformation.

A shape can be classified either as static or dynamic. A static (or "rigid" shape) is one that does not change over time by deformation. An example of such a shape is a car model. A dynamic shape deforms over time: for example, a human face undergoes changes when speaking or smiling. Various techniques have been designed to describe shapes, and each has its strengths and its limitations. These techniques aim at providing a simplified representation of the shape under consideration while preserving its main characteristics.

The literature is rich with shape representation techniques. These techniques can generally be categorized as parametric (such as Fourier descriptors and spherical harmonics), or non-parametric (such as landmark-based techniques, medial axes, and distance transform). In many applications, in particular in image-based morphological studies in the field of medical imaging, the analysis starts with the extraction of a quantitative description of the anatomical shapes of interest from the input images. The following section overviews the two families of shape descriptors (parametric and non-parametric) and explains how they are extracted from the images.

14.2.1 Parametric representations

Within this family, the techniques fit a parametric model to a curved outline in a 2D image or a bounding surface in a 3D image. The model parameters are typically derived from segmented images and are used to describe the shape being considered. This family of descriptors includes, among others, the following:

- *Geometric moments.* The mathematical concept of moments has been around for many years and has been utilized in several fields, including mechanics, statistics, pattern recognition, and image understanding. Historically, the first significant work considering moments for pattern recognition was introduced by Hu in 1962 [14.14]. In general, the three-dimensional $(p+q+r)$th geometric moment, $\mathcal{M}_{pqr}$, of a function $f(x,y,z)$ (an image intensity or a density distribution function) is defined as

$$\mathcal{M}_{pqr} = \int_{-\infty}^{+\infty}\int_{-\infty}^{+\infty}\int_{-\infty}^{+\infty} x^p y^q z^r f(x,y,z) dx dy dz, \qquad (14.1)$$

where $p,q,r \in \mathbb{N}$. Geometric moments are not orthogonal since their basis functions, the monomials $x^p y^q z^r$, are not orthogonal. Moreover, according to the uniqueness theorem, the moment set($\mathcal{M}_{pqr}$) is uniquely determined for a given image function f, and the existence theorem states that the moments of all orders exist. These two theorems give rise to the reconstruction property of moments.

Finally, note that if the function f is a binary function with a value 1 inside the region enclosed by the shape, and 0 outside, then the zeroth order moment is equal to the area enclosed by the shape.

Hu [14.14] derived a set of seven moment invariants, using non-linear combinations of geometric moments. These invariants remain the same under image translation, rotation, and scaling. Foulonneau et al. [14.15] used moments in affine-invariant shape-based segmentation using active contours. Mathematically, moments have the advantage of being concise, but it is difficult to correlate high-order moments with shape features.

- *Spherical harmonics (SPHARM).* Surfaces in 3D can be represented by a series expansion of parametric coordinate functions in 2D parameter space (e.g., Brechbühler et al. [14.16]). The surface voxels are projected onto the unit sphere S^2 with its origin located at the center of mass of the object and the surface. $v(\theta,\phi) = (v_1(\theta,\phi), v_2(\theta,\phi), v_3(\theta,\phi))$ is expressed as a linear combination of its harmonics as follows:

$$v_i(\theta,\phi) = \sum_{l \geq 0} \sum_{|m| \leq l} C_{lm}^i Y_l^m(\theta,\phi), \text{ with } \theta \in [0,\pi], \text{ and } \phi \in [0,2\phi] \quad (14.2)$$

where C_{lm}^i are the expansion coefficients given by

$$C_{lm}^i = \int_{S^2} v_i(\theta,\phi) Y_l^m(\theta,\phi) \sin\theta d\theta d\phi,$$

and $Y_l^m(\theta,\phi)$ are the harmonic of degree l and order m, which are defined as solutions to the normal Laplace equation in spherical coordinates. Truncating this expansion at a given frequency l allows the reconstruction of the original surface at the different levels.

Kazhdan et al. [14.17] used spherical harmonics for obtaining rotation-invariant representations of 3D shapes and for 3D shape-matching scenarios. Chung et al. [14.18] used a modified spherical harmonics representation for various MRI studies of the cortex. This representation of $v(\theta,\phi)$ at different scales σ is given by

$$v_i(\theta,\phi) = \sum_{l \geq 0} \sum_{m=-l}^{l} e^{l(l+1)\sigma} C_{lm}^i Y_l^m(\theta,\phi). \quad (14.3)$$

Note that the weighted SPHARM corresponds to the traditional SPHARM for the particular case $\sigma = 0$.

14.2.2 Landmark-based representation

The boundary of a shape (a curve in 2D or surface in 3D) can be represented by a set of points known as landmarks. Such points can be manually placed by a knowledgeable user of the underlying anatomy to determine *"special locations,"* or can be detected

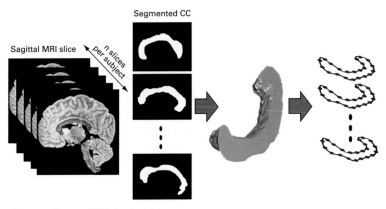

Figure 14.2 Corpus callosum (CC) landmarks

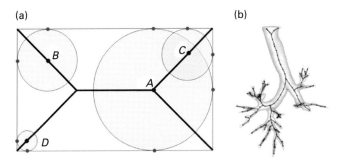

Figure 14.3 (a) Illustration of maximal disks in 2D. (b) Curve skeleton of a synthetic 3D shape.

automatically using some geometric features of the boundary, such as curvature (e.g., [14.19], [14.20]). Both manual and automatic landmarks can be extracted either from grayscale or segmented images. Figure 14.2 illustrates an example of the shape of the corpus callosum represented by landmarks (e.g. [14.21]).

14.2.3 Medial axes representation

A medial axis or skeleton of a shape was initially defined by Blum [14.22] as the locus of centers of disks in 2D or spheres in 3D of maximal size that fit in the domain occupied by the shape (see Figure 14.3a). Medial axes have been extensively used in computer vision and medical imaging applications. Each point on the medial axis has at least two equidistant points on the shape's outline, and is associated with a radius of the corresponding maximal disk or sphere. This allows the shape to be represented using less information, and the shape can be fully recovered from its medial axis. Note that in the 3D case, the skeleton can be a medial surface or, in the case of tubular structures, a set of medial curves as shown in Figure 14.3b. This dimension reduction plays a major role in several applications, such as shape matching and retrieval (e.g. [14.23], [14.24]), segmentation of tubular-like structures (e.g. [14.25]), and virtual endoscopy (e.g. [14.26]).

Several techniques have been proposed for medial axis extraction. The algorithms in Fritsch et al. [14.27] and Pizer et al. [14.28] simultaneously estimate the boundary and the medial axis from the input grayscale image. Hassouna and Farag [14.29] developed an approach for extraction skeleton in 2D and 3D using gradient vector flow. This approach requires a prior segmentation of the surface or volume.

14.2.4 Implicit representation using the vector distance function

A shape representation in vector form was proposed by Faugeras and Gomes [14.30], and has been popular in various image analysis applications. Called the vector distance function (VDF) method, it uses the vector that connects any point in space to its closest point on the object of interest. Given a manifold $\mathcal{M}$ in $\mathbb{R}^n$, ($n = 2,3$), let $d(\mathbf{x}) = \text{dist}(\mathbf{x}, \mathcal{M})$ denote the distance from a point $\mathbf{x} \in \mathbb{R}^n$ to $\mathcal{M}$; that is, $d(\mathbf{x}) = \|\mathbf{x} - \mathbf{x}_0\|$ with $\mathbf{x}_0$ being the closet point to $\mathbf{x}$ on $\mathcal{M}$. The function $d(\mathbf{x})$ is Lipschitz-continuous and hence is differentiable, and so is the squared distance function defined by

$$\mathbb{D}(\mathbf{x}) = \frac{1}{2} d^2(\mathbf{x}). \quad (14.4)$$

The vector distance function $V(\mathbf{x})$ is defined as the derivative of $\eta(\cdot)$. That is,

$$V(\mathbf{x}) = \nabla \mathbb{D}(\mathbf{x}) = d(\mathbf{x}) \nabla d(\mathbf{x}). \quad (14.5)$$

The VDF, $V(\cdot)$, is an implicit representation of the manifold $\mathcal{M}$, with $\mathcal{M} = V^{-1}(0)$, and for each $\mathbf{x} \in \mathbb{R}^n$, $V(\mathbf{x})$ is a vector of length $d(\mathbf{x})$ since $d(\cdot)$ satisfies the Eikonal equation $\|\nabla d(\mathbf{x})\| = 1$. In addition, let $\mathbf{x}$ be a point where $d(\cdot)$ is differentiable, and let $\mathbf{x}_0 = P_\mathcal{M}(\mathbf{x})$ be the unique projection of $\mathbf{x}$ onto $\mathcal{M}$, i.e., $d(\mathbf{x}) = \|\mathbf{x} - \mathbf{x}_0\|$. If $\mathcal{M}$ is smooth at $\mathbf{x}$, then the VDF to $\mathcal{M}$ at $\mathcal{M}$ is given by (e.g. [14.30]):

$$V(\mathbf{x}) = \mathbf{x} - \mathbf{x}_0 = \mathbf{x} - P_\mathcal{M}(\mathbf{x}). \quad (14.6)$$

Figure 14.4 shows examples of the x- and y-components of the VDFs corresponding to different 2D shapes.

14.2.5 Implicit representation using distance transform

The distance transform, or the distance map, of a given shape assigns to each point $\mathbf{x}$ in the image its minimal Euclidean distance, $D(\mathbf{x})$, from the shape boundary. Some two-dimensional examples of such representations are shown in Figure 14.5.

The boundary is modelled as the zero-level set of the distance transform. In many applications, including the present work, a signed variant of the distance transform is considered. This variant negates the values of the distance transform either inside or outside the region enclosed by the shape. Let S denote an imaged shape in $\mathbb{R}^n$ which defines a partition of the image domain Ω into two regions: the region enclosed by S, Ω_S, and its complement in Ω, $\Omega \setminus \Omega_S$. The shape S can be implicitly defined by the following signed distance transform

$$\Phi_S(\mathbf{x}) = \begin{cases} 0, & \text{if } \mathbf{x} \in S, \\ +\text{dist}(\mathbf{x}, S), & \text{if } \mathbf{x} \in \Omega_S, \\ -\text{dist}(\mathbf{x}, S), & \text{if } \mathbf{x} \in \Omega \setminus \Omega_S, \end{cases} \qquad (14.7)$$

where dist($\mathbf{x}$, S) refers to the minimum Euclidean distance between an image point $\mathbf{x}$ and the shape S. Examples of such representation are presented in Figure 14.6 for the 2D shapes in Figure 14.5.

The signed variant has the advantage of eliminating the singularities at the shape outline and leads to a linear transition as one crosses the object boundary. The implicit representation using distance transforms has been used previously in several shape registration techniques (e.g., [14.1]–[14.4]). In this work, we chose to represent shapes using the signed distance transform for different reasons. First and foremost, this representation provides a feature space in which the registration energy functionals that can be optimized using gradient descent can be conveniently and efficiently used. Indeed, Huang et al. [14.2] stated that this representation satisfies a sufficient condition for the convergence of gradient descent methods. Second, the signed distance representation is invariant to rotations and translations. Third, in the context of shape-based segmentation, since this representation is set in an Eulerian framework, it does not require point correspondences during the phase of building a shape model from a set of training samples. In addition, it can handle topological changes such as merging and breaking. This ability is of great value for segmenting medical images where organs or lesions can present as one confluent object or as a union of disconnected islands.

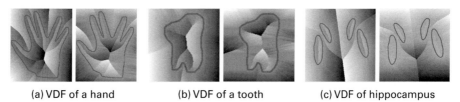

(a) VDF of a hand (b) VDF of a tooth (c) VDF of hippocampus

Figure 14.4 Shape representation using the VDF of hand; tooth; and hippocampus. Left: *x*-component; right: *y*-component.

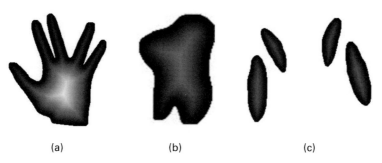

(a) (b) (c)

Figure 14.5 Examples of the distance map inside of 2D shapes. (a) Hand. (b) Tooth. (c) Hippocampus.

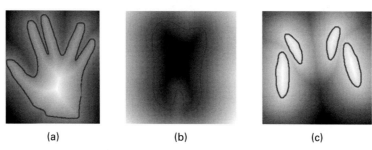

Figure 14.6 Examples of the signed distance representation of 2D shapes by negating the distance outside the shapes. (a) Hand. (b) Tooth. (c) Hippocampus.

The only concern about the implicit signed distance representation is that it has one dimension higher than the original shapes. This problem has been addressed thoroughly in the level-set segmentation literature using a narrow band implementation. In the context of shape registration, one can reduce the sample domain for registration to a narrow band around the input shape in the embedding space.

14.3 Global registration of shapes in implicit spaces

This section focuses on the specific implicit representation of shapes using signed distance transforms and how this representation can be used for global shape alignment. The implicit representation of shapes using the signed distance map has been used previously to achieve global alignment of shapes (e.g., [14.1]–[14.4]). This representation is invariant to rotations and translations, and can be efficiently used in the case of homogeneous scaling. In this chapter, we present a cost function which measures the disparity between the implicit representations of the two input shapes. This measure leads to accurate results even when dealing with anisotropic scales.

14.3.1 Global matching of shapes

Global transformation models are usually defined by a small set of parameters. These models include, among others, the rigid transformation (translations and rotations), the similarity transformation (translations, rotations, and isotropic scaling), and the affine transformation, which in addition to translations and rotations accounts for anisotropic scaling and/or shearing. Such a transformation can be used alone to efficiently align two shapes, or it can be used as a pre-step for a local matching algorithm. Several techniques have been proposed to achieve global alignment between shapes. Some of these techniques are feature-based (e.g. [14.31]) and proceed by extracting salient features and using them to match a set of corresponding points. Finally, the matched points are used to recover the transformation parameters. Other methods, in contrast, recover these parameters by directly optimizing a similarity/dissimilarity criterion between the two shape representations. For instance, in Huang *et al.* [14.2], an approach is proposed to achieve global registration of shapes by maximizing the MI between the SDF representation of the input shapes.

Fahmi [14.32] introduced a new SSD criterion expressed in the space of signed distance transforms to globally align shapes. This new criterion can handle both rigid and affine transformations and leads to more accurate results than other criteria. The treatment below follows Fahmi's dissertation work [14.32].

14.3.1.1 Similarity and affine registration

The implicit representation of shapes using the signed distance map has been employed in many applications in order to achieve global alignment of shapes. This representation is proven to be invariant to rotation and translations, and can be efficiently used in the case of homogeneous scaling. Two different types of transformations will be considered to achieve shape alignment.

Case 1: Similarity alignment
To simplify the representation, let us limit the discussion to the two-dimensional case, and let us consider two shapes, S and T, that are implicitly represented by their corresponding signed distance maps, Φ_S and Φ_T, respectively. Assume that the target shape, $\mathcal{J}$, is a deformed version of the source shape S, according to a similarity transformation $\mathcal{A} \doteq \mathcal{A}(s, \mathcal{R}, \mathcal{J})$, given by:

$$\mathcal{A}\mathbf{x} = s\mathcal{R}\mathbf{x} + \mathcal{J}, \tag{14.9}$$

$$= s \begin{pmatrix} \cos\theta & \sin\theta \\ -\sin\theta & \cos\theta \end{pmatrix} \cdot \begin{pmatrix} x \\ y \end{pmatrix} + \begin{pmatrix} \mathcal{J}_x \\ \mathcal{J}_y \end{pmatrix}, \tag{14.10}$$

where S is a scaling factor, $\mathcal{R} = \mathcal{R}(\theta)$ is a rotation matrix, and $\mathcal{J} = [\mathcal{J}_x, \mathcal{J}_y]^T$ is a translation vector. The question is how to recover these parameters and then align the two given shapes.

First, note that if we denote by $\hat{\Phi}_S$ the level set function Φ_S transformed by $\mathcal{A}$, then one can show that the zero crossing of $\hat{\Phi}_S$ gives a new shape, $\hat{S}$, that corresponds, up to the scale $\hat{S}$, to the transformation of the original shape S by $\mathcal{A}$.

Indeed, let $\mathbf{x}$ be an image point, and let $\hat{\mathbf{x}}$ denote its image by $\mathcal{A}$, i.e., $\hat{\mathbf{x}} = \mathcal{A}\mathbf{x}$. Then we have:

$$\text{dist}(\hat{\mathbf{x}}, \hat{S}) = \min_{\hat{\mathbf{y}} \in \hat{S}} \|\hat{\mathbf{x}} - \hat{\mathbf{y}}\| = \min_{\mathbf{y} \in S} \|(s\mathcal{R}\mathbf{x} + \mathcal{T}) - (s\mathcal{R}\mathbf{y} + \mathcal{T})\| \tag{14.11}$$

$$= \min_{\mathbf{y} \in S} s\|\mathbf{x} - \mathbf{y}\| = s\,\text{dist}(\mathbf{x}, S). \blacksquare \tag{14.12}$$

Considering this property of the signed distance function under similarity transformation, one way of recovering the parameters of the transformation $\mathcal{A}$, is by minimizing the following SSD similarity criterion as was proposed in Paragios et al. [14.1]:

$$D(s, \mathcal{R}, \mathcal{T}) = \int_{\Omega} (s\Phi_S(\mathbf{x}) - \Phi_T(\mathcal{A}\mathbf{x}))^2 d\mathbf{x}, \tag{14.13}$$

which measures the dissimilarity between the distance values of image points on one image and that of the transformed points by A on the other image. For computational considerations, one can consider a narrow band formed of points that are a distance ε away from the source shape and their projections on the target:

$$D(s, \mathcal{R}, \mathcal{T}) = \int_\Omega d_\varepsilon(\Phi_S(\mathbf{x}), \Phi_T(\mathcal{A}\mathbf{x})) \cdot [s\Phi_S(\mathbf{x}) - \Phi_T(\mathcal{A}\mathbf{x})]^2 d\mathbf{x}, \qquad (14.14)$$

where

$$d_\varepsilon(a, b) = \begin{cases} 0 & \text{if } \min(|a|, |b|) > \varepsilon, \\ 1 & \text{otherwise.} \end{cases}$$

The corresponding Euler–Lagrange equations for each transformation parameter are given by:

$$\begin{aligned}
\frac{d}{dt}s &= 2 \int_\Omega d_\varepsilon(\Phi_S, \Phi_T) \left[\Phi_S(\mathbf{x}) - \nabla \Phi_T^T(\mathcal{A}\mathbf{x}) \begin{pmatrix} x\cos\theta + y\sin\theta \\ -x\sin\theta + y\cos\theta \end{pmatrix} \right] \cdot \mathbf{r} d\mathbf{x}, \\
\frac{d}{dt}\theta &= 2 \int_\Omega d_\varepsilon(\Phi_S, \Phi_T) \left[s\nabla \Phi_T^T(\mathcal{A}\mathbf{x}) \begin{pmatrix} -x\sin\theta + y\cos\theta \\ -x\cos\theta - y\sin\theta \end{pmatrix} \right] \cdot \mathbf{r} d\mathbf{x}, \\
\frac{d}{dt}T_x &= 2 \int_\Omega d_\varepsilon(\Phi_S, \Phi_T) \frac{\partial \Phi_T}{\partial x}(\mathcal{A}\mathbf{x}) \cdot \mathbf{r} d\mathbf{x}, \\
\frac{d}{dt}T_y &= 2 \int_\Omega d_\varepsilon(\Phi_S, \Phi_T) \frac{\partial \Phi_T}{\partial y}(\mathcal{A}\mathbf{x}) \cdot \mathbf{r} d\mathbf{x},
\end{aligned} \qquad (14.15)$$

where $\mathbf{r}(\mathbf{x}) = s\Phi_S(\mathbf{x}) - \Phi_T(\mathcal{A}\mathbf{x})$. A gradient descent scheme can be used to solve these equations. Figures 14.12b and 14.10b show examples of global alignment of different shapes using this model.

Case 2: Affine alignment

Consider a more general transformation (to be recovered) $A \doteq A(S, R, T)$, defined by:

$$\mathcal{A}\mathbf{x} = \mathcal{S}\mathcal{R}\mathbf{x} + \mathcal{T} \qquad (14.16)$$

$$= \begin{pmatrix} s_x & 0 \\ 0 & s_y \end{pmatrix} \begin{pmatrix} \cos\theta & \sin\theta \\ -\sin\theta & \cos\theta \end{pmatrix} \begin{pmatrix} x \\ y \end{pmatrix} + \begin{pmatrix} T_x \\ T_y \end{pmatrix}. \qquad (14.17)$$

The minimization of the cost function given by Eq. (14.14) fails to produce accurate results in this case because of the anisotropic scales (different scales in the x- and y-directions). One way of coping with this issue is to represent the input shapes using the VDF representation. In this work, we use a new dissimilarity criterion and show its potential when compared with the homogeneous scale-based and the VDF-based criteria (see Eq. (14.14) and Eq. (14.21), respectively).

14.3.2 VDF-based dissimilarity measure

Let V_S and V_T be the VDFs of the shapes S and T, respectively. First, it is clear that the VDF representation is invariant to translation. Now, let us denote by $\hat{V}_S$ the "VDF" obtained after transforming V_S by $\mathcal{A}$. The set $\hat{V}_S^{-1}(0)$ implicitly represents a shape $\hat{S}$ which corresponds to the warped shape $\mathcal{A}(S)$, up to a rotation and some scale effects. Given an image point $\mathbf{x} \in \Omega_S$ on the source shape, let $\hat{\mathbf{x}}$ be its transform by $\mathcal{A}$, i.e., $\hat{\mathbf{x}} = \mathcal{A}\mathbf{x}$, and let $\mathbf{x}^0 = V_S(\mathbf{x})$ be the closest point to $\mathbf{x}$ on S. One can easily show that

$$V_T(\mathcal{A}(\mathbf{x})) = V_T(\hat{\mathbf{x}}) = \hat{\mathbf{x}} - \hat{\mathbf{x}}_0 \tag{14.18}$$

$$= \mathcal{SR}(\mathbf{x} - \mathbf{x}_0) = \mathcal{SR}V_S(\mathbf{x}). \tag{14.19}$$

Based on this property of the VDF representation under affine transformation, one can consider the following SSD criterion to achieve global alignment of the two input shapes:

$$D(\mathcal{S}, \mathcal{R}, \mathcal{T}) = \int_\Omega (\mathcal{SR}V_S(\mathbf{x}) - V_T(\mathcal{A}\mathbf{x}))^2 d\mathbf{x}. \tag{14.20}$$

To reduce the computational complexity of minimizing this criterion, one can limit the matching space to a narrow band around the two given shapes

$$D(\mathcal{S}, \mathcal{R}, \mathcal{T}) = \int_\Omega \delta_s(V_S(\mathbf{x}), V_T(\mathcal{A}\mathbf{x})) \cdot (\mathcal{S}.\mathcal{R}.V_S(\mathbf{x}) - V_T(\mathcal{A}\mathbf{x}))^2 d\mathbf{x}, \tag{14.21}$$

where δ_ε is given by

$$d_\varepsilon(\mathbf{a}, \mathbf{b}) = \begin{cases} 0, & \text{if} \min(\|\mathbf{a}\|, \|\mathbf{b}\|) > \varepsilon, \\ 1, & \text{if } \min(\|\mathbf{a}\|, \|\mathbf{b}\|) \le \varepsilon. \end{cases} \tag{14.22}$$

The corresponding Euler–Lagrange equations for each parameter of the transformation $\mathcal{A}$ are given by:

$$\frac{d}{dt}s = 2\int_\Omega \delta_s(V_S, V_T)\mathbf{r}^T [\nabla_s \mathcal{SR}V_S(\mathbf{x}) - \nabla V_T^T(\mathcal{A}\mathbf{x})\nabla_s(\mathcal{A}\mathbf{x})], \tag{14.23.a}$$

$$\frac{d}{dt}\theta = 2\int_\Omega \delta_s(V_S, V_T)\mathbf{r}^T [\mathcal{S}\nabla_\theta \mathcal{R}V_S(\mathbf{x}) - \nabla V_T^T(\mathcal{A}\mathbf{x})\nabla_\theta(\mathcal{A}\mathbf{x})], \tag{14.23.b}$$

$$\frac{d}{dt}t = 2\int_\Omega \delta_s(V_S, V_T)\mathbf{r}^T [\nabla V_T^T(\mathcal{A}\mathbf{x})\nabla_t(\mathcal{A}\mathbf{x})], \tag{14.23.c}$$

where $\mathbf{r}(\mathbf{x}) = \mathcal{SR}V_s(\mathbf{x}) - V_T(\mathcal{A}\mathbf{x})$, $s \in \{s_x, s_y\}$, and $t \in \{\mathcal{T}_x, \mathcal{T}_y\}$. Each of these equations is solved using the gradient method.

14.3.3 SDF-based dissimilarity measure

Let Φ_S and Φ_T be the signed distance representations of the shapes S and T, respectively. Consider an image point $\mathbf{x}$, whose transform by $\mathcal{A}$ is denoted by $\hat{\mathbf{x}}$, and let $\hat{\Phi}_S$ be the level set function obtained by transforming Φ_S by $\mathcal{A}$.

Fahmi [14.32] introduced a new sum-of-squared-differences criterion in order to recover the parameters of the transformation $\mathcal{A}$. We derive the formulas for that measure for 2D and 3D cases below.

14.3.3.1 Two-dimensional case

The dissimilarity measure is defined as follows:

$$D(\mathcal{S}, \mathcal{R}, \mathcal{T}) = \int_\Omega (\|\mathcal{S}\|\Phi_S(\mathbf{x}) - \Phi_T(\mathcal{A}\mathbf{x}))^2 d\mathbf{x}, \qquad (14.24)$$

where $\|\mathcal{S}\| = \max(|s_x|,|s_y|)$ is the infinity norm of the matrix $\mathcal{S}$. Note that in the absence of scale variations, our measure coincides with that proposed in Paragios et al. [14.1]. For computational and technical considerations, one can consider a narrow band formed of points that are a distance ε from the source shape and their projections on the target shape:

$$D(\mathcal{S}, \mathcal{R}, \mathcal{T}) = \frac{1}{2}\int_\Omega d_\varepsilon(\Phi_S(\mathbf{x}), \Phi_T(\mathcal{A}\mathbf{x}))[\|\mathcal{S}\|\Phi_S(\mathbf{x}) - \Phi_T(\mathcal{A}\mathbf{x})]^2 d\mathbf{x}, \qquad (14.25)$$

where $d_\varepsilon(a, b) = \begin{cases} 0, & \text{if } \min(|a|, |b|) > \varepsilon, \\ 1, & \text{otherwise.} \end{cases}$

Each parameter of the transformation $\mathcal{A}$ is recovered by solving its corresponding Euler–Lagrange equations using a gradient descent scheme:

$$\frac{ds_x}{dt} = \int_\Omega \left[\frac{d\|\mathcal{S}\|}{ds_x}\Phi_S(\mathbf{x}) - \nabla\Phi_T^T(\mathcal{A}\mathbf{x})\begin{pmatrix} x\cos\theta + y\sin\theta \\ 0 \end{pmatrix}\right]\mathbf{r}(\mathbf{x})d\mathbf{x}, \qquad (14.26a)$$

$$\frac{ds_y}{dt} = \int_\Omega \left[\frac{d\|\mathcal{S}\|}{ds_y}\Phi_S(\mathbf{x}) - \nabla\Phi_T^T(\mathcal{A}\mathbf{x})\begin{pmatrix} 0 \\ -x\sin\theta + y\cos\theta \end{pmatrix}\right]\mathbf{r}(\mathbf{x})d\mathbf{x}, \qquad (14.26b)$$

$$\frac{d\theta}{dt} = \int_\Omega \left[\nabla\Phi_T^T \cdot \begin{pmatrix} s_x(-x\sin\theta + y\cos\theta) \\ s_y(-x\cos\theta - y\sin\theta) \end{pmatrix}\right]\mathbf{r}(\mathbf{x})d\mathbf{x}, \qquad (14.26c)$$

$$\frac{dT_x}{dt} = \int_\Omega \frac{\partial\Phi_T}{\partial x}(\mathcal{A}\mathbf{x})\mathbf{r}(\mathbf{x})d\mathbf{x}, \qquad (14.26d)$$

$$\frac{dT_y}{dt} = \int_\Omega \frac{\partial\Phi_T}{\partial y}(\mathcal{A}\mathbf{x})\mathbf{r}(\mathbf{x})d\mathbf{x}, \qquad (14.26e)$$

where $\mathbf{r}(\mathbf{x}) = d_\varepsilon(\Phi_S(\mathbf{x}),\Phi_T(\mathbf{x}))(\|\mathcal{S}\|\Phi_S(\mathbf{x})-\Phi_T(\mathcal{A}\mathbf{x}))$, and ∇ denotes the gradient operator. Note that, since we are considering positive scale values, the terms $\frac{d\|\mathcal{S}\|}{ds_{x;y}}$ equal either 0 or 1.

14.3.3.2 Three-dimensional case

For the three-dimensional case, the similarity transform $\mathcal{A}$ is defined by $\mathcal{A}\mathbf{x} = \mathcal{SRx} + \mathcal{T}$ where:

$$\mathcal{S} = \begin{pmatrix} s_x & 0 & 0 \\ 0 & s_y & 0 \\ 0 & 0 & s_z \end{pmatrix}, \quad \mathcal{T} = \begin{pmatrix} T_x \\ T_y \\ T_z \end{pmatrix} \quad (14.27)$$

and $\mathcal{R} = \mathcal{R}(\theta_x, \theta_y, \theta_z) = \mathcal{R}_x \mathcal{R}_y \mathcal{R}_z$, with:

$$\mathcal{R}_x = \begin{pmatrix} 1 & 0 & 0 \\ 0 & \cos\theta_x & \sin\theta_x \\ 0 & -\sin\theta_x & \cos\theta_x \end{pmatrix}, \quad \mathcal{R}_y = \begin{pmatrix} \cos\theta_y & 0 & -\sin\theta_y \\ 0 & 1 & 0 \\ \sin\theta_y & 0 & \cos\theta_y \end{pmatrix},$$

$$\mathcal{R}_z = \begin{pmatrix} \cos\theta_z & \sin\theta_z & 0 \\ -\sin\theta_y & \cos\theta_z & 0 \\ 0 & 0 & 1 \end{pmatrix}. \quad (14.28)$$

In this case, the cost function to be minimized in order to recover the nine parameters of the transformation $\mathcal{A}$ is given by:

$$D(\mathcal{S}, \mathcal{R}, \mathcal{T}) = \frac{1}{2} \int_\Omega (\|\mathcal{S}\| \Phi_S(\mathbf{x}) - \Phi_T(\mathcal{A}\mathbf{x}))^2 d\mathbf{x}, \quad (14.29)$$

where $\|\mathcal{S}\| = \max(|s_x|, |s_y|, |s_y|)$ is the infinity norm of the matrix $\mathcal{S}$.

As was done in the 2D case, we can consider a narrow band formed of points that are a distance ε away from the source shape and their projections on the target shape, and solve the following Euler–Lagrange equations for each of the nine parameters of $\mathcal{A}$ using a gradient descent scheme:

$$\frac{ds_x}{dt} = \int_\Omega \left[\frac{d\|\mathcal{S}\|}{ds_x} \Phi_S(\mathbf{x}) - \nabla\Phi_T^T(\mathcal{A}\mathbf{x}) \begin{pmatrix} R_{11}x + R_{12}y + R_{13}z \\ 0 \\ 0 \end{pmatrix} \right] r(\mathbf{x}) d\mathbf{x}, \quad (14.30)$$

$$\frac{ds_y}{dt} = \int_\Omega \left[\frac{d\|\mathcal{S}\|}{ds_y} \Phi_S(\mathbf{x}) - \nabla\Phi_T^T(\mathcal{A}\mathbf{x}) \begin{pmatrix} 0 \\ R_{21}x + R_{22}y + R_{23}z \\ 0 \end{pmatrix} \right] r(\mathbf{x}) d\mathbf{x}, \quad (14.30)$$

$$\frac{ds_z}{dt} = \int_\Omega \left[\frac{d\|\mathcal{S}\|}{ds_z} \Phi_S(\mathbf{x}) - \nabla\Phi_T^T(\mathcal{A}\mathbf{x}) \begin{pmatrix} 0 \\ 0 \\ R_{31}x + R_{32}y + R_{33}z \end{pmatrix} \right] r(\mathbf{x}) d\mathbf{x}, \quad (14.31)$$

Similarly,

$$\frac{d\theta_x}{dt} = \int_\Omega \left[\nabla\Phi_T^T(A\mathbf{x})S\mathcal{R}'_x\mathcal{R}_y\mathcal{R}_z\mathbf{x}\right]\mathbf{r}(\mathbf{x})d\mathbf{x},$$

$$\frac{d\theta_y}{dt} = \int_\Omega \left[\nabla\Phi_T^T(A\mathbf{x})S\mathcal{R}_x\mathcal{R}'_y\mathcal{R}_z\mathbf{x}\right]\mathbf{r}(\mathbf{x})d\mathbf{x},$$

$$\frac{d\theta_z}{dt} = \int_\Omega \left[\nabla\Phi_T^T(A\mathbf{x})S\mathcal{R}_x\mathcal{R}_y\mathcal{R}'_z\mathbf{x}\right]\mathbf{r}(\mathbf{x})d\mathbf{x},$$

$$\frac{dT_x}{dt} = \int_\Omega \frac{\partial \Phi_T}{\partial x}(A\mathbf{x})\mathbf{r}(\mathbf{x})d\mathbf{x},$$

$$\frac{dT_y}{dt} = \int_\Omega \frac{\partial \Phi_T}{\partial y}(A\mathbf{x})\mathbf{r}(\mathbf{x})d\mathbf{x},$$

$$\frac{dT_z}{dt} = \int_\Omega \frac{\partial \Phi_T}{\partial z}(A\mathbf{x})\mathbf{r}(\mathbf{x})d\mathbf{x},$$

where $\mathbf{r}(\mathbf{x}) = d_\varepsilon(\Phi_S(\mathbf{x}), \Phi_T(\mathbf{x}))(\|_S\|\Phi_S(\mathbf{x}) - \Phi_T(A\mathbf{x}))$, ∇ denotes the gradient operator, and

$$\mathcal{R}'_x = \begin{pmatrix} 0 & 0 & 0 \\ 0 & -\sin\theta_x & \cos\theta_x \\ 0 & -\cos\theta_x & -\sin\theta_x \end{pmatrix}, \mathcal{R}'_y = \begin{pmatrix} -\sin\theta_y & 0 & -\cos\theta_y \\ 0 & 0 & 0 \\ \cos\theta_y & 0 & -\sin\theta_y \end{pmatrix},$$

$$\mathcal{R}'_z = \begin{pmatrix} -\sin\theta_z & \cos\theta_z & 0 \\ -\cos\theta_y & -\sin\theta_z & 0 \\ 0 & 0 & 0 \end{pmatrix}.$$

Note that, since we are considering positive scale values, the terms $\frac{d\|S\|}{ds_{x;y;z}}$ equal either 0 or 1.

14.3.4 Examples

Before testing and comparing the performance of the SSD criteria given by Eq. (14.25) against the other two criteria (Eqs. (14.14) and (14.21)), an empirical evaluation of the proposed criterion was performed for the "hand" example (first column of Figure 14.6) in the space of two unknown parameters of the transformation $\mathcal{A}$, while the remaining three parameters are fixed. We considered the following ranges for each parameter: $\theta \in [-\pi/3, \pi/3]$, $S_x, S_y \in [0.7, 1.25]$, and $T_x, T_y \in [-20, 20]$. For each test, the unknown parameter ranges were quantized using uniform sampling. The corresponding results (Figure 14.7) show that, for each case, the cost function exhibits nice smoothness and convexity properties. This indicates that the proposed minimization criterion is well behaved.

To quantitatively validate the model in Eq. (14.25), we perform several registration experiments. For each trial, the source shape is fixed and the target shape is generated by deforming the source using a known transformation $\mathcal{A} = \mathcal{A}(\mathcal{S}, \mathcal{R}, \mathcal{T})$ which will be considered as the ground truth (GT). Then we use our model to recover the optimal

14.3 Global registration of shapes in implicit spaces

Table 14.1 Comparison of recovered parameters when using our model **M1** (Eq. 14.29) and when using a similarity-based model (**M2**), i.e. $s_x = s_y = s$ (Paragios et al. [1]). Results are for the examples presented in the second and last columns of Figure 14.8; **GT** stands for ground truth.

Transformation	Corpus callosum			Fish #1		
	GT	M1	M2	GT	M1	M2
s_x	1.5	1.50	0.99	0.6	0.60	0.71
s_y	0.9	0.90	–	1.0	1.00	–
$\Theta(°)$	10	10	22.75	60	60	52.03
t_x	2.5	1.61	0.14	−3.5	−4.17	−5.82
t_y	0.0	−0.6	2.50	−5	−5.16	−7.52

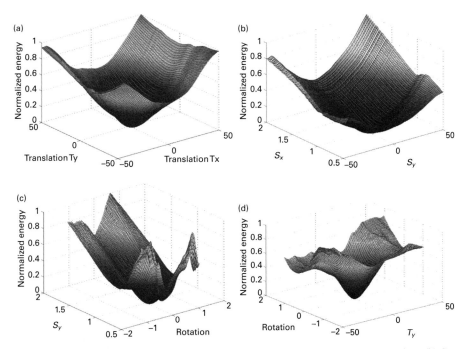

Figure 14.7 Empirical evaluation of the proposed criterion (Eq. 14.27). Unknowns are: (a) T_x and T_y; (b) S_x and S_y; (c) S_y and rotation; (d) θ and T_y.

alignment parameters. The recovered parameters are compared with the GT and with those obtained when using a homogeneous scale-based measure; for the case in which $s_x = s_y = s$, the matrix S reduces to the scalar s, and the measure given by Eq. (14.25) is changed accordingly, as well as the Euler–Lagrange equations, as presented in [14.1].

In each case, the algorithm leads to more accurate results, and one can see that the isotropic scale-based criterion completely fails when the difference between s_x and s_y is large (see for example the last two columns of Figure 14.8). Table 14.1 summarizes some of these results. More results and simulations are in [14.32].

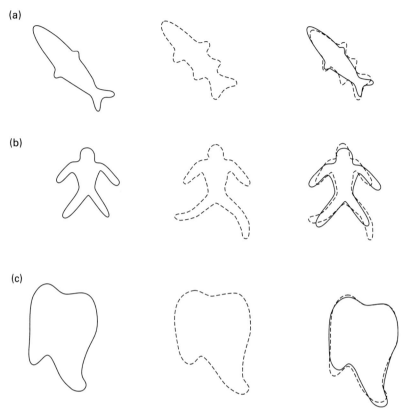

Figure 14.8 Global registration. (a) Input shapes (source and target). (b) Registration results using the isotropic-scale based model. (c) Registration using the proposed model (Eq. 14.25).

Another set of experiments was carried out to compare the registration performance of the proposed criterion with the other two criteria by registering pairs of arbitrary shapes that belong to the same class. Some of these results are presented in Figure 14.9 and 14.10. One can easily see from these figures that the proposed method outperforms the other two models.

Figure 14.11 stresses how the proposed criterion outperforms the isotropic scale-based one. This figure shows the history of the SSD measure in Eq. 14.25 and that of the isotropic scale-based measure vs. iteration for the example shown on the first row of Figure 14.9. One can clearly see that the value of the proposed distance functional drops faster at each iteration step.

In addition, contrary to the SSD measure, the isotropic scale-based measure stops decreasing at a value far from the ideal minimum, leading to less accurate results than to the one developed by Fahmi [14.32], which is used in this work.

Finally, several 3D experiments were carried out to test the proposed global alignment algorithm. Figure 14.12 shows registration of two pairs of teeth. For each pair, a 3D tooth shape of size $117 \times 117 \times 125$ is used as the target shape. This shape is used to generate various deformed instances by randomly assigning different values to the transformation parameters $(s_x, s_y, s_z, \theta_x, \theta_y, \theta_z, t_x, t_y,$ and $t_z)$. For each trial, the deformed shape is used as

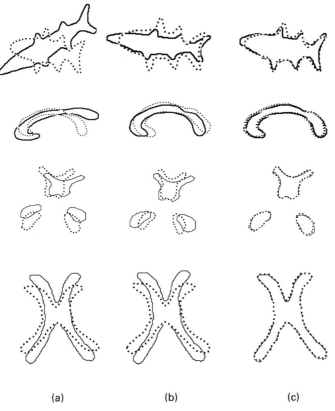

(a) (b) (c)

Figure 14.9 Global registration. (a) Input shapes. (b) Registration using homogeneous scale-based measure. (c) Registration using the proposed registration model (Eq. 14.25).

the source and is registered to the target shape using the proposed algorithm. Some of the corresponding results are shown in Figure 14.12. For each trial, note the high accuracy of the registration results.

14.4 Local shape registration

In many applications, the global matching has to be completed by dense one-to-one correspondences in the presence of local deformations (e.g., [14.33]). Explicitly determining the displacement field plays a key role in various medical applications. Complementary to the global registration field, the local coordinate transformation between the two globally aligned shapes is explicitly estimated by minimizing an energy functional, similar to what was proposed by Fahmi [14.32]. This functional consists of three terms, the first of which is a discrepancy measure between the two shape representations. The second term penalizes the deviation of the distance map representation of

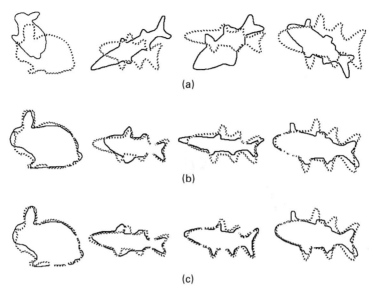

Figure 14.10 Global matching: proposed signed distance vs. VDF-based affine registrations. A color version of this figure is available online at www.cambridgeorg/farag. (a) Input shapes. (b) Affine registration using the VDF representation (Eq. 14.21). (c) Affine registration using our new SSD criterion (Eq. 14.25).

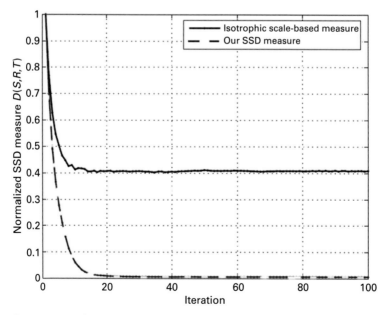

Figure 14.11 Convergence of the new SSD measure (Eq. 28) and comparison to rigid matching case for the examples shown on the first row of Figure 14.9. History of $D(S;R;T)$ for both cases: the new measure (lower) and isotropic scale-based measure (upper).

14.4 Local shape registration

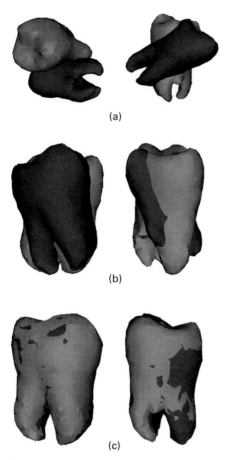

Figure 14.12 Three-dimensional global registration of two pairs of teeth. (a) Input shapes. (b) An intermediate state. (c) Registration using the proposed registration model (Eq. 14.27).

the globally warped source shape from a signed distance function, while the local displacement field, which aims at aligning it with the target shape, is being updated. The last term is a regularization term that enforces the smoothness of the recovered deformations. This leads to a set of coupled equations that are simultaneously minimized through a gradient descent scheme.

14.4.1 Local alignment

Various applications may benefit from explicitly establishing dense point correspondences between two or more shapes. For instance, given a training set of anatomical shapes, the established point correspondences can be used to build a point distribution model (PDM) (e.g. [14.34]) to capture the statistics of the corresponding elements across the training data. Many techniques have also been published using shape priors for the segmentation of medical imagery. A major component in learning such priors is the alignment of the training shapes (see for instance [14.34], [14.35]). In this section, we propose a new variational framework to recover a dense local displacement field between two globally aligned shapes.

14.4.1.1 Variational formulation

Given two shapes, a source S and a target T, assume that these two shapes are globally aligned according to an affine transformation model A. Let $\hat{S} = A(S)$ denote the corresponding transformed source shape. To complement the global matching model, we must recover a pixel-wise displacement field $\mathbf{u} = [u_1, \cdots, u_n]^T : \mathbb{R}^n \to \mathbb{R}^n$, with $n = 2,3$ in practice, in such a way that $\Phi_T \circ g$ (the deformed distance map of the target) matches $\Phi_{\hat{S}}$, where $\Phi_{\hat{S}}$ and Φ_T are the implicit distance map representations of $\hat{S}$ and T, respectively, and where $g(\mathbf{x}) = \mathbf{x} + \mathbf{u}(\mathbf{x})$ is the geometric deformation. The most common way of solving this problem is through the minimization of the following functional w.r.t. $\mathbf{u}$:

$$E_1(\mathbf{u}) = \int_\Omega (\Phi_{\hat{S}}(\mathbf{x}) - \Phi_T(g(\mathbf{x})))^2 d\mathbf{x}. \quad (14.32)$$

This measure, the SSD, has been extensively used for image and shape matching. Its limitations are well established, especially when dealing with images with different modalities, and other criteria have been proposed to cope with this issue. When dealing with shapes, we know that the registration in the presence of scale variations is analogous to aligning different modality images (e.g. [14.1]). However, we have already shown that the proposed global alignment model yields accurate results in the presence of scale variations. Hence, in order to recover the local displacement field, the SSD criterion (14.32) is adopted in this work, but in a different setting. Instead of directly minimizing the functional $E_1(\cdot)$ w.r.t. $\mathbf{u}$, we initialize a function $\Phi(\cdot)$ to be the signed distance representation of the globally aligned source shape $\hat{S}$ when there is no displacement (i.e., $\mathbf{u} = 0$). Then, once we start updating $\mathbf{u}$, we propose to simultaneously penalize the deviation of the corresponding deformed shape representation, $\Phi(g(\cdot))$, from a signed distance function.

14.4.1.2 Reinitialization of a distance function

In most scenarios of moving interface-based methods, it is impossible to maintain the level set function as a signed distance function to the moving front. As the interface moves, flat and/or step regions develop, introducing computational inaccuracies. For this practical reason, as well as for theoretical reasons (e.g. [14.36]), one needs to keep the level set function close to a signed distance function (i.e., $|\nabla \phi| \approx 1$) from time to time during the course of its evolution. This process is known as the distance reinitialization of the level set function. The standard reinitialization method is to compute the embedding function, $\phi(\cdot)$, as the steady state of the following PDE equation:

$$\phi_t = \text{sign}(\phi_0)(1 - |\nabla \phi|) \text{ and } \phi(\mathbf{x}, 0) = \phi_0(\mathbf{x}), \quad (14.33)$$

where ϕ_0 is the function to be reinitialized and $\text{sign}(\cdot)$ is the sign function. The idea of using this equation is that at steady state, the solution will correspond to a signed distance function ($|\nabla \phi| = 1$) with the same zero-level set as the initial function Φ_0. Hence, every few steps of the evolution process, the embedding function Φ is rebuilt with the above equation. However, as has been reported by various authors (e.g., [14.37]), if the initial condition Φ_0 is not smooth or if it is much steeper on one side of the embedded interface, the resulting function, Φ, can be moved incorrectly with respect to the original function. In addition, this reinitialization may fail if the level set function is initially far from a signed distance function. Practically, the reinitialization process can be complicated, expensive and have subtle side effects. Li et al. [14.38] proposed a new variational level set formulation that forces the level-set function to be close to a signed distance and hence eliminates the need for the reinitialization process. This was done in the context of level-set-based segmentation, by incorporating the following internal energy term into their segmentation energy:

$$\mathcal{T}(\Phi) = \frac{1}{2} \int_\Omega (|\nabla \Phi(\mathbf{x})| - 1)^2 d\mathbf{x}. \tag{14.34}$$

Owing to this energy, the level-set function is automatically kept close to a signed distance function during the evolution process. The numerical advantages of this new reinitialization technique were highlighted in [14.38]. In this work, we use the same reinitialization approach and propose a new variational formulation for non-rigid registration of shapes.

14.4.1.3 Energy formulation

Instead of directly minimizing the functional $E_1(\cdot)$ in Eq. (14.32) with respect to the unknown displacement field $\mathbf{u}$, we initialize a function $\Phi(\cdot)$ to be the signed distance representation of the globally aligned source shape $\hat{S}$ when there is no displacement (i.e., when $\mathbf{u} = 0$). Then, once we start updating $\mathbf{u}$, we propose to simultaneously penalize the deviation of the corresponding deformed shape representation, $\Phi(g(\cdot))$, from a signed distance function following the idea proposed by Li et al. [14.38]. Adding the following energy term into the functional E_1:

$$E_2(\Phi, \mathbf{u}) = \int_\Omega (|\nabla \Phi(g(\mathbf{x}))| - 1)^2 d\mathbf{x} \tag{14.35}$$

will ensure that the source shape is kept implicitly represented by a signed distance function while it is being warped by the updated displacement field $\mathbf{u}$. With the two functionals, E_1 and E_2, we propose to minimize the following data-driven energy in order to explicitly determine the geometric transformation between the two shapes:

$$\begin{aligned} E_{\text{data}}(\Phi, \mathbf{u}) &= \alpha E_1(\Phi, \mathbf{u}) + \beta E_2(\Phi, \mathbf{u}) \\ &= \alpha \int_\Omega \left(\Phi(\mathbf{x}) - \Phi_T(g(\mathbf{x})) \right)^2 d\mathbf{x} + \beta \int_\Omega \left(|\nabla \Phi(g(\mathbf{x}))| - 1 \right)^2 d\mathbf{x}, \end{aligned} \tag{14.36}$$

where α and β are two real parameters that balance the contribution of the two terms.

To further measure and constrain the "irregularity" of $\mathbf{u}$, we propose to add a regularization term inspired from the equilibrium equations of linearized elasticity (we refer the reader to Ciarlet [14.39]) for a formal study of 3D elasticity theory. If we assume that the geometric deformation $g(\mathbf{x}) = \mathbf{x} + \mathbf{u}(\mathbf{x})$ corresponds to the strain of an elastic and isotropic material, then the strain energy is given by:

$$E_{\text{smoothness}}(\mathbf{u}) = \int_{\Omega} \left(\frac{\lambda}{2} (\operatorname{div} \mathbf{u})^2 + \mu \sum_{i,j=1}^{n} \left(\varepsilon_{ij}(\mathbf{u})\right)^2 \right) d\mathbf{x}, \qquad (14.37)$$

where μ, λ are the Lamé coefficients of the material, and $\varepsilon_{ij}(\mathbf{u}) = \frac{1}{2}\left(\frac{\partial u_i}{\partial x_j} + \frac{\partial u_j}{\partial x_i}\right)$ is the deformation tensor. This regularization term is chosen over others for the flexibility gained by the relative weight which one can give to the operators $\Delta \mathbf{u}$ and $\nabla(\nabla \mathbf{u})$ (divergence of Jacobian of $\mathbf{u}$). Valadez [12] has in-depth studies of this and other regularization operators. Integration of all the energy functionals defined above leads to minimizing the following total energy in order to recover $\mathbf{u}$:

$$E_{\text{total}}(\Phi, \mathbf{u}) = E_{\text{data}}(\Phi, \mathbf{u}) + \gamma E_{\text{smoothness}}(\mathbf{u}). \qquad (14.38)$$

14.4.2 Gradient descent flows and numerical implementation

In order to recover the displacement field $\mathbf{u}$, we simultaneously minimize the total energy E_{total} in Eq. (14.38) with respect to $\mathbf{u}$ and Φ. We use the standard gradient descent (or steepest descent) method to minimize this energy. By calculus of variations, the Gateaux derivatives of the functional E_{total} with respect to Φ and to the displacement field $\mathbf{u}$ can be found as detailed below.

14.4.2.1 Gradient flow with respect to Φ

Finding a minimizer Φ of E_{total} is equivalent to numerically solving the following PDE:

$$\Phi_t = -\frac{\partial E_{\text{total}}}{\partial \Phi}, \text{ and initial condition } \Phi_0. \qquad (14.39)$$

The derivatives of the total energy w.r.t. Φ can be calculated as follows:

$$\frac{\partial E_{\text{total}}}{\partial \Phi} = \alpha \frac{\partial E_1}{\partial \Phi} + \beta \frac{\partial E_2}{\partial \Phi} + \gamma \frac{\partial E_{\text{smoothness}}}{\partial \Phi}, \qquad (14.40)$$

where

$$\frac{\partial E_1}{\partial \Phi} = 2(\Phi(\mathbf{x}) - \Phi_T(g(\mathbf{x}))), \qquad (14.41)$$

$$\frac{\partial E_2}{\partial \Phi} = 2\left[\Delta\Phi(g(\mathbf{x})) - \operatorname{div}\left(\frac{\nabla\Phi(g(\mathbf{x}))}{|\Phi(g(\mathbf{x}))|}\right)\right], \qquad (14.42)$$

$$\frac{\partial E_{\text{smoothness}}}{\partial \Phi} = 0. \qquad (14.43)$$

14.4.2.2 Gradient flow with respect to the displacement field u

Similarly, finding a minimizer Φ of E_{total} is equivalent to numerically solving the following PDE:

$$\mathbf{u}_t = -\frac{\partial E_{\text{total}}}{\partial \mathbf{u}}, \text{ and initial condition } \mathbf{u}_0. \tag{14.44}$$

The derivatives of the total energy with respect to $\mathbf{u}$ can be found as follows:

$$\frac{\partial E_{\text{total}}}{\partial \mathbf{u}} = \alpha \frac{\partial E_1}{\partial \mathbf{u}} + \beta \frac{\partial E_2}{\partial \mathbf{u}} + \gamma \frac{\partial E_{\text{smoothness}}}{\partial \mathbf{u}}, \tag{14.45}$$

where

$$\frac{\partial E_1}{\partial \mathbf{u}} = 2\left[\Phi(\mathbf{x}) - \Phi_T\big(g(\mathbf{x})\big)\right] \cdot \nabla \Phi_T(g(\mathbf{x})), \tag{14.46}$$

and

$$\frac{\partial E_2}{\partial \mathbf{u}} = 2(|\nabla \Phi(\mathbf{x})| - 1) \cdot \frac{\partial}{\partial \mathbf{u}}(|\nabla \Phi(\mathbf{x})|). \tag{14.47}$$

Let us evaluate the term $\frac{\partial}{\partial \mathbf{u}}|\nabla \Phi(g(\mathbf{x}))| = \left[\frac{\partial}{\partial u_1}(|\nabla \Phi(g(\mathbf{x}))|) \ldots \frac{\partial}{\partial u_n}(|\nabla \Phi(g(\mathbf{x}))|)\right]^T$, in the last equation. Let us define the following quantities: $\mathbf{x} = (x_1, \cdots, x_n)$, $\mathbf{u}(\mathbf{x}) = (u_1(\mathbf{x}), \cdots, u_n(\mathbf{x}))$, and let $\nabla \Phi(g(\mathbf{x})) = \left[\frac{\partial}{\partial x_1}\Phi(\mathbf{x} + \mathbf{u}(\mathbf{x})), \ldots, \frac{\partial}{\partial x_n}\Phi(\mathbf{x} + \mathbf{u}(\mathbf{x}))\right]^T$. With these notations, we have $|\nabla \Phi(g(\mathbf{x}))| = \left(\sum_{i=1}^{n} \frac{\partial}{\partial x_i}\Phi(\mathbf{x} + \mathbf{u}(\mathbf{x}))^2\right)^{\frac{1}{2}}$. Hence, the derivative of $|\nabla \Phi(g(\mathbf{x}))|$ with respect to the jth component, u_j, of the displacement field $\mathbf{u}$, is given by

$$\frac{\partial}{\partial u_j}|\nabla \Phi(g(\mathbf{x}))| = \frac{1}{2}\left|\nabla \Phi\big(g(\mathbf{x})\big)\right|^{-1} \sum_{i=1}^{n} 2\frac{\partial}{\partial x_i}\Phi(\mathbf{x} + \mathbf{u}(\mathbf{x})) \cdot \frac{\partial}{\partial u_j}\left(\frac{\partial}{\partial x_i}\Phi(\mathbf{x} + \mathbf{u}(\mathbf{x}))\right)$$

$$= |\nabla \Phi(g(\mathbf{x}))|^{-1} \sum_{i=1}^{n} \frac{\partial}{\partial x_i}\Phi(\mathbf{x} + \mathbf{u}(\mathbf{x})) \cdot \frac{\partial}{\partial x_i}\left(\frac{\partial}{\partial u_j}\Phi(\mathbf{x} + \mathbf{u}(\mathbf{x}))\right) \tag{14.48}$$

Note that $\frac{\partial}{\partial u_j}\Phi(\mathbf{x} + \mathbf{u}(\mathbf{x}))) = \frac{\partial}{\partial x_j}\Phi(\mathbf{x} + \mathbf{u}(\mathbf{x})))$, hence:

$$\frac{\partial}{\partial u_j}(|\nabla \Phi(g(\mathbf{x}))|) = |\nabla \Phi(g(\mathbf{x}))|^{-1} \sum_{i=1}^{n} \frac{\partial}{\partial x_i}\Phi(\mathbf{x} + \mathbf{u}(\mathbf{x})) \cdot \frac{\partial}{\partial x_i}\left(\frac{\partial}{\partial x_j}\Phi(\mathbf{x} + \mathbf{u}(\mathbf{x}))\right)$$

$$= \Phi(g(\mathbf{x}))|^{-1} \sum_{i=1}^{n} \frac{\partial}{\partial x_i}\Phi(g(\mathbf{x})) \cdot \frac{\partial^2}{\partial x_i \partial x_j}\Phi \circ g(\mathbf{x}) \tag{14.49}$$

The above equation can be put together in a matrix form as:

$$\frac{\partial}{\partial \mathbf{u}}|\nabla \Phi(\mathbf{x})| = \left[\frac{\partial}{\partial u_i}|\nabla \Phi(\mathbf{x})|, \ldots \frac{\partial}{\partial u_n}|\nabla \Phi(\mathbf{x})|\right]^T,$$

$$= |\nabla \Phi(g(\mathbf{x}))|^{-1} \begin{bmatrix} \frac{\partial^2 \Phi \circ g}{\partial x_1 \partial x_1}(\mathbf{x}) & \cdots & \frac{\partial^2 \Phi \circ g}{\partial x_1 \partial x_n}(\mathbf{x}) \\ \vdots & \ddots & \vdots \\ \frac{\partial^2 v}{\partial x_n \partial x_1}(\mathbf{x}) & \cdots & \frac{\partial^2 \Phi \circ g}{\partial x_n \partial x_n}(\mathbf{x}) \end{bmatrix} \cdot \begin{pmatrix} \frac{\partial \Phi \circ g}{\partial x_1}(\mathbf{x}) \\ \vdots \\ \frac{\partial \Phi \circ g}{\partial x_n}(\mathbf{x}) \end{pmatrix} \quad (14.50)$$

$$= |\nabla \Phi(g(\mathbf{x}))|^{-1} \mathcal{H}(\Phi \circ g)(\mathbf{x}) \cdot \nabla \Phi(g(\mathbf{x})).$$

Then, the derivative of the energy term E_2 (see Eq. (14.49)) can be written as

$$\frac{\partial E_2}{\partial \mathbf{u}} = 2(|\nabla \Phi(\mathbf{x})| - 1)|\nabla \Phi(g(\mathbf{x}))|^{-1} \mathcal{H}(\Phi \circ g)(\mathbf{x}) \cdot \nabla \Phi(g(\mathbf{x}))$$

$$= 2\left(1 - \frac{1}{|\nabla \Phi(\mathbf{x})|}\right) \mathcal{H}(\Phi \circ g)(\mathbf{x}) \cdot \nabla \Phi(g(\mathbf{x})) \quad (14.51)$$

where $\mathcal{H}(\Phi \circ g)(\mathbf{x})$ is the Hessian matrix of $\Phi \circ g$ as defined in Eq. (14.50). Finally, the derivative of the smoothness energy $E_{\text{smoothness}}$ with respect to $\mathbf{u}$ leads to the following operator:

$$\frac{\partial}{\partial \mathbf{u}} E_{\text{smoothness}} \doteq \mathcal{R}(\mathbf{u}) = 2 \begin{pmatrix} \mu \Delta u_1(\mathbf{x}) + (\lambda + \mu) \sum_{i=1}^n \frac{\partial^2}{\partial x_1 \partial x_i} u_i(\mathbf{x}) \\ \vdots \\ \mu \Delta u_n(\mathbf{x}) + (\lambda + \mu) \sum_{i=1}^n \frac{\partial^2}{\partial x_n \partial x_i} u_i(\mathbf{x}) \end{pmatrix}, \quad (14.52)$$

where $\Delta = \sum_{i=1}^n \frac{\partial^2}{\partial x_i^2}$ denotes the Laplace operator. Combining equations (14.40) and (14.45) results in the following set of $(n+1)$ coupled evolution equations:

$$\begin{cases} \Phi_t = -\frac{\partial E_{\text{total}}}{\partial \Phi} - 2\left[\alpha(\Phi(\mathbf{x}) - \Phi_T(g(\mathbf{x})) + \beta\left(\Delta \Phi(g(\mathbf{x})) - \text{div}\left(\frac{\nabla \Phi(g(\mathbf{x}))}{|\nabla \Phi(g(\mathbf{x}))|}\right)\right)\right], \\ \mathbf{u}_t = -\frac{\partial E_{\text{total}}}{\partial \mathbf{u}} \\ \quad = -2\left[\alpha(\Phi(\mathbf{x}) - \Phi_T(g(\mathbf{x}))) \cdot \nabla \Phi_T(g(\mathbf{x})) - \beta\left(1 - \frac{1}{|\nabla \Phi(g(\mathbf{x}))|}\right) \cdot \mathcal{H}(\Phi \circ g)(\mathbf{x}) \cdot \nabla \Phi(g(\mathbf{x})) + \gamma \mathcal{R}(\mathbf{u})\right] \\ \Phi(\mathbf{x}, 0) = \Phi_{\hat{S}}(\mathbf{x}), \\ \mathbf{u}(\mathbf{x}, 0) = 0. \end{cases}$$

$$(14.53)$$

14.4 Local shape registration

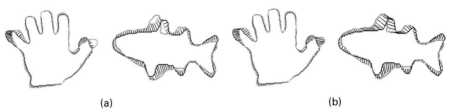

(a)   (b)

Figure 14.13 Established point-wise correspondences after local registration. (a), Without penalizing energy $E(\cdot)$; (b) using the model in Eq. (14.52). A color version of this figure is available online at www.cambridgeorg/farag. Source shape is blue, locally deformed source green; target red.

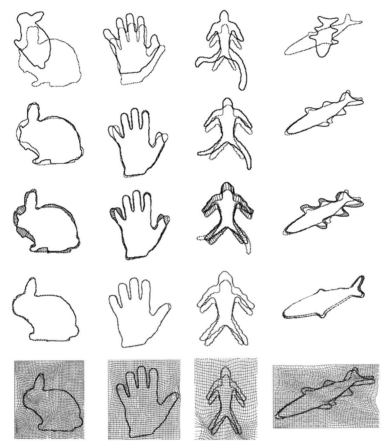

Figure 14.14 Sample registration results. A color version of this figure is available online at www.cambridgeorg/farag. (a) Initial positions of the source shape (blue) and target (red). (b) Global alignment using our new global matching model. (c) Established shape correspondences after local matching. (d) Locally deformed source (green) overlaid on target (red). (e) Space warping with globally deformed source (blue), locally deformed source (green), and target (red). Adapted from Fahmi [14.32].

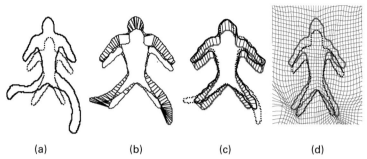

Figure 14.15 Example of registration in presence of large deformations. (a) Initial poses of source relative to target shape. (b) Point correspondences using the ICP algorithm. (c) Point correspondences using the proposed registration method. (d) Deformation field corresponding to results in (c).

14.4.2.3 Numerical implementation

The following finite difference schemes were used to discretize the continuous non-rigid matching Eq. (14.53).

- The gradient terms were approximated using central differences.
- Standard second-order approximations were used to compute $\frac{\partial^2 u}{\partial x_i^2}$.
- The four-point approximation with truncation order d^2 was used to approximate $\frac{\partial^2 u}{\partial x_i \partial x_j}$, with d being the isotropic grid spacing in each direction.
- Bilinear (for 2D cases) and trilinear interpolation (for 3D cases) schemes were used to estimate data values (such as distance maps of transformed shapes) at positions other than grid points. Finally, the Lamé constants were set to $\mu = 0.5$ and $\lambda = 0$ for all experiments.

First, Figure 14.13b illustrates one of the advantages of using the penalty factor expressed by the functional $E_2(\cdot)$ (Eq. 14.44). The effect of this energy helps in guiding the transformed shape in the right direction even where the deformation is large. In contrast, more iterations were used for the results shown in Figure 14.13a, when the penalty term is dropped, with less accurate results. More 2D examples are shown in Figure 14.14 to demonstrate the overall performance of the proposed non-rigid registration framework. Figure 14.15 shows how accurate the registration results are even in the presence of very large deformations. The results shown are compared with those obtained using the iterative closest point (ICP) method. The proposed approach clearly outperforms the ICP.

In Figure 14.14, we compare the accuracy of our algorithm to that presented in Haung et al. [14.2], which also uses the signed distance-based implicit representation for shape registration. In Huang et al. [14.2], the authors maximize the MI between the two implicit representations, where the probability density functions are approximated using non-parametric Gaussian kernels with empirical width value. Regarding the local deformation (Figure 14.14d), the competing method used in [14.2] recovers the registration field by iteratively minimizing a regularized energy with respect to each component of each control point, using the gradient descent method.

Finally, Figure 14.15 shows the accuracy of the registration results even in the presence of very large deformations. The results are compared with those obtained using the iterative closest point (ICP) method. The proposed approach clearly outperforms the ICP.

As a quantitative evaluation of both the global and the local registration models can be in terms of the root-mean-square error (RMS), which is computed between the implicit representations of the two input shapes before and after global and local alignments. The RMS error is denoted as ζ and is given by:

$$\zeta = \sqrt{\frac{\sum \left(\Phi_1^2(\mathbf{x}_i) - \Phi_2^2(\mathbf{x}_i) \right)}{N}}, \quad (14.54)$$

where Φ_i, $i = 1, 2$, refers to the implicit representation of the two shape being registered; $\mathbf{x}_i$ are the image voxels; and N is the total number of voxels.

14.5 Summary

This chapter has presented a self-contained variational framework for dense global-to-local registration of shapes. Implicit shape representation through sign distance function was considered to represent the input shapes. The SSD criterion developed by Fahmi [14.32] was used to globally align the input shapes. This criterion supports both rigid and affine transformations. Various experiments were presented to show the effectiveness of this new measure. Comparisons with the isotropic scale-based SSD criterion and with the VDF-based criterion show that the proposed measure outperforms both of these.

The local deformation field is explicitly established between the two globally aligned shapes, by minimizing a new energy functional that incrementally and simultaneously updates the displacement field while keeping the corresponding distance map representation of the globally warped source shape as close to a signed distance function as possible. The resulting paradigm is validated using a novel technique based on the finite element method. Given a shape S, we simulate a finite element deformation of S which is considered as the target T. The simulated displacement field is used as the ground truth to validate our non-rigid matching model. The accuracy of our registration model is assessed by registering the simulated deformed shape with the original one, and comparing the magnitude of the recovered displacement field at the points located on the source shape with the bio-mechanically simulated one. Various experiments were presented to show the potential of the proposed framework, and a comparison with the latest published results was presented.

It is only fair to mention, though, that our local registration model may not output accurate results in the presence of highly local non-rigid deformations. This limitation may be overcome by incorporating more information about the two shapes in the evolutive model. One attractive way of doing so, which we are currently investigating, is to exploit the local geometric features of the signed distance transform in order to determine point correspondences in the target and the source shapes, and then integrate this new information into our framework. This may also help when dealing with spurious structures.

References

[14.1] N. Paragios, M. Rousson and V. Ramesh, Non-rigid registration using distance functions, *Comp. Vis. Image Understand.* **89** (2003) 142–165.

[14.2] X. Huang, N. Paragios and D. N. Metaxas, Shape registration in implicit spaces using information theory and free form deformations. *IEEE Trans. Pattern Anal. Mach. Intel.* **28**(8) (2006) 1303–1318.

[14.3] H. AbdEl-Munim and A. A. Farag, A variational approach for shapes registration using vector maps. *Proc. IEEE Int. Conf. Image Processing (ICIP'06)* April 12–16 (2006), Washington, DC, USA 337–340.

[14.4] H. AbdEl Munim, A. A. Farag and A. A. Farag, Shape representation and registration in vector implicit spaces: adopting a closed-form solution in the optimization process. *IEEE Trans. Pattern Anal. Mach. Intel.* **35** (2013) 763–768.

[14.5] S. Belongie, J. Malik, and J. Puzicha, Shape matching and object recognition using shape contexts. *IEEE Trans. Pattern Anal. Mach. Intel.* **24**(24) (2002) 509–522.

[14.6] T. B. Sebastian, P. N. Klein and B. B. Kimia, Recognition of shapes by editing their shock graphs. *IEEE Trans. Pattern Anal. Mach. Intel.* **26**(5) (2004) 550–571.

[14.7] L. H. Staib and J. S. Duncan, Boundary finding with parametrically deformable models. *IEEE Trans. Pattern Anal. Mach. Intel.* **14**(11) (1992) 1061–1075.

[14.8] H. Li, T. Shen and X. Huang, Approximately global optimization for robust alignment of generalized shapes. *IEEE Trans. Pattern Anal. Mach. Intel.* **33** (6) (2011) 1116–1131.

[14.9] H. Abd El Munim and A. A. Farag, A new variational approach for 3D shape registration. *Proc. Int. Symp. Biomedical Imaging (ISBI'07)*, April 12–15 (2007), Metro, Washington, DC, 1324–1327.

[14.10] R. Fahmi and A. A. Farag, A global-to-local 2D shape registration in implicit spaces using level sets. *Proc. IEEE Int. Conf. Image Processing (ICIP'07)*, September 16–19 (2007), St Antonio, Texas, VI-237–VI-240.

[14.11] R. Fahmi and A. A. Farag, A novel shape registration framework and its application to 3D face recognition in the presence of expressions. *4th Int. Symp. Visual Computing (ISVC-08)*, December 1–3 (2008), Las Vegas, 287–296.

[14.12] G. Hermosillo Valadez, Variational methods for multimodal image matching. Unpublished PhD thesis, Université de Nice – Sophia Antipolis (2002).

[14.13] C. Goodall, Procrustes methods in the statistical analysis of shape. *J. Roy. Stat. Soc.* **53**(2) (1991) 285–339.

[14.14] M-K. Hu, Visual pattern recognition by moment invariants. *IRE Trans. Inform. Theory* **49**(8) (1962) 179–189.

[14.15] A. Foulonneau, P. Charbonnier and F. Heitz, Affine-invariant geometric shape priors for region-based active contours. *IEEE Trans. Pattern Anal. Mach. Intel.*, **28**(8) (2006) 1352–1357.

[14.16] C. Brechbühler, G. Gerig and O. Kübler, Surface parametrization and shape description. *Comp. Vis. Image Understand.* **61**(2) (1995) 154–170.

[14.17] M. Kazhdan, T. Funkhouser and S. Rusinkiewicz, Rotation invariant spherical harmonic representation of 3D shape descriptors. In H. Hoppe L. Kobbelt, P. Schröder (eds.) *Eurographics Symposium on Geometry Processing'03* June 22–25 (2003) Aire-la-Ville, Switzerland.

[14.18] M. K. Chung, K. M. Dalton, L. L. Shen, A. C. Evans and R. J. Davidson, Weighted Fourier series representation and its application to quantifying the amount of gray matter. *IEEE Trans. Med. Imag. (Special Issue on Computational Neuroanatomy)* **26** (2007).

[14.19] X. Pennec, N. Ayache and J-P. Thirion, Landmark-based registration using features identified through differential geometry. In I. Bankman, ed., *Handbook of Medical Imaging*, Waltham, MA: Academic Press (2000) ch. 31, 499–513.

[14.20] P. Laskov and C. Kambhamettu, Curvature-based algorithms for nonrigid motion and correspondence estimation. *IEEE Trans. Pattern Anal. Mach. Intel.*, **25**(10) (2003) 1349–1354.

[14.21] A. Farag, S. Elhabian, M. Abdelrahman et al., Shape modeling of the corpus callosum. *Proc. 32nd IEEE Engineering in Medicine and Biology Society (EMBC)* (2010) Buenos Aires, 4288–4291.

[14.22] H. Blum, A transformation for extracting new descriptors of shape. In W. Wathen-Dunn (ed.), *Models for the Perception of Speech and Visual Form*. Cambridge: MIT Press (1967) 362–380.

[14.23] A. Brennecke and T. Isenberg, 3D shape matching using skeleton graphs. In *Simulation and Visualization*, March 4–5 (2004) Magdeburg, 299–310.

[14.24] M. Hilaga, Y. Shinagawa, T. Kohmura and T. L. Kunii, Topology matching for fully automatic similarity estimation of 3D shapes. In *SIGGRAPH'01: Proc. 28th Annual Conf. Computer Graphics and Interactive Techniques* August 12–17 (2001), Los Angeles, CA, 203–212.

[14.25] R. Fahmi, A. Jerebko, M. Wolf and A. A. Farag, Robust segmentation of tubular structures in medical images. Proc. SPIE'08, San Diego, CA (2008).

[14.26] M. Sabry Hassouna and A. A. Farag, PDE-based three dimensional path planning for virtual endoscopy. *Proc. Information Processing in Medical Imaging 2005 (IPMI'05)*. Glenwood Springs, CO, July (2005) 529–540.

[14.27] D. S. Fritsch, S. M. Pizer, B. S. Morse, D. H. Eberly and A. Liu, The multiscale medial axis and its applications in image registration. *Pattern Recogn. Lett.* **15**(5) (1994) 445–452.

[14.28] S. M. Pizer, D. S. Fritsch, V. E. Johnson and E. L. Chaney, Segmentation, registration, and measurement of shape variation via image object shape. *IEEE Trans. Med. Imaging*, **18**(10) (1999) 851–865.

[14.29] M. Sabry Hassouna and A. A. Farag, Variational curve skeletons using gradient vector flow. *IEEE Trans. Pattern Anal. Mach. Intel.* **31** (12), (2009) 2257–2274.

[14.30] O. D. Faugeras and J. Gomes, Dynamic shapes of arbitrary dimension: The vector distance functions. *Proc. 9th IMA Conf. Mathematics of Surfaces*. London: Springer (2000). 227–262.

[14.31] R. Fahmi, A. Abdel-Hakim Aly, A. El-Baz and A. Farag, New deformable registration technique using scale space and curve evolution theory and a finite element based validation framework. *28th Annual Int. Conf. IEEE Engineering in Medicine and Biology Society*, New York, August 31–Sept 3 (2006), 3041–3044.

[14.32] R. Fahmi, Variational methods for shape and image registrations. Unpublished PhD dissertation, Computer Vision and Image Processing Laboratory, University of Louisville (2008).

[14.33] J. Feldmar and N. Ayache, Rigid, affine and locally affine registration of free-form surfaces. *Int. J. Comput. Vision* **18**(2) (1996) 99–119.

[14.34] T. F. Cootes, C. J. Tayor, D. H. Cooper and J. Graham, Active shape models – their training and application. *Comp. Vis. Image Understand.* **61**(1) (1995) 38–59.

[14.35] A. Tsai, A. Yezzi Jr., W. Wells *et al.*, A shape-based approach to the segmentation of medical imagery using level sets. *IEEE Trans. Med. Imag.*, **22**(2) (2003) 137–154.

[14.36] J. Gomes and O. Faugeras, Reconciling distance functions and level sets. *J. Vis. Commun. Image Repres.* **11** (2000) 209–223.

[14.37] D. Peng, B. Merriman, S. Osher, H. Zhao and M. Kang, A PDE-based fast local level set method. *J. Comp. Phys.*, **155** (1999) 410–438.

[14.38] C. Li, C. Xu, C. Gui and M. D. Fox, Level set evolution without re-initialization: A new variational formulation. *Proc. IEEE Comp. Vis. Pattern Recog. (CVPR'2005)*, Vol. **1** (2005) 430–436.

[14.39] P. G. Ciarlet, *Mathematical Elasticity*: Volume I: *Three Dimensional Elasticity*. North Holland: Elsevier (1988).

15 Statistical models of shape and appearance

15.1 Introduction

In this chapter, statistical models, derived from the shape and texture of an object in an image or volume, are studied. Statistical shape and appearance models can capture patterns of variability in shape and gray-level appearance. They form the basis of two of the most powerful tools for object analysis – active shape models (ASM) and active appearance models (AAM) – and are very popular in the computer vision and biomedical imaging analysis literature. This chapter reviews the basic foundation of these two statistical models and provides illustrative examples of their effectiveness in object modeling. The chapter builds upon various ideas studied in previous chapters.

15.2 Statistical shape models

The shape of an object can be represented by a set of n points, which can be in any dimension (i.e., 2D or 3D). Adopting Kendall's definition [15.1][15.2], shape is formally defined as:

DEFINITION 15.1 *A shape embodies all the geometrical information that remains when location, scale, and rotational effects are filtered out from an object.* ∎

Shapes may be represented by various methods, mostly starting from certain landmarks that best describe the object. A landmark can be formally defined as:

DEFINITION 15.2 *A landmark is a point of correspondence on each object that matches between and within populations.* ∎

Real-world objects may take various forms, and may be linear, planar, or three dimensional. In [15.4], Dryden and Mardia define anatomical landmarks as points assigned by an expert that correspond between organisms in some biologically meaningful way; mathematical landmarks as points located on an object according to some mathematical or geometrical property, e.g. high curvature or an extremum point; and pseudo-landmarks as constructed points on an object either on the outline or between landmarks. Figure 15.1 illustrates examples of landmark points for various objects.

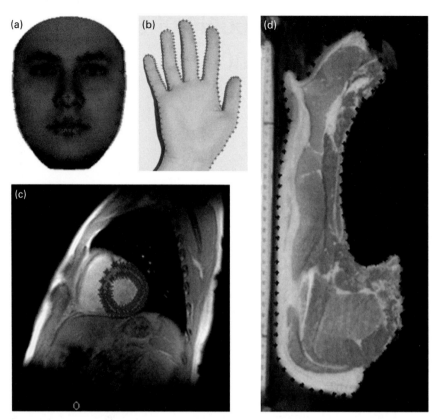

Figure 15.1 Examples of landmark points for hand, heart, and meat objects.

A shape is considered to be a set of n vertices $x \in R^k$; for the 2D case:

$$x = [x_1, x_2, \ldots, x_n, y_1, y_2, \ldots, y_n]^T \tag{15.1}$$

The shape ensemble (collection of shapes) is to be adjusted (aligned) against the same reference to enable filtering of scale, orientation and translation among the ensemble, as in the shape definition. This alignment generates the so-called shape space, which is the set of all possible shapes of the object in question, formally defined as follows:

DEFINITION 15.3 *The* shape space *is the orbit shape of the non-coincident* n *point set configurations in* R^k *under the action of the* Euclidean *similarity transformations.* ∎

To align the shapes in an ensemble, various procedures may be used (see previous chapter). The *generalized Procrustes analysis* procedure [15.3], which is the most common approach for rigid shape alignment, is discussed below. The alignment process removes the redundancies of scale, translation, and rotation using a similarity measure that provides the minimum Procrustes distance. The Procrustes distance between two shapes s_1 and s_2 is the sum of squared difference (SSD)

15.2 Statistical shape models

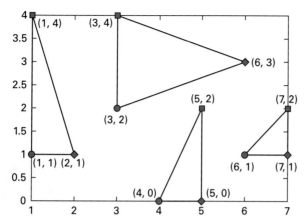

Figure 15.2 A collection of triangular shapes before alignment using generalized Procrustes analysis.

$$P_d^2 = \sum_{j=1}^{n} (x_{j_1} - x_{j_2})^2 + (y_{j_1} - y_{j_2})^2 \qquad (15.2)$$

The generalized Procrustes analysis alignment procedure may be accomplished by the following steps in Pseudocode 15.1.

Example 15.1 This example will illustrate how to perform generalized Procrustes analysis on the collection of shapes shown in Figure 15.2. Each vertex is denoted by a circle, diamond, or square, which denotes corresponding vertices across the ensemble of shapes. Code 15.1 shows the code snippet in MATLAB to perform generalized Procrustes analysis. Note the comments in the code snippet indicating the association between the steps in Pseudocode 15.1 and Code 15.1. Figures 15.3a and 15.3b visualize the collection of shapes at pre-alignment and post-alignment, respectively.

15.2.1 Construction of statistical shape model using PCA

Annotated data of an ensemble of shapes of a certain object carries redundancies due to imprecise definitions of landmarks, and due to errors in the annotations. To perform proper shape alignment these redundancies may be reduced by a transformation step that flags the important features and filters out the highly correlated ones. Principal component analysis (PCA) is a technique for data reduction that has been widely used because of its computational efficiency and theoretical appeal (global registration may be executed by level set methods as in the previous chapter. See also [15.12], [15.13]).

In a nutshell, PCA involves linearly transforming the original data such that the important features may be weighted heavily with respect to the eigenvectors of the transformation. In PCA, the original shape vector *xxx* is linearly transformed by a

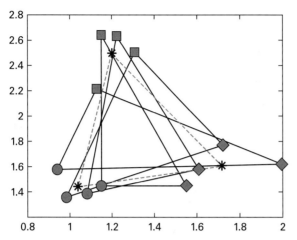

Figure 15.3 Visualization of the ensemble of shapes at (a) pre-alignment and (b) post-alignment using generalized Procrustes analysis.

mapping $\mathbf{M}$ such that $\mathbf{z} = \mathbf{Mx}$ has less correlated and highly separable features. The mapping $\mathbf{M}$ is derived for an ensemble of N shapes as follows:

$$\bar{\mathbf{x}} = \frac{1}{N} \sum_{i=1}^{N} \mathbf{x}_i \text{ and } \Sigma_\mathbf{x} = \frac{1}{N} \sum_{i=1}^{N} (\mathbf{x}_i - \bar{\mathbf{x}})(\mathbf{x}_i - \bar{\mathbf{x}})^T \qquad (15.3)$$

are the mean and covariance of $\mathbf{x}$. Therefore, the mean and covariance of $\mathbf{z}$ would be:

$$\bar{\mathbf{z}} = \frac{1}{N} \sum_{j=1}^{N} \mathbf{z}_j \text{ and } \Sigma_\mathbf{z} = \frac{1}{N} \sum_{i=1}^{N} (\mathbf{z}_i - \bar{\mathbf{z}})(\mathbf{z}_i - \bar{\mathbf{z}})^T = \mathbf{M}\Sigma_\mathbf{x}\mathbf{M}^T \qquad (15.4)$$

If the linear transformation $\mathbf{M}$ is chosen to be orthogonal, i.e., $\mathbf{M}^{-1} = \mathbf{M}^T$, and is selected to be the eigenvectors of the symmetric matrix $\Sigma_\mathbf{x}$, this would make $\Sigma_\mathbf{z}$ a diagonal matrix of the eigenvalues of $\Sigma_\mathbf{x}$. The eigenvectors corresponding to the small eigenvalues can be eliminated, which provides the desired reduction. Therefore, $\mathbf{x}$ may be expressed as:

$$\mathbf{x} = \bar{\mathbf{x}} + \mathbf{Pb} \qquad (15.5)$$

where $\mathbf{P} = (\mathbf{p}_1|\mathbf{p}_2|\ldots|\mathbf{p}_m)$ is the matrix of m largest eigenvectors of $\Sigma_\mathbf{x}$ and $\mathbf{b}$ is the $m \times 1$ vector given by

$$\mathbf{b} = \mathbf{P}^T(\mathbf{x} - \bar{\mathbf{x}})$$

The equation in (15.5) is the statistical shape model which is derived using PCA.

By varying the elements of $\mathbf{b}$ one can vary the synthesized shape $\mathbf{x}$ in Eq. (15.5). The variance of the ith parameter $b_i \in \mathbf{b}$ can be shown across the training set to be equal to the eigenvalue λ_i [15.5]. The distribution of the PCA reduction is optimal if the training shapes have a Gaussian distribution – the *modes* of the $b_i \in \mathbf{b}$ may be limited to within three times the standard deviation; i.e., $\pm 3\sqrt{\lambda_i}$, which will provide an adequate synthesized shape model. Of course, not all of these modes may be needed to generate a synthesized shape model; depending on the complexity of the shape ensemble at hand, a few modes may be enough. An adequate number of modes may be selected either by visual inspection or by SSD error measure. The fact that the generated (synthesized) shape is mode-dependent makes it deformable.

Example 15.2 This example will demonstrate how to generate the shape model in Eq. (15.5) from the resulting aligned shapes in Example 15.1, as shown in Figure 15.3b. Pseudocode 15.2 summarizes the discussion in Section 15.1.1 and is implemented in MATLAB in Code 15.1.2., The resulting shape model is $\mathbf{x} = \bar{\mathbf{x}} + \mathbf{P}\,\mathbf{b}$, where

$$\bar{\mathbf{x}} = (0.91, 1.18, 1.91, 1.23, 3.22, 1.54)^T \text{ and } P = \begin{bmatrix} -0.53 & 0.35 \\ 0.22 & 0.30 \\ 0.31 & -0.65 \\ -0.30 & -0.47 \\ -0.32 & 0.11 \\ 0.62 & 0.36 \end{bmatrix}$$

---

assuming that the first two modes are chosen. Note that the matrix $\mathbf{P}$ is related to the eigenvectors from the eigenvalue analysis performed within the PCA framework.

15.2.2 Fitting a model to new points

Given the shape model (15.5) constructed from the previous section, an instance of this model is described by the shape parameters b, together with the transformation from the model coordinate frame to the input image frame. A model instance $\mathbf{x}$ can then be represented as

$$\mathbf{x} = T_{X_t, Y_t, s, \theta}(\bar{\mathbf{x}} + \mathbf{P}\,\mathbf{b}) \tag{15.6}$$

where $T_{X_t, Y_t, s, \theta}$ performs rotation, translation, and scaling.

Suppose it is necessary to find the best pose (X_t, Y_t, s, θ) and shape parameters $\mathbf{b}$ to match the model instance $\mathbf{x}$ to a novel shape $\mathbf{Y}$ in the image domain; this problem is equivalent to minimizing the expression

$$|\mathbf{Y} - T_{X_t, Y_t, s, \theta}(\bar{\mathbf{x}} + \mathbf{P}\,\mathbf{b})|^2 \tag{15.7}$$

A simple iterative approach can solve this, illustrated in Pseudocode 15.1.3 and Example 15.3.

Example 15.3 Suppose there is a novel input shape, shown in Figure 15.4, which needs to be described by the generated shape model from the previous examples. Code 15.1.3 provides a code snippet in MATLAB to do this task. Note that in Code 15.1.3, steps (2)–(5) are performed by the MATLAB function procrustes. The solved shape

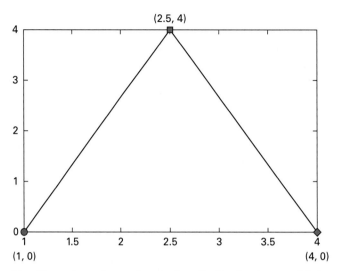

Figure 15.4 Novel input shape that needs to be described by the shape model derived from Example 14.2.

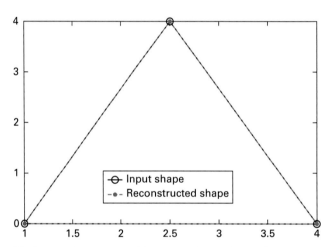

Figure 15.5 The input and reconstructed shape superimposed on each other. Note the close reconstruction of the input shape by the statistical shape model.

parameters, for each iteration, are constrained to within $\pm 3\sqrt{\lambda_i}$ as discussed in Section 15.1.1. Figure 15.5 shows the reconstructed shape from the statistical shape model, superimposed with the original input shape.

15.2.3 Statistical modeling of structures

A major application that may greatly benefit from an image, shape or volume registration model consists of building compact representations of anatomical structures from a set of

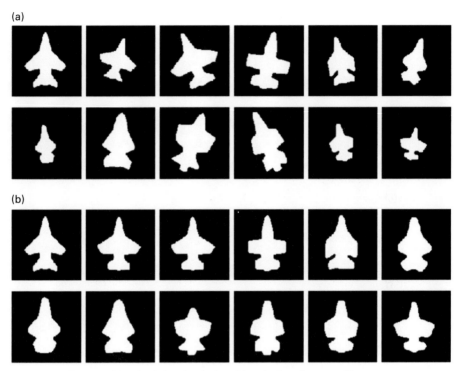

Figure 15.6 Twelve 2D shape models of a fighter jet, before (a) and after alignment (b).

training samples, where redundancies are reduced using statistical analysis methods such as PCA. The alignment process allows one to capture shape variations in the databases without interference from pose variations. As an example, we show the statistical modeling of two different shapes: a fighter jet and the number four (e.g., [15.13]). Training sets consisting of 12 binary representations of these two shapes are presented in Figures 15.6 and 15.7 respectively. The global registration approach discussed in the previous chapter is first applied to align the shapes in each training set. To this end, the first shape within each database is chosen as reference. The alignment results are shown in Figures 15.6b and 15.7b.

To qualitatively assess the accuracy of the alignment results, the overlap images before and after alignment for each of these shapes are shown in Figure 15.8 for both the fighter jets and the digit 4 databases. These overlap images are generated by stacking all the binary images within each group and adding them together pixel by pixel. The clear increase in overlap between after alignment illustrates the effectiveness of the process.

Quantitatively, the correlation coefficient is computed as a measure of similarity between these shapes before and after alignment. This measure is given by:

$$\gamma = \frac{E[(\Phi_1 - \mu_1)(\Phi_2 - \mu_2)]}{\sigma_1 \sigma_2}, \tag{15.8}$$

where, Φ_1 and Φ_2 are the implicit representations of the input shapes to be compared, and μ_i and σ_i denote the mean and standard deviations of each of these representations over the

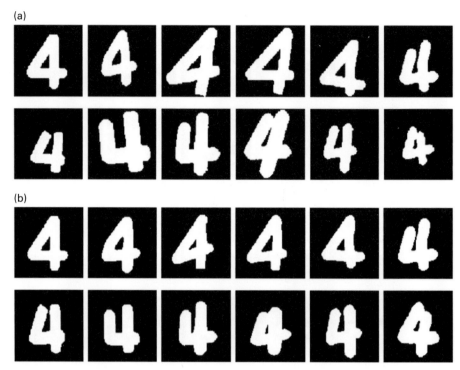

Figure 15.7 Twelve 2D shape models of the number 4 before (a) and after (b) alignment.

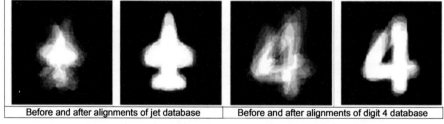

Figure 15.8 Superposition of shapes before and after alignment to show effect of global registration on the fighter jet and digit 4 databases.

image domain occupied by the shapes. Finally, $E(\cdot)$ stands for the mathematical expectation. The closer the correlation coefficient is to 1, the closer are the two shapes to each other. For each database, the correlation coefficients before and after alignments are plotted and shown in Figure 15.9a–b. Note how the proposed registration algorithm leads to accurate alignments.

15.2.4 Modeling shape variations

As we indicated before, shapes may be represented in various forms, including the outer contour of the object, its center line or medial axis, its Fourier descriptors, and the sign square distance. In this section, we use the shape representation using the sign square distance, and

15.2 Statistical shape models

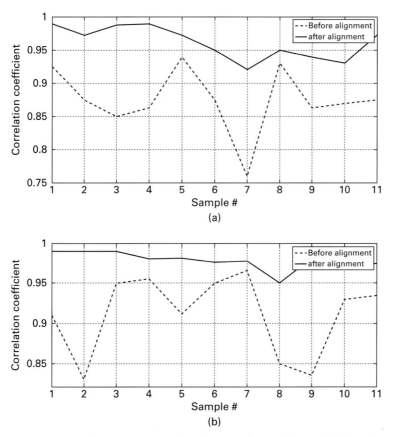

Figure 15.9 Correlation coefficients before and after alignments for the fighter jet database (a) and the number 4 database (b). Note that the sample number runs from 2 to 12 for each database.

apply global alignment of multiple shapes using the PCA approach which is at the heart of various rigid registration approaches as indicated before. We assume the availability of a training set (also denoted by realizations or database) of a particular object. For each training data set, let $\Psi_1, \Psi_2, \ldots, \Psi_N$ denote the signed distance representations of the N aligned shapes. These representation form a distribution in the Nd-dimensional space in which they reside, where $d = r \times c$ is the size of the image domain occupied by each shape. Modeling this distribution allows one to generate new and plausible shapes "similar" to those in the original training set. The PCA reduces the dimensionality of the data by computing the main axes of the cloud of points represented by each point in the training set. By convention, the first principal component accounts for as much of the variability in the data as possible. As discussed before, the PCA approach can be summarized in the following steps:

1. Compute the mean of the data

$$\overline{\Phi} = \frac{1}{N} \sum_{i=1}^{N} \Psi_i. \tag{15.9}$$

2. Compute the mean offsets, $\widetilde{\Psi}_i$, to capture the shape variabilities

$$\widetilde{\Psi} = \Psi_i - \overline{\Phi}. \tag{15.10}$$

3. Represent each mean-offset, $\widetilde{\Psi}_i$, as a column vector, $\widetilde{\psi}_i$, by stocking its column vectors on top of one another (recall that $\widetilde{\Psi}_i$ are 2D matrices of size $d = r \times c$). Then form the shape variability matrix as follows:

$$S = [\widetilde{\psi}_1 \widetilde{\psi}_2 \ldots \widetilde{\psi}_N]. \tag{15.11}$$

Note that S is of size $d \times N$.

4. Perform an eigenvalue decomposition to factor the following covariance matrix of the data

$$\frac{1}{N} SS^T = U\Sigma U^T, \tag{15.12}$$

where U is an $d \times N$ matrix whose columns are the d orthogonal modes of variations in the shape, and Σ is an $d \times d$ diagonal matrix whose entries are the corresponding eigenvalues.

We note that the ith principal mode, also known as the ith eigenshape and denoted by Y_i, can be determined by rearranging the column vectors of the matrix U back into the structure of a r-by-c rectangular grid. A maximum of N such eigenshapes are then generated, and will be denoted $\Phi_1, \Phi_2, \cdots, \Phi_N$. From a computational view point, the eigenvalues and eigenvectors of the covariance matrix $\frac{1}{N} SS^T$ can be efficiently computed from the following smaller matrix of size $N \times N$

$$T = \frac{1}{N} S^T S. \tag{15.13}$$

One can easily show that if X_i is an eigenvector of T corresponding to the eigenvalue λ_i, then $Y_i = SX_i$ is an eigenvector of $\frac{1}{N} SS^T$ associated with the same eigenvalue λ_i. Indeed,

$$\begin{aligned}\frac{1}{N} SS^T Y_i &= \frac{1}{N} SS^T (SX_i) \\ &= S\left(\frac{1}{N} S^T SX_i\right) \\ &= S(\lambda_i X_i) = \lambda_i SX_i \\ &= \lambda Y_i\end{aligned} \tag{15.14}$$

We note the following with respect to the PCA approach:

(a) The eigenvector associated with the largest eigenvalue has the same direction as the first principal component; the eigenvector associated with the second largest eigenvalue determines the direction of the second principal component and so forth.

(b) Each eigenvalue λ_i reflects the amount of variance of shape variability associated with the corresponding eigenshape.

(c) The number of models, k, to be used to capture the prominent shape variations present in the training set can be chosen in different ways. The most common way of choosing k is as follows. Let $\vartheta_T = \sum_i \lambda_i$ denote the total variance of the data about the mean shape in the direction of the corresponding eigenshapes. Then, if one wishes to retain a proportion, p_v, of the total variance ϑ_T, the number k can be chosen such that

$$\sum_i^k \lambda_i \geq p_v.\vartheta_T. \tag{15.15}$$

(d) Once the number of modes to be retained for the shape representation has been decided, new shapes can be generated. The signed distance representation of such a shape is expressed as:

$$\Phi(\mathbf{x}) = \overline{\Phi(\mathbf{x})} + \sum_{i=1}^{k} \omega_i \Phi_i(\mathbf{x}), \tag{15.16}$$

where $\mathbf{w} = (\omega_i)_i$ is the weight vector.

(e) By varying the elements of $\mathbf{w}$, various instances of the model represented by the training shapes can be generated. This can be seen in Figures 15.10 and 15.11, where three modes are shown with a variation from $-2\sqrt{\lambda_i}$ to $2\sqrt{\lambda_i}$.

To illustrate the encoding of the shape variability for both data sets, Figures 15.10 and 15.11 show the mean shape and its shape variations based on varying the first four principal modes from $-2\sqrt{\lambda_i}$ to $-2\sqrt{\lambda_i}$ for $i = 1,\ldots, 4$ for the fighter jet and the number 4 data sets respectively. One can see that the model captures the variations in each training set very well, and new plausible shapes similar to the ones in the training sets are generated. This is due mainly to the effectiveness of the proposed registration model.

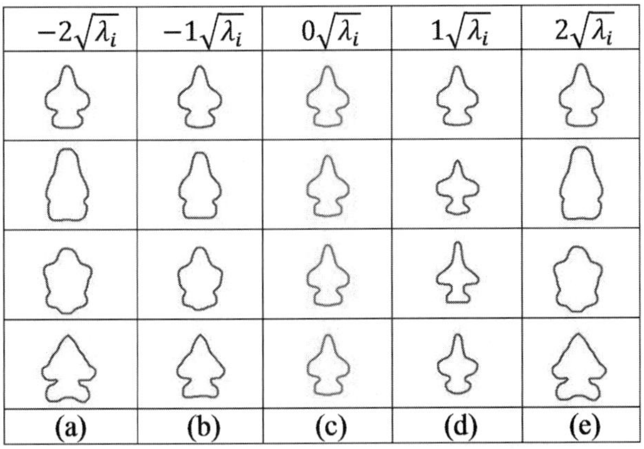

Figure 15.10 Illustration of shape variabilities in the fighter jet data base. The first four modes are shown from top to bottom, with respect to the average shape shown in the middle column. For each row, from left to right the mode changes from $-2\sqrt{\lambda_i}$ to $-2\sqrt{\lambda_i}$.

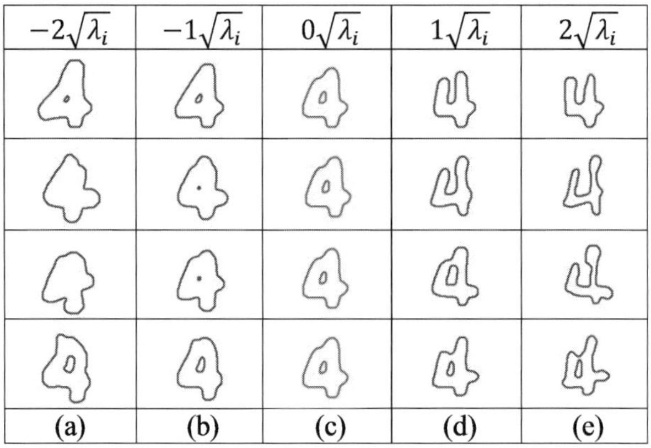

$-2\sqrt{\lambda_i}$	$-1\sqrt{\lambda_i}$	$0\sqrt{\lambda_i}$	$1\sqrt{\lambda_i}$	$2\sqrt{\lambda_i}$
⌀	⌀	⌀	⌀	⌀
⌀	⌀	⌀	⌀	⌀
⌀	⌀	⌀	⌀	⌀
⌀	⌀	⌀	⌀	⌀
(a)	(b)	(c)	(d)	(e)

Figure 15.11 Illustration of the shape variabilities in the number four data base. The first four modes are shown from top to bottom w.r.t. to the average shape shown in the middle column. From left to right the mode changes from $-2\sqrt{\lambda_i}$ to $-2\sqrt{\lambda_i}$.

15.3 Statistical appearance models

To synthesize a meaningful instance of an object in an image or volume, it is necessary to model both its shape and its texture. Texture can be defined as the pattern of intensity or color across the region of the object [15.6]. In the previous section, it was discussed how to generate a statistical shape model. This section will focus on the construction of the statistical appearance model.

It is necessary to have a training set of labeled images, similar to Figure 15.1, where crucial landmarks are marked on each training sample. The next step is to generate a statistical shape model, as discussed in the previous section. Each training example will then be warped to the mean shape, from the statistical model, to come up with a *shape-free* patch. PCA will then be used to generate the statistical appearance model.

15.3.1 Image warping

A crucial step in constructing the appearance model is to warp the training image to the mean shape. This can be achieved by a variety of approaches, e.g., piecewise affine warping [15.6] or thin-plate splines warping [15.7]. This section will focus on the thin-plate splines approach owing to its simplicity of implementation, with warp parameters solved through a series of matrix operations.

To warp an image **I** such that the set of control points $\{x_i\}$ are mapped to new positions, $\{x'_i\}$, a continuous vector-valued mapping function, f, is needed such that

$$f(x_i) = x'_i \tag{15.17}$$

To avoid holes and interpolation problems in reality, it is practical to find the reverse mapping function, f', that maps $\{x'_i\}$ to $\{x_i\}$. In this section, $\{x_i\}$ refers to the landmark points in the training image and $\{x'_i\}$ refers to the mean shape. For each pixel in the

15.3 Statistical appearance models

shape-free warped image, I', it is possible to determine where it corresponds to in the original training image I through the reverse map f' and fill it in with the corresponding pixel.

15.3.2 One-dimensional thin-plate splines

In the 1D case, let $(r) = r^2 \log(r^2)$; then the 1D thin-plate spline is

$$f_{1D}(x) = \sum_{i=1}^{n} w_i U(\|x - x_i\|) + a_0 + a_1 x \qquad (15.18)$$

where $\|\cdot\|$ refers to the Euclidean L_2 norm. The weights (w_i, a_0, a_1) are chosen such that $f_{1D}(x_i) = x'_i$. To simplify notation, let $\boldsymbol{u}_1 = (U(\|x-x_1\|), \cdots, U(\|x-x_n\|), 1, x)^T$ and $\boldsymbol{w}_1 = (w_1, \cdots, w_n, a_0, a_1)$; then (15.18) becomes

$$f_{1D}(x) = \boldsymbol{w}_1^T \boldsymbol{u}_{1D} \qquad (15.19)$$

Using all pairs of corresponding landmark points $\{x'_i\}$ and $\{x_i\}$, there will be n linear equations of the form

$$x'_j = \sum_{i=1}^{n} w_i U(x_j - x_i) + a_0 + a_1 x_j \qquad (15.20)$$

The terms U_{ij} and U_{ji} are symmetric, i.e., $U_{ij} = U_{ji} = U(\|x_j - x_i\|)$. Let $\boldsymbol{K}$ be a $n \times n$ matrix whose elements are $\{U_{ij}\}$. Define additional matrices $\boldsymbol{Q}_1$ and $\boldsymbol{L}_1$ to be

$$\boldsymbol{Q}_1 = \begin{bmatrix} 1 & x_1 \\ 1 & x_2 \\ \vdots & \vdots \\ 1 & x_n \end{bmatrix}, \quad \boldsymbol{L}_1 = \begin{bmatrix} \boldsymbol{K} & \boldsymbol{Q}_1 \\ \boldsymbol{Q}_1^T & 0_{2 \times 2} \end{bmatrix} \qquad (15.21)$$

where $0_{2 \times 2}$ is a 2×2 zero matrix. Let $\boldsymbol{X}'_i = (x'_1, \ldots, x'_n, 0, 0)^T$. The last rows of $\boldsymbol{L}_1$ are included to ensure that the coefficients (w_i) sum is zero and that its cross-product with the control points $\{x_i\}$ is zero. The weights for the 1D spline, $\boldsymbol{w}_1 = (w_1, \cdots, w_n, a_0, a_1)$, can be solved from the linear equation

$$\boldsymbol{L}_1 \boldsymbol{w}_1 = \boldsymbol{X}'_1 \qquad (15.22)$$

15.3.3 N-dimensional thin-plate splines

It is straightforward to extend the 1D thin-plate splines into the n-dimensional case. In place of $\boldsymbol{u}_1$, the n-dimensional analog is $\boldsymbol{u}_d(\boldsymbol{x}) = (U(\|\boldsymbol{x} - \boldsymbol{x}_1\|), \cdots, U(\|\boldsymbol{x} - \boldsymbol{x}_n\|), 1 | \boldsymbol{x}^T)^T$. The thin-plate spline for this case is

$$f(\boldsymbol{x}) = \boldsymbol{W} \boldsymbol{u}_d(\boldsymbol{x}) \qquad (15.23)$$

where w is a $d \times (n + d + 1)$ matrix. The matrices Q_d and L_d are

$$Q_1 = \begin{bmatrix} 1 & x_1^T \\ 1 & x_2^T \\ \vdots & \vdots \\ 1 & x_n^T \end{bmatrix}, \quad L_1 = \begin{bmatrix} K & Q_d \\ Q_d^T & 0_{d+1} \end{bmatrix} \quad (15.24)$$

where 0_{d+1} is a 2×2 zero matrix. The equivalent of X'_1 from the previous section is the $(n + d + 1) \times d$ matrix

$$X'_d = \begin{bmatrix} x'_1 \\ \vdots \\ x'_n \\ 0_d \\ \vdots \\ 0_d \end{bmatrix} \quad (15.25)$$

The matrix of weights can be solved, via pseudo-inverse, through the linear equation

$$L_d^T W_d^T = X'_d \quad (15.26)$$

Example 15.4 This example will illustrate how to use the thin-plate spines algorithm to perform image warping. Figures 15.12a and 15.12b show the source and target image frames, respectively. The goal is to warp the source image to the target image using the indicated control points (landmarks). From the above discussion, the first step is to get the warp parameters from the target image to the source image. Code 15.2.1 contains the MATLAB code to obtain the warp parameters. The solved parameters are then used to

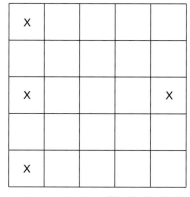

Figure 15.12 Image warping example. (a) Source image with control points, $\{(1, 1), (3, 3), (1, 5), (5, 3)\}$ and (b) target image frame with landmarks, $\{(1, 1), (1, 3), (1, 5), (5, 3)\}$.

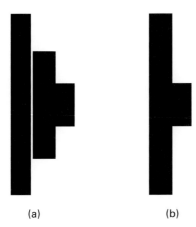

Figure 15.13 Image warping example. (a) Source image and (b) target image after image warping.

reconstruct the target control points (Line 21 of Code 15.2.1) to see if they are superimposed to the source control points after the application of warp parameters.

After solving for the warp parameters, Code 15.2.2 will do the actual image warping from the source image to the target image using the MATLAB function *interp*. Figure 15.13a is the original source image and Figure 15.13b is the image warped to the target frame.

15.3.4 Statistical appearance model construction using PCA

To create a statistical model of appearance, it is necessary to warp each training image such that its landmarks match that of the mean shape. The previous section on thin-plate spines warping can be used in this process. This step is needed to eliminate texture variation due to shape differences that would affect the construction of the statistical appearance model. Figure 15.14 illustrates an example of a facial image warped to its mean shape, creating a shape-free patch.

Before creating the statistical appearance model, it may be helpful to perform global illumination normalization on each training shape-free patch. The most common approach is to apply scaling and offset values such that the mean of the resulting image vector is zero and that its variance is unity, i.e.,

$$g = \frac{g - \mu}{\sigma} \tag{15.27}$$

The next step is to construct the actual statistical appearance model. The method outlined in Section 15.2.1 may work well with shape vectors with relatively small numbers of elements but may cause problems with large image vectors, owing to the formation of extremely huge covariance matrices. To illustrate this point, consider training images of size 64×64. This leads to a data matrix of size $4096 \times m$, where m is the number of

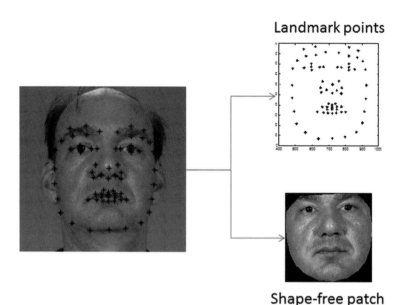

Figure 15.14 A training facial image from the FRGC database sample split into two components: (a) shape from landmark points and (b) shape-free patch obtained by warping the training image to the mean shape from the statistical shape model.

training images, and a covariance matrix of size 4096 × 4096. Performing eigenvalue analysis on covariance matrices of this size is computationally expensive. To overcome this problem, Turk and Pentland [15.8] used the snapshot method of eigenspace projection, which performs eigenvalue analysis on the smaller matrix, $X^T X$, where X is the data matrix. The snapshot method is justified by the following manipulations of the classical equations for eigenvalue decomposition.

Consider the eigenvectors v_i of $X^T X$ such that $X^T X v_i = \lambda_i v_i$. Multiplying both sides of the equation with X, we have $XX^T(Xv_i) = \lambda_i(Xv_i)$, where we can infer that the eigenvectors of $C = XX^T$ are the eigenvectors v_i of $X^T X$ but transformed by X, i.e., Xv_i. Therefore, we can perform eigenvalue analysis on the smaller matrix $X^T X$ and just multiply the resulting eigenvectors with the data matrix X to obtain the equivalent eigenvectors from the bigger covariance matrix, $C = XX^T$. After obtaining the eigenvectors, the constructed statistical appearance model has the form of

$$\mathbf{g} = \bar{\mathbf{g}} + \mathbf{P_g}\, \mathbf{b_g} \qquad (15.28)$$

where P_g refers to the texture eigenvectors, $\bar{g}$ is the mean texture vector and $\mathbf{b_g}$ are the texture parameters.

Example 15.5 This example will illustrate how to generate a statistical appearance model from four training images, assuming that the preliminary image warping steps have already been performed. Figure 15.15 shows the four training images, corresponding to pixelated versions of the digits 1, 2, 4 and 0. Code 15.6 lists the MATLAB code to do this

250	3	230		5	3	25		21	249	10		2	7	6
245	10	253		240	15	235		11	8	9		14	255	19
252	30	249		8	8	9		255	220	6		7	7	10

Figure 15.15 Four training images corresponding to pixelated versions of the digits 1, 2, 4, and 0.

task. The first part of the code uses the original approach to get the appearance model while the later parts of the code use the snapshot approach to obtain the model. Both methods give the same results and the statistical appearance model is of the form $\mathbf{g} = \bar{\mathbf{g}} + \mathbf{P_g}\,\mathbf{b_g}$, where

$$\bar{\mathbf{g}} = \begin{bmatrix} 69.5 \\ 127.5 \\ 130.5 \\ 65.5 \\ 72.0 \\ 66.25 \\ 67.75 \\ 129.0 \\ 68.5 \end{bmatrix}, \quad \mathbf{P_g} = \begin{bmatrix} -0.40 & -0.15 & -0.33 \\ -0.43 & 0.18 & 0.38 \\ -0.19 & -0.61 & -0.15 \\ 0.22 & -0.49 & 0.18 \\ 0.24 & 0.31 & -0.60 \\ 0.15 & -0.44 & 0.14 \\ -0.37 & -0.09 & -0.26 \\ -0.44 & 0.18 & 0.34 \\ -0.40 & -0.11 & -0.35 \end{bmatrix}$$

15.3.5 Combined appearance models

One may combine the ASM and AAM equations above. Let $\mathbf{b}_s$ (Eq. 15.6) and $\mathbf{b}_g$ represent the shape and intensity vectors. The two representations may be concatenated as follows:

$$\mathbf{b} = \begin{pmatrix} \mathbf{W}_s\mathbf{b}_s \\ \mathbf{b}_g \end{pmatrix} = \begin{pmatrix} \mathbf{W}_s{\mathbf{P}_s}^T(x - \bar{\mathbf{x}}) \\ {\mathbf{P}_g}^T(g - \bar{\mathbf{g}}) \end{pmatrix}. \tag{15.29}$$

where $\mathbf{W}_s$ is a diagonal matrix of weights for each shape parameters, allowing for the difference in units between the shape and intensity models [15.6]. Further application of PCA on the concatenated representation may reduce the redundancies. The results would be the following model:

$$\mathbf{b} = \mathbf{Qc} \tag{15.30}$$

where $\mathbf{Q}$ are the eigenvectors and $\mathbf{c}$ the vector of appearance parameters controlling both the shape and intensity of the model [15.6]. The shape and intensity models can still be expressed, i.e.,

$$\mathbf{x} = \bar{\mathbf{x}} + \mathbf{P}_s \mathbf{W}_s \mathbf{Q}_s \mathbf{c} \ , \quad \mathbf{g} = \bar{\mathbf{g}} + \mathbf{P}_g \mathbf{Q}_g \mathbf{c} \tag{15.31}$$

where

$$\mathbf{Q} = \begin{pmatrix} \mathbf{Q}_s \\ \mathbf{Q}_g \end{pmatrix} \tag{15.32}$$

The above representation can be used to synthesize an image for a given appearance parameters **c** by generating the shape-free intensity image vector g and warping it using the features or control points described by **x**.

Example 15.6 This example shows how to build an active appearance model for representing the vertebrae. Figure 15.16 shows an ensemble of vertebral bodies, which constitute the training set for building active appearance models. Figure 15.17

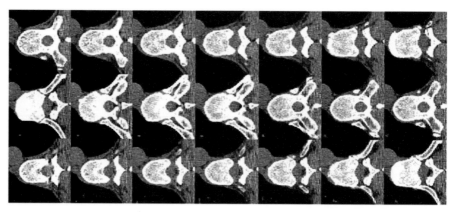

Figure 15.16 Training images of the human vertebrae. Statistical shape and appearance models will be built using these images.

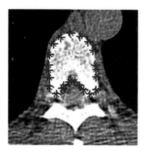 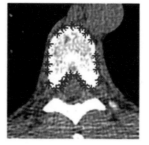 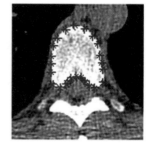

Figure 15.17 Sample annotations of the data in Figure 15.10. The annotated points represent the shape of the object and determine the region of interest for texture information on the object.

15.3 Statistical appearance models

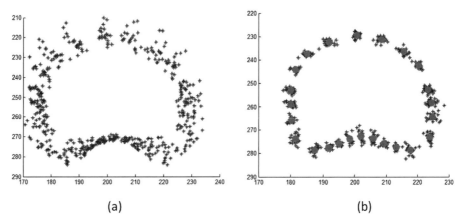

Figure 15.18 Scatter plot of training shapes (a) before and (b) after alignment using generalized Procrustes analysis (GPA). A color version of this figure is available online at www.cambridgeorg/farag. The red circles in (b) refer to the computed mean shape.

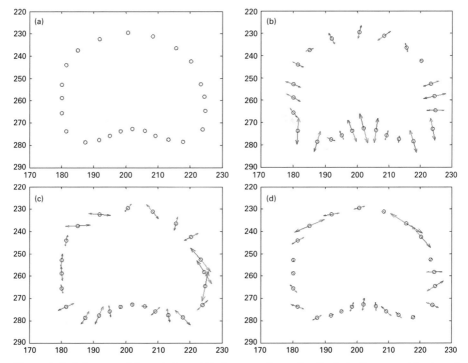

Figure 15.19 The statistical shape model consisting of (a) the mean shape plus (b–d) the linear combination of n shape eigenvectors, visualized as quiver plots superimposed on the mean shape.

shows some annotated vertebral bodies marking their outside contours. Figure 15.18 shows the scatter plot of the vertebral shapes as represented by their contours. Figure 15.18a is unaligned shapes and Figure 15.18b is the aligned shapes by global registration. Figure 15.19 shows the results of the shape modeling process described

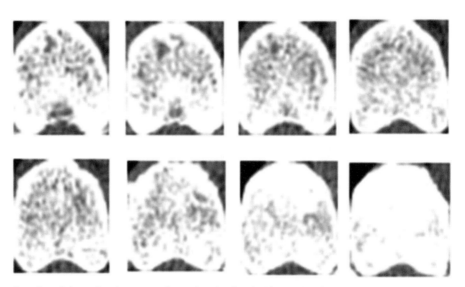

Figure 15.20 Samples of shape-free image patches using the data in Figure 15.16.

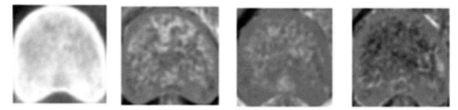

Figure 15.21 Statistical appearance model consisting of the (a) mean image plus the linear combination of n (b–d) image eigenvectors, visualized as 2D images.

before. Finally, Figures 15.20 and 15.21 show the results of the appearance-only modeling of the vertebral bodies. Aslan *et al.* [15.14] used the active appearance modeling to generate shape priors for statistical-based segmentation of the vertebral bodies. Aslan [15.15] has detailed analysis and algorithmic evaluations of AAM methods as applied to analysis of the vertebral bodies from low-resolution CT imaging. These techniques may be applicable to analysis of bone diseases and calcium absorption.

15.4 Analysis of lung nodules in low-dose CT (LDCT) scans

We provide another example for the effectiveness of the active appearance approaches for small-size random objects. These objects are hard to identify from their contours or their salient features. The most notable examples of such objects are small-size nodules

15.4 Analysis of lung nodules in low-dose CT (LDCT) scans

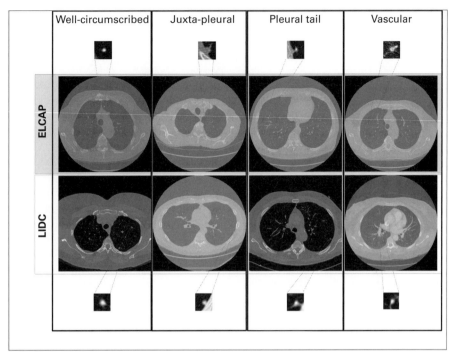

Figure 15.22 Examples of lung nodules of size below 10 mm from the ELCAP and LIDC clinical studies. The upper and lower rows show zoomed pictures of the nodules.

that appear in low-dose CT (LDCT) scans. The treatment below is based on the work of Farag et al. [15.19][15.20]. Farag [15.21] has theoretical and algorithmic details of modeling small-size objects under uncertainty.

15.4.1 Lung nodules in low-dose CT

Figure 15.22 shows examples of small-size nodules (≤ 1 cm) from four categories of nodules: well-circumscribed, juxta-pleural, pleural tail, and vascular nodules, according to the categorization of Kostis et al. [15.16]. These nodules are obtained from two clinical studies, the ELCAP and LIDC [15.17][15.18]. Notice the ambiguities associated with shape definition, location in the lung tissues, and lack of crisp discriminatory features.

Another difficulty with small nodules lies in the lack of exact boundary definition. For example, radiologists may differ in outlining the lung nodules' spatial area as shown in Figure 15.23. Difference in manual annotation is common for small objects that have no well-defined description. This adds another dimension of difficulty to automatic approaches, as they are supposed to provide outputs that mimic human experts. In other words, if human experts differ among themselves, how would they judge a computer output?

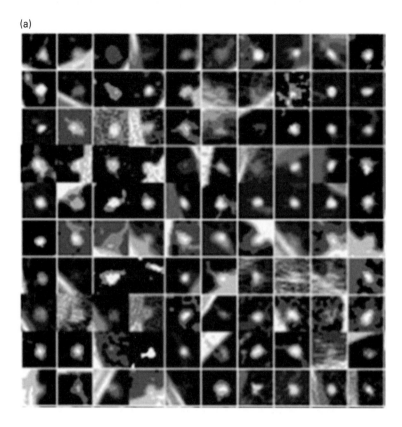

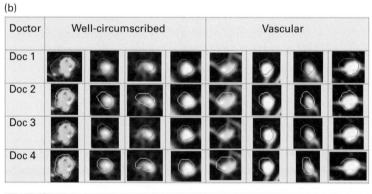

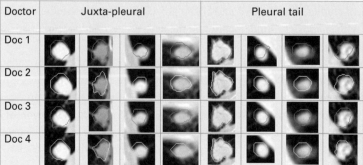

Figure 15.23 (a) An ensemble of small-sized lung nodules, less than 1 cm diameter, from the LIDC clinical study. (b) Manual annotation of the main portion of the spatial support of lung nodules by four radiologists from the LIDC study [15.18].

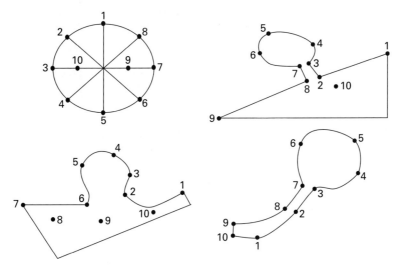

Figure 15.24 Definition of control points (landmarks) for well-circumscribed nodules (top left), pleural-tail (top right), juxta-pleural (bottom left), and vascularized (bottom left).

Lung nodule modeling

In order to construct the active appearance or active tensor models, we need an annotated ensemble of objects. In the case of random objects, the annotation process becomes extremely difficult; it acquires yet another level of difficulty with small size. We used the fuzzy description of lung nodules from Kostis *et al.* [15.16] to devise a feature definition approach for the four categories of nodules mentioned above: *well-circumscribed*, *vascularized*, *juxta-pleural*, and *pleural-tail* nodules. Figure 15.24 illustrates the landmarks that correspond to the clinical definition of these four nodule categories. Using these definitions, we create a manual approach to annotate the nodules. First, we take the experts' annotation, zoom it, and manually register it to a template defining the nodule type/category, and then we select the control points on the actual nodule using the help of the template.

This annotation enables the creation of active appearance models (AAM), which mimic the physical characteristics of lung nodules that cannot be modeled otherwise. Figure 15.25 shows examples of nodule models generated by ensembles from the ELCAP and LIDC clinical lung screening studies. The average nodules capture the main features of real nodules. Details of this modeling process are in Farag *et al.* [15.19][15.20].

Nodule detection

The modeling approach above offers tremendous promise in three subsequent steps of lung nodule analysis: detection, segmentation, and categorization (e.g., Farag [15.22]). We briefly show the results of lung nodule detection using AAM nodule models. We report only a basic detection approach that is based on template matching with normalized cross-correlation (NCC) as similarity measure, defined as follows:

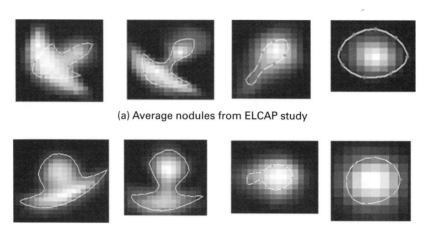

(a) Average nodules from ELCAP study

(b) Average nodule from LIDC study

Figure 15.25 Average nodules from co-registration of 24 nodules per nodule type. (a) ELCAP nodules, (b) LIDC nodules. The models possess the physical characteristics of real nodules.

$$\text{NCC} = \frac{\sum_{(i,j)\in W} I_t(i,j) * I_i(x+i, y+j)}{\sqrt[2]{\sum_{(i,j)\in W} I_t^2(i,j) * \sum_{(i,j)\in W} I_i^2(x+i, y+j)}} \quad (15.33)$$

where $I_t(i,j)$ represents the template, $I_i(x,y)$ is the image slice or input image, W is the region of interest on which the similarity measure is evaluated, $\overline{I_t}(.)$ is the mean of the template image, and $\overline{I_i}(.)$ is the mean of the input image slice. Farag [15.22] examined nine similarity measures for nodule detection, and discussed various issues related to nodule detection, segmentation, and categorization. In Figure 15.26 we show the outcome of the nodule detection process through construction of the classical receiver operating characteristics (ROC) curve, showing the overall *sensitivity* and (1 – *specificity*) of the detection process. These parameters are defined as follows:

$$\text{Sensitivity} = \frac{\text{True positives}}{\text{True positives} + \text{false negatives}} \quad (15.34)$$

$$\text{Specificity} = \frac{\text{True negatives}}{\text{True negatives} + \text{false positives}} \quad (15.35)$$

For comparison purposes, we show the results of the AAM-based nodules vs. parametric nodules (e.g., circular, semicircular), in Figure 15.26. Details of the design process of these nodules and more results are given in Farag et al. [15.19] to [15.20]. The results show that the AAM models provided better detection results than the parametric models. In generating these ROCs, we used the mean in the AAM models as the nodule template.

This example illustrates the process of nodule annotation and the steps to create AAM nodule models. The models resemble the real nodules, and provide a huge advantage for

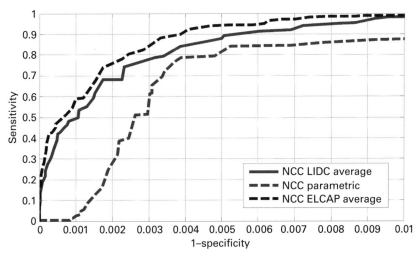

Figure 15.26 ROC curves for nodule detection on the ELCAP and LIDC databases, using AAM-based nodule models versus the parametric models.

nodule detection, segmentation, and categorization over the non-realistic parametric models used before (e.g., Lee *et al.* [15.22]). Nodule models based on the AAM approach offer two further improvements over the parametric approaches: they can automate the processes of nodule segmentation and categorization (e.g., Farag [15.21]).

15.5 Appearance-based approach for complete human jaw reconstruction

There has been a long-standing effort to construct models of the human jaw using non-ionizing radiation. Starting from a series of images obtained by an intraoral camera, we have employed a number of methods to extract the shape of the human jaw (e.g., [15.23]). As we have discussed in this chapter, we can use rigid registration methods to co-register shapes in various dimensions. In Chapter 13, we showed how to use image-based registration to co-register multiple images as well. In this example, we describe an approach, based on a single captured optical image combined with statistical shape recovery, which makes use of a small number of measured points, in order to construct a plausible 3D model of the jaw. The purpose is to show a complete example of the application of the methodologies described in this chapter and throughout the book. Figure 15.27 illustrates the components of the jaw reconstruction approach:

(a) An aligned ensemble of the shapes and albedos of human jaws is used to build 3D shape and albedo models. This is to be performed off-line in a direct application of methods in this chapter.

(b) Given the albedo and surface normals of a certain jaw in the ensemble, appearance bases are constructed. Spherical harmonics is used to compute the illumination spectrum of a database of environment maps while an approach based on

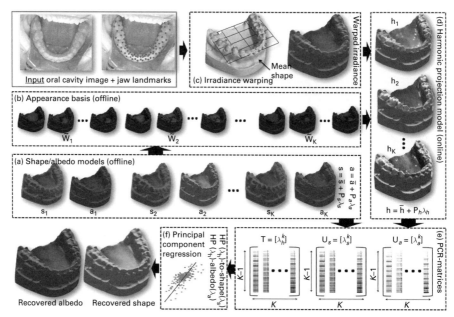

Figure 15.27 Block diagram of model-based human jaw shape recovery. (a) An aligned ensemble of the shapes and albedos of human jaws is used to build the 3D shape and albedo models. (b) Given the albedo and surface normals of a certain jaw in the ensemble, appearance bases are constructed. (c) Dense correspondence is established between the input irradiance and the mean jaw shape using 3D thin-plate splines. (d) The input image, in the reference frame, is projected onto the subspace spanned by the appearance basis of each jaw sample which are scaled and summed to construct the harmonic projection (HP) irradiance that encodes the illumination and reflectance conditions of the input image. Such images are then used to construct an HP model of the input image. The inherent relation between the HP irradiance and the corresponding shape and albedo is cast into a regression framework to recover the shape and albedo of the input image.

Helmholtz hemispherical harmonics (HSH) is used to compute the reflectance spectrum of a database of teeth reflectance [15.24].

We uniformly sample the roughness and the enamel's refractive index (1.62 ± 0.02) domain, following the work of Wang *et al.* [15.25]. Image irradiance harmonics are computed based on the visible surface normals of the object of interest and then sorted according to their average power content. The illumination and reflectance spectrum components are sorted accordingly to provide a single index-based notation. Now given an input oral cavity image, under general unknown illumination, and a set of human jaw anatomical landmark points, we proceed as follows:

(c) We establish dense correspondence between the input irradiance and the mean jaw shape using 3D thin-plate splines.
(d) The input image, in the reference frame, is projected onto the subspace spanned by the appearance basis of each jaw sample. These projections are scaled and summed

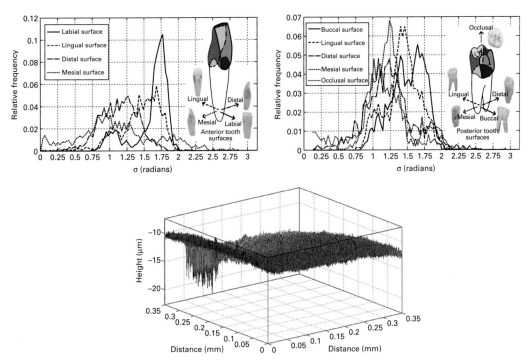

Figure 15.28 The roughness parameter is estimated by measurement of microscopic height variation of 0.35 mm^2 surface patches of different surface types for incisor and molar teeth (see left for a sample). According to the distribution, the parameter tends to lie between 0.7 and 2 radians regardless of the tooth surface type.

to construct the harmonic projection (HP) irradiance that encodes the illumination and reflectance conditions of the input image. Such images are then used to construct an HP model of the input image. The inherent relation between the HP irradiance and the corresponding shape and albedo is cast into a regression framework to recover the shape and albedo of the input image.

This example could be treated by direct application of statistical models to relate a given shape to basis functions obtained by PCA, as we did in previous examples. The example of a tooth in Figure 15.28, however, adds an angle on how to incorporate some of the recent approaches in facial information modeling into the application to the jaw. The theoretical foundation of this subject matter can be found in the work of Elhabian [15.26].

We used a 3D optical surface profiler (Zygo NewView 700s) to measure the height variations of different visible tooth surfaces over an area of 0.35 mm^2 using 10× optical zoom (see Figure 15.28). The average surface profiles provide a physical validation that the appearance of a tooth surface can be modeled using the microfacet-theory, which assumes that the surface consists of a large number of small flat facets. Microfacet reflectance models tend to be intuitive with tractable analytical expressions.

15.5.1 Jaw prior models

The model-based shape recovery in [15.27] involves the construction of three models, namely the shape, albedo (also referred to as texture), and appearance (net result of illumination and reflectance) models. While the first two models are constructed in an offline stage, the appearance model is constructed at runtime when an input image is presented to our shape recovery framework.

Shape model: full 3D

The jaw shape model is constructed from a training data ensemble of 3D triangular meshes where each mesh is obtained from a high-resolution CT scan of human jaw molds. We follow the work by Patel *et al.* [15.28] in obtaining dense correspondence between different jaw surfaces where a finite set of sparse landmark points are manually annotated for all the database samples. Generalized Procrustes analysis (GPA) [15.6] is then performed to provide an initial rigid alignment of the dense shapes to a common reference frame. The 3D thin-plate spline [15.7] is then applied in an iterative manner in order to obtain a dense correspondence between all shapes in the database. PCA is then performed on the set of shape vectors, where the resulting shape model can be written as $\mathbf{s} = \bar{\mathbf{s}} + \mathbf{P}_s \lambda_s$ where $\mathbf{P}_s = [\mathbf{s}_1, \mathbf{s}_2, \cdots]$ are the shape eigenvectors and λ_s is the set of shape coefficients.

Albedo model: color incorporated

Shadows due to non-convex jaw regions and non-uniform distribution of illumination inhibit using occlusal images as albedo. As such, we factor out the reflectance information (albedo) from the given texture using the intrinsic image decomposition proposed by Barron and Malik [15.29]. We use 3D thin-plate spline to provide a warping function between image pixels (assumed to be on the *xy*-plane in the 3D space) and surface points using image landmarks and surface landmarks as control points. Mapping ambiguities are resolved using a least-squares plane fit to the cervical landmark points. In order to incorporate color information, we use the Lab color space instead of the RGB one since the latter suffers from strong correlation among its color channels as well as non-linearity. PCA is then performed on the set of albedo vectors, where the resulting albedo model can be written as $\mathbf{a} = \bar{\mathbf{a}} + \mathbf{P}_a \lambda_a$ where $\mathbf{P}_a = [\mathbf{a}_1, \mathbf{a}_2, \cdots]$ are the albedo eigenvectors and λ_a is the set of albedo coefficients.

Harmonic projection (HP) model

While the shape model and the albedo model are constructed in a pre-processing (offline) step, the HP model is constructed when the input irradiance is given to our framework in order to incorporate the illumination and reflectance conditions of the given irradiance into the prior information. In order to handle specularity and non-convex regions presented in the input image, the pixel-corruption spatial support $\mathbf{f}_k$ for each computed HP image $\mathbf{h}_k$ is used to determine the overall error spatial support $\mathbf{f}$ where the projection coefficients $\hat{\mathbf{y}}_k$ are computed using non-corrupted pixels from both the input image and the appearance basis. The resulting HP model can be written as $\mathbf{h} = \bar{\mathbf{h}} + \mathbf{P}_h \lambda_h$ where $\mathbf{P}_h$ are the HP eigenvectors and λ_h is the set of HP coefficients.

15.5.2 Model-based shape and albedo recovery

Given a jaw occlusal image, we use its sparse landmarks to infer a warping function between image pixels and the vertices of the mean jaw shape $\bar{s}$ using a 3D thin-plate spline, where the landmarks are assumed to be located on the *xy*-plane in the 3D space. The cervical least-squares plane is then used to remove mapping ambiguity in a similar manner to that used in constructing the albedo model. When the light source and the viewer are far from the object compared with the object size, the image irradiance E from surface point x can be defined as the surface radiance being modulated by the surface albedo $\rho(x)$, i.e. $E(x) = \rho(x)\mathcal{R}(\vec{n}(x))$. The classical brightness constraint in SFS measures the total brightness of the reconstructed image irradiance compared with the input irradiance. It can be defined as:

$$\varepsilon = \int\int \left(E(\mathbf{x}) - \rho(\mathbf{x})\mathcal{R}(\vec{n}(x))\right)^2 d\mathbf{x} \tag{15.36}$$

where $\rho(\cdot)$ is the surface albedo at point $\mathbf{x}$ while $\mathcal{R}(\cdot)$ is the radiance of the surface patch with unit normal $\vec{n}(x) = cart(\alpha, \beta)$, also known as the *surface reflectance function* [15.30]. The brightness constraint in Eq. (15.36) can be rewritten in the discrete domain as a linear combination of pre-computed basis resulted from the harmonic expansion of the reflectance function. Thus the image intensity *xxx* can be expressed as:

$$E(\mathbf{x}) = \sum_{s=1}^{S} y_s \mathcal{W}_s(\vec{n}(x)) \tag{15.37}$$

where $\mathcal{W}_s$ is the sth column of $\widetilde{\mathbf{W}}$ and $\{y_s\}$ is the weighting vector which results from projecting E onto the subspace spanned by $\{\mathcal{W}_s\}$. In matrix notation, let $\mathbf{e} \in R^D$ be an image vector with D pixels, $\widetilde{\mathbf{W}} = [\mathcal{W}_1(\vec{n}(x)), \ldots, \mathcal{W}_S(\vec{n}(x))] \in R^{D \times S}$ be the subspace projection matrix having appearance basis as its columns, where S is the number of bases, and $\mathbf{y} \in R^S$ be a vector of irradiance coefficients. Hence the discrete version of the brightness constraint becomes:

$$\varepsilon = \sum_{\mathbf{x}} \left[E(\mathbf{x}) - \widetilde{\mathbf{W}}(\vec{n}(x))\mathbf{y}\right]^2 = \|\mathbf{e} - \widetilde{\mathbf{W}}\mathbf{y}\| \tag{15.38}$$

While Eq. (15.36) can be solved in an iterative manner to infer the underlying shape as in [15.31], the inherent relation between the HP irradiance $\mathbf{h}$ and the corresponding shape $\mathbf{s}$ and albedo $\mathbf{a}$ can be cast into a regression framework resulting into the HP-to-shape and HP-to-albedo models. In this case, the shape and albedo is solved for using a series of matrix operations guaranteeing faster shape recovery than its iterative counterpart. This was proven to yield comparable results in terms of reconstruction accuracy [15.32]. Building the regression models is now based on the K-set of shape/albedo/HP coefficients $\{\lambda_s^k, \lambda_a^k \text{ and } \lambda_h^k\} \, \forall k \in [1, K]$ instead of using the high-dimensional vectors $\{\mathbf{s}_k, \mathbf{a}_k \text{ and } \mathbf{h}_k\}$ where the HP coefficients are considered the independent variable while the shape and albedo coefficients are the dependent variables. We use principal component regression (PCR) [15.33] to avoid random noise which might exist in the dependent and independent variables. It also deals with the small-sample-size (SSS) problem where the ratio between observations and variables is usually low. Again, we refer to Figure 15.27 which shows the offline/online processes for the shape/albedo recovery approach.

15.5.3 Sample results

In this section, we show experiments to evaluate the performance of the proposed framework in recovery 3D models for human jaws. Upper jaw models are constructed from 52 upper jaw molds belonging to 33 males and 19 females, with average age 20 years old; lower jaw models are constructed from 58 lower jaw molds belonging to 33 males and 25 females, with average age 19 years old. There are two samples per subject, one *pre-repair* jaw and another *post-repair* jaw, referring to the jaw status before and after applying an orthodontic teeth alignment process, respectively. The statistical priors (shape, albedo and appearance models) are trained using out-of-training samples with pre- and post-repair instances using the oral cavity images and the CT-scan of the respective molds (lower and upper jaws).

In order to share the same metric coordinate frame, the average jaw shape $\bar{\mathbf{s}}$ (along with its anatomical landmarks) is used as a reference to establish a dense correspondence between the ground-truth CT scan of the jaw mold corresponding to each testing image and the reconstructed shape. The alignment proceeds as follows. Procrustes-based rigid registration is used to filter out translation, scale, and rotation, and is followed by 3D thin-plate splines for non-rigid registration. We assess the reconstruction accuracy using the RMS error between the 3D points from the CT scan and the corresponding reconstructed surface points. Note that errors are computed based on the surface points of the visible crowns, to exclude errors which might rise from the reconstruction of the mold base.

To evaluate the proposed approach, out-of-training jaw samples are reconstructed and compared against the ground-truth CT scan. Four types of samples are considered: (a) pre-repair and (b) post-repair lower jaw, (c) pre-repair and (d) post-repair upper jaw. Along with the ground-truth shapes, Figure 15.29 shows a sample of shape and albedo reconstruction of a lower jaw. It important to note that SFS only recovers a height map (2.5D) of the input image where there is no metric information reserved. With the metric prior used to train the offline shape model, our approach reconstructs the triangular mesh (3D) corresponding to the input image. This emphasizes the role of incorporating prior information for shape recovery as well as appearance modeling. Figure 15.30 shows sample reconstructions for human jaws with tooth fillings versus those without fillings. Note that our approach is able to reconstruct teeth with fillings, which present a source of corruption (occlusion) in the input image.

Table 15.1 reports the RMS error (in mm) between the 3D points from the CT scan and the corresponding reconstructed surface points. For comparison, we also include results in the case where we assume Lambertian reflectance [15.34], where the second column

15.5 Appearance-based approach for complete human jaw reconstruction

Table 15.1 Average whole jaw surface reconstruction accuracy (RMS) in mm

Jaw type	Non-Lambertian SSFS	Lambertian SSFS – Mesh	Lambertian SSFS height map [15.26]	SFS [15.34]
Upper, Pre-repair, 12 teeth	1.3246	1.3413	2.08999	14.4351
Upper, Post-repair, 12 teeth	0.6124	0.6738	2.02334	15.6815
Lower, Pre-repair, 12 teeth	0.7171	0.7416	3.11911	11.4926
Lower, Post-repair, 14 teeth	0.7831	0.7970	2.57112	11.8562
Upper, Pre-repair, 14 teeth	0.7842	0.7532	1.5644	15.1874
Upper, Post-repair, 14 teeth	0.7937	0.7781	2.1485	16.6482
Lower, Pre-repair, 14 teeth	0.8238	0.8581	2.1485	12.5489
Lower, Post-repair	0.8124	0.8293	2.3152	13.7707

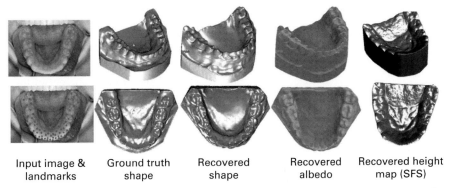

Input image & landmarks | Ground truth shape | Recovered shape | Recovered albedo | Recovered height map (SFS)

Figure 15.29 Sample reconstruction result of a lower (post-repair) jaw (bottom row shows the top view of the occlusal surface).

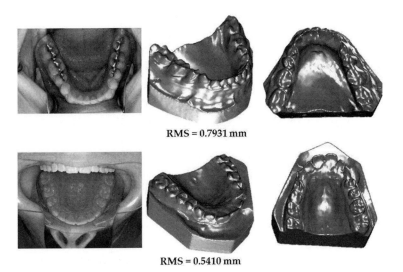

RMS = 0.7931 mm

RMS = 0.5410 mm

Figure 15.30 Sample reconstructions of human jaw with filling versus without filling. Note that our approach can still reconstruct filled regions.

reports the results for a mesh-based shape model and the third column reports the results when using height maps in the shape model. Note that the error values of our reconstructions are minimal when compared with SFS-based reconstruction. Pre-repair error values are comparable to post-repair values in most of the samples, indicating the capability of capturing irregular tooth shapes and locations. These results illustrate the importance of invoking prior information as well as object reflectance characteristics into surface reconstruction. In particular, on the average, our approach reduces the error metric by 0.0151 mm compared with the Lambertian counterpart and by 13.12 mm compared with the SFS counterpart. While the improvements due to non-Lambertian appearance are fractions of a millimeter, this is considered significant for dental-related applications such as tooth implant and surface analysis.

A natural question arises where even smaller reconstruction errors are needed for medical applications. To that end we need to point out that these results are based on a model that is being trained on a relatively small ensemble of jaws. With a large enough ensemble of objects, credible shape, albedo, and appearance models would be possible, which when morphed to the crown reconstructions would produce a more realistic jaw.

15.6 Summary

The goal of this chapter has been to study the basic aspects of object modeling in terms of constructing the statistical shape and appearance models that are precursors to more elaborate approaches for computer vision and biomedical image analysis. Active shape models (ASM) and active appearance models (AAM) are used together with various types of automatic fitting framework, to actively describe objects in an image or volume. Important concepts such as principal component analysis (PCA) and image warping were discussed, since they are crucial in the formation of the statistical models. Practical numerical examples were provided to give the reader an intuitive feeling for the implementation aspect of these models. In particular, two approaches of PCA were provided to acquaint the reader with the challenges in dealing with high-dimensional data. The chapter also covered detailed examples of applying global shape registration for co-registering of shapes.

References

15.1 D. G. Kendall, The diffusion of shape. *Adv. Appl. Prob.*, **9** (1977) 428–430.
15.2 D. G. Kendall, Shape manifolds, Procrustean metrics, and complex projective spaces. *Bull. Lond. Math. Soc.* **16** (2) (1984) 81–121.
15.3 C. Goodall, Procrustes methods in the statistical analysis of shape. *J. Roy. Stat. Soc.* **53**(2) (1991) 285–339.
15.4 L. Dryden and K. V. Mardia, *Statistical Shape Analysis*. Wiley (1998).
15.5 T. Cootes, An introduction to active shape models. In Baldock, R. and Graham, J., eds. *Model-Based Methods in Analysis of Biomedical Images*, Chapter 7, Oxford University Press (2000) 223–248.

15.6 T. Cootes and C. J. Taylor, Statistical models of appearance for computer vision. Tech. Report, Imaging Science and Biomedical Engineering, University of Manchester, UK (2004).

15.7 F. L. Bookstein, Principal warps: thin-plate splines and the decomposition of deformations. *IEEE Trans. Pattern Anal. Mach. Intel.* **2** (6) (1989) 567–585.

15.8 M. Turk and A. Pentland, Eigenfaces for recognition. *J. Cogn. Neurosci.* **3** (1): (1991) 71–86.

15.9 S. Milborrow and F. Nicolls, Locating facial features with an extended active shape model. *Proc. Eur. Conf. Computer Vision (ECCV)* (2008) Berlin: Springer, 504–513.

15.10 I. Matthews and S. Baker, Active appearance models revisited. *Int. J. Comp. Vis.* **60**(2) (2004) 135–164.

15.11 Face Recognition Grand Challenge (FRGC) Database: http://www.nist.gov/itl/iad/ig/frgc.cfm

15.12 R. Fahmi and A. A. Farag, A global-to-local 2D shape registration in implicit spaces using level sets. *Proc. IEEE Int. Conf. Image Processing (ICIP'07)*, St. Antonio, Texas, September 16–19 (2007) VI-237–VI-240.

15.13 R. Fahmi, Variational methods for shape and image registrations. Unpublished PhD dissertation, Computer Vision and Image Processing Laboratory, University of Louisville (2008).

15.14 M. S. Aslan, A. Ali, A. A. Farag *et al.*, A new segmentation and registration approach for vertebral body analysis. *Proc. 2011 IEEE Int. Symp. Biomedical Imaging (ISBI)*, March (2011) 2006–2009.

15.15 M. S. Aslan, Probabilistic and geometric shape based segmentation methods. Unpublished PhD dissertation, Computer Vision and Image Processing Laboratory, University of Louisville (2012).

15.16 W. J. Kostis, D. F. Yankelevitz, A. P. Reeves *et al.*, Small pulmonary nodules: reproducibility of three-dimensional volumetric measurement and estimation of time to follow-up. *Radiology* **231** (2004) 446–452.

15.17 The United States Department of Health and Human Services (NIH): www.nih.gov

15.18 G. Armato, G. McLennan, M. F. McNitt-Gray *et al.*, Lung image database consortium: developing a resource for the medical imaging research community. *Radiology,* **232** (3) (2004) 739–748. (LIDC)

15.19 A. Farag, J. Graham, A. Farag, S. Elshazly and R. Falk, Parametric and non-parametric nodule models: design and evaluation, *Proc. Third Int. Workshop Pulmonary Image Processing in conjunction with MICCAI* (2010) 151–162.

15.20 A. Farag, H. Abdelmunim, J. Graham *et al.*, An AAM-based detection approach of lung nodules from LDCT scans. *Int. Symp. Biomedical Imaging (ISBI-12)*, Barcelona, Spain, May 1–3 (2012) 1040–1043

15.21 A. Farag, Modeling small objects under uncertainties: novel algorithms and applications. Unpublished PhD dissertation, Computer Vision and Image Processing Laboratory, University of Louisville (2012).

15.22 Y. Lee, T. Hara, H. Fujita *et al.*, Automated detection of pulmonary nodules in helical CT images based on an improved template matching technique, *IEEE Trans. Med. Imaging* **20** (2001) 595–604.

15.23 S. M. Yamany, A. A. Farag, D. Tasman and A. G. Farman, A 3-D reconstruction system for the human jaw using a sequence of optical images, *IEEE Trans. Med. Imaging* **19** (5) (2000) 538–547.

15.24 S. Elhabian, H. Rara, and A. Farag, Towards efficient and compact phenomenological representation of arbitrary bidirectional surface reflectance. In *Proc. British Machine Vision Conf. (BMVC)*, BMVA Press (2011) 89.1–89.11.

15.25 X.-J. Wang, T. E. Milner, J. F. de Boer et al., Characterization of dentin and enamel by use of optical coherence tomography. *Appl. Opt.* **38**(10) (1999) 2092–2096.

15.26 A. Farag, S. Elhabian, A. Abdelrahim et al., Model-based human teeth shape recovery from a single optical image with unknown illumination. In *MICCAI Medical Computer Vision Workshop (MCV)*, (2012), Berlin: Springer, 263–272.

15.27 S. Elhabian, Phenomenological modeling of image irradiance for non-lambertian surfaces under natural illumination. PhD dissertation, Computer Vision and Image Processing Laboratory, University of Louisville, December, (2012).

15.28 A. Patel and W. A. P. Smith, 3D morphable face models revisited. *Proc. IEEE Computer Society Conf. Computer Vision and Pattern Recognition, Miami, FL, 20–25 June* (2009) 1327–1334.

15.29 J. T. Barron and J. Malik, Color constancy, intrinsic images, and shape estimation. In *12th Eur. Conf. Computer Vision, Florence, Italy*, October 7–13 (2012) 57–70.

15.30 R. Basri and D. W. Jacobs, Lambertian reflectance and linear subspaces. *IEEE Trans. Pattern Anal. Mach. Intel.*, **25**(2) (2003) 218–233.

15.31 H. Rara, S. Elhabian, T. Starr, and A. Farag, Model-based shape recovery from single images of general and unknown lighting. In *16th IEEE Int. Conf. Image Processing (ICIP2009)*, 7–10 Nov. (2009) 517–520.

15.32 H. Rara, S. Elhabian, T. Starr and A. Farag, 3D face recovery from intensities of general and unknown lighting using partial least squares. In *Proc. 17th IEEE Int. Conf. Image Processing (ICIP2010)*, Sept. (2010) 4041–4044.

15.33 M. Castelan and J. Van Horebeek, Relating intensities with three-dimensional facial shape using partial least squares. *Computer Vision, IET*, **3** (2009) 60–73.

15.34 A. Ahmed and A. Farag, Shape from shading under various imaging conditions. In *Proc. IEEE Conference on Computer Vision and Pattern Recognition (CVPR'07)*, Minneapolis, MN, June 18–23 (2007) X1–X8.

Appendix 15.1 Pseudocodes and MATLAB realizations

Pseudocode 15.1 Steps to generate the statistical shape model using principal component analysis

1. Collect an ensemble of training shapes.
2. Map each n-dimensional shape sample into a one-dimensional column vector; i.e., a $(n \times d)$ 2D shape will be mapped to a vector $x \in R^{nd}$
3. Obtain mean of training shapes.
4. Center data: The training shape must be centered by subtracting the mean from each.
5. Create data matrix: After centering, the training samples are combined into a $(N \times P)$ data matrix, where P is the number of training images and $N = nd$.
6. Create covariance matrix: The data matrix is multiplied by its transpose to create a covariance matrix as shown in [15.6].

7. Compute the eigenvalues and eigenvectors: The eigenvalues and corresponding eigenvectors are computed for the covariance matrix.
8. Order eigenvectors: Order the eigenvectors according to their corresponding eigenvalues from high to low. Keep only the first m eigenvectors, where m is a predetermined value.

Pseudocode 15.2 Steps to fit the statistical shape model to new points in the image frame

Algorithm: Matching model points to target points

1. Initialize the shape parameters, **b**, to zero (the mean shape).
2. Generate the model point positions using $\mathbf{x} = \bar{\mathbf{x}} + \mathbf{P}\mathbf{b}$
3. Find the pose parameters (X_t, Y_t, s, θ) which best align the model points **x** to the current found points $\mathbf{x_t}$
4. Project $\mathbf{x_t}$ into the model coordinate frame by inverting the transformation $T: \mathbf{y} = T^{-1}_{X_t, Y_t, s, \theta}(\mathbf{x_t})$
5. Project $\mathbf{y}$ into the tangent plane to $\bar{\mathbf{x}}$ by scaling: $\mathbf{y}' = \mathbf{y}/(\mathbf{y} \cdot \bar{\mathbf{x}})$.
6. Update the model parameters to match to $\mathbf{y}'$ $\mathbf{b} = \mathbf{P}^T(\mathbf{y}' - \bar{\mathbf{x}})$
7. Return to step 2 if not converged.

Code 15.1 MATLAB code snippet to perform generalized Procrustes analysis on an ensemble of shapes

```
function mainGenProcrustesAnalysis()
clear all
clc
close all

x{1} = [1, 1; 1, 4; 2, 1];
x{2} = [3, 4; 6, 3; 3, 2];
x{3} = [4, 0; 5, 2; 5, 0];
x{4} = [6, 1; 7, 2; 7, 1];

% Visualize shapes before GPA
figure, hold on
for ii = 1:length(x)
    x_ii = x{ii};
    plot( x_ii(:,1),x_ii(:,2),'*-' )
end
hold off

xMod = x;
nIter = 20;
refShape = x{1}; % Step 1
for ii = 1:nIter
```

```
        for jj = 1:length(xMod) % Step 2
            [d, Z] = procrustes (refShape, xMod{jj});
            xMod{jj} = Z;
        end

        % Step 3
        aveShape = zeros(size(refShape));
        for jj = 1:length(xMod)
            aveShape = aveShape+xMod{jj};
        end
        aveShape = aveShape/length(xMod);

        % Step 4
        if norm(aveShape(:)-refShape(:)) < 0.05
            break;
        else
            refShape = aveShape;
        end
    end

    % Visualize shapes after GPA
    figure, hold on
    for ii = 1:length(xMod)
        x_ii = xMod{ii};
        plot( x_ii(:,1),x_ii(:,2),'*-' )
    end
    hold off
    %%%%%%%%%%%%%%%%%%%%%%%%%%%%%%%%%
    % Code block from Example 1.1
    %%%%%%%%%%%%%%%%%%%%%%%%%%%%%%%%%

    for ii = 1:length(xMod)
        x_ii = xMod{ii};
        X(:,ii) = x_ii(:); % Step 2
    end
    m = mean(X,2); % Step 3
    Xm = X – repmat(m, [1, size(X,2)]); % Step 4

    C = Xm*Xm'; % Step 6
    [V,D] = eig(C); % Stcp 7
    % Step 8
    nEig = 2;
    D = diag(D);
    [y,I] = sort(D,'descend');
    D = D(I);
    V = V(:,I);
    V = V(:,1:nEig);
```

Code 15.2 MATLAB code snippet to generate the statistical shape model via Principal Component Analysis (PCA)

```
%%%%%%%%%%%%%%%%%%%%%%%%%%%%%%%
% Code block from Example 1.2
%%%%%%%%%%%%%%%%%%%%%%%%%%%%%%%

% Example3
inpShape = [1,0; 2.5,4; 4,0];
inpShape2 = inpShape(:);

b = zeros(1,nEig);
for iter = 1:2

    modShape = m + V*b';
    modShape2 = reshape(modShape,[3,2]);
    [d, Z] = procrustes(modShape2, inpShape);

    Z2 = Z(:);
    b = V'*(Z2 - m);
    b = ConstrainParam(b, D);
    b = b';
end

% Reconstructed shape
[d, R] = procrustes (inpShape, Z);
figure, plot ( inpShape(:,1),inpShape (:,2),'r*-' ), hold on
plot (R(:,1), R(:,2),'go-'), hold off
test = 0;

function b = ConstrainParam (b, D)

for ii = 1:length(b)
    limit = 3*sqrt(D(ii));
    if b(ii) > limit
        b(ii) = limit;
    elseif b(ii) < -limit
        b(ii) = - limit;
    else, end
end
```

Code 15.3 MATLAB code snippet to fit a model to a novel input shape

```
function mainGetTPSParam()

clear all
x = [1,1; 1,3; 1,5; 5,3]; % Target landmarks
xp = [1,1; 3,3; 1,5; 5,3]; % Source landmarks
imXp = [0, 255, 255, 255, 255 % Source image
        0, 0, 255, 255, 255
        0, 0, 0, 255, 255
        0, 0, 255, 255, 255
        0, 255, 255, 255, 255];

% Warp x to xp (Sec 2.1)
% (a) Construct matrices
K = matrixK(x);
Q = matrixQ(x);
L = matrixL(K, Q);
Xd = matrixXd(xp);

% (b) Get warp parameters
W = pinv(L)*Xd;
xr = reconsPts(x, x, W); % Verify parameters (xr == xp)

function U = funcU(r) % Eq 10
r(r == 0) = 1;
U = (r.^2).*log(r.^2);

function K = matrixK(x) % Eq 13,16
K = zeros (size(x,1),size(x,1));
for ii = 1:size(x,1)
  for jj = 1:size(x,1)
    if (ii==jj)
      K(ii,jj) = 0;
      continue;
    end
    K(ii,jj) = funcU(norm(x(ii,:)-x(jj,:)));
  end
end

function K = matrixRK(pixPts, x) % Eq 13,16
K = zeros( size (pixPts,1), size(x,1));
for ii = 1:size (pixPts,1)
  for jj = 1:size (x,1)
    K(ii,jj) = funcU (norm(pixPts(ii,:)-x(jj,:)));
  end
end

function Q = matrixQ(x) % Eq 13,16
Q = [ones(size(x,1),1),x];
```

```
function L = matrixL(K, Q) % Eq 13,16

L = [K, Q; Q', zeros(3,3)];

function Xd = matrixXd(xp) % Eq 17
Xd = [xp; zeros(3,2)];

function xr = reconsPts (pixPts, x, W) % Eq 11
K = matrixRK(pixPts, x);
Q = matrixQ (pixPts);
xr = [K, Q]*W;
```

Code 15.4 MATLAB code snippet to obtain the thin-plate splines warp parameters

```
%%%%%%%%%%%%%%%%%%%%%%%%%%%%%%%
% Code block from Code 2.1 (Example 2.1)
%%%%%%%%%%%%%%%%%%%%%%%%%%%%%%%

sizeX = size(imXp,2);
sizeY = size(imXp,1);
[X,Y] = meshgrid(1:sizeX,1:sizeY);
pts = [X(:),Y(:)];

xr = reconsPts(pts, x, W);
imr = interp2(imXp, xr(:,1), xr(:,2),'nearest');
imr = reshape(imr,size(imXp));

figure, imshow(uint8(imXp))
figure, imshow(uint8(imr))
```

Code 15.5 MATLAB code snippet to do the actual image warping after solving for the warp parameters in Code 15.2.1

```
function mainTexturePCA()

clear all
clc
close all

x{1} = [250,3,230; 245, 10, 253; 252, 30, 249];
x{2} = [5, 3, 25; 240, 15, 235; 8, 8, 9];
x{3} = [21, 249, 10; 11, 8, 9; 255, 220, 6];
x{4} = [2, 7, 6; 14, 255, 19; 7, 7, 10];

for ii = 1:length(x)
    x_ii = x{ii};
```

```
    X(:,ii) = x_ii(:); % Step 2
end

m = mean(X,2);
Xm = X – repmat(m, [1, size(X,2)]); % Step 4

% Original approach
C = Xm*Xm';
[V,D] = eig(C);
D = diag(D);
[y,I] = sort(D,'descend');
D = D(I);
V = V(:,I);

% Snapshot
C2 = Xm'*Xm;
[V2,D2] = eig(C2);

D2 = diag(D2);
[y2,I2] = sort(D2,'descend');
D2 = D2(I2);
V2 = V2(:,I2);

V3 = Xm*V2;
for ii = 1:3
    V3(:,ii) = V3(:,ii)/norm( V3(:,ii) );
end

test = 0;
```

Code 15.6 MATLAB code snippet to construct the statistical appearance model from training images in Figure 15.15

```
function mainTexturePCA()

clear all
clc
close all

x{1} = [250,3,230; 245, 10, 253; 252, 30, 249];
x{2} = [5, 3, 25; 240, 15, 235; 8, 8, 9];
x{3} = [21, 249, 10; 11, 8, 9; 255, 220, 6];
x{4} = [2, 7, 6; 14, 255, 19; 7, 7, 10];

for ii = 1:length(x)
    x_ii = x{ii};
    X(:,ii) = x_ii(:); % Step 2
end
```

```
m = mean(X,2);
Xm = X - repmat(m, [1, size(X,2)]); % Step 4

% Original approach
C = Xm*Xm';
[V,D] = eig(C);

D = diag(D);
[y,I] = sort(D,'descend');
D = D(I);
V = V(:,I);

% Snapshot
C2 = Xm'*Xm;
[V2,D2] = eig(C2);

D2 = diag(D2);
[y2,I2] = sort(D2,'descend');
D2 = D2(I2);
V2 = V2(:,I2);

V3 = Xm*V2;
for ii = 1:3
   V3(:,ii) = V3(:,ii)/norm( V3(:,ii) );
end

test = 0;
```

Index

1-ring neighborhood 203
2D digital filter 31
2-manifold 201
3D Gaussian filters 257
3D SIFT 264

a priori information 299
abdominal scans 184
active appearance models (AAM) 417, 436, 440, 448
active contours 3, 275, 316
    formulations 318
active shape models (ASM) 417, 448
admissible functions 347
affine 348
    affine intensity transformations 234
    affine-invariant 221, 223
    affine tangent 280
    affine transformation 245, 280, 352, 369
albedo model 444
albedo recovery 445
alignment 346, 361
amplitude-sampling 10
analog signal 10
anisotropic 353
    anisotropic diffusion filtering 33
    anisotropic Gibbs energy function 148
    anisotropic model 146
    anisotropic pairwise interaction model 149
arc-length 279
area 201
artificial markers 368
ASIFT 213, 239
autocorrelation 100
    autocorrelation function 118
autobinomial model 147, 157
autocovariance function 120
average 91
axial planes 369
axioms 80

band-limited signals 10
bandpass filter 33
band-reject filters 33
bandwidth 18, 24, 67, 166
barycentric coordinates 201
biased estimator 167
basis functions 190, 191
Bayes' rule 328
Bayesian maximum-*a-posteriori* (MAP) 301
Bayesian network 137
Bernstein polynomials 191, 192
bimodal image segmentation 342
binomial theorem 192
biological tissue 9
biomedical images 300
blood vessel segmentation 312
Boolean operators 186
Borel sets 85
boundary 185
Bremsstrahlung 41

Canny edge detector 215, 221
canonical orientation 262, 263
Cartesian space 190
categories 213
Cauchy theorem 31
causality 232
centroid 362
Chan and Vese model 319, 342
Chapman–Kolmogorov theorem 139
characteristic function 93
Chebyshev inequality 91
circular convolution 28, 29
classical deformable model 279
coding patterns 154
collimators 44, 50
composite product 359
computational geometry 183, 204
computed tomography (CT) 3, 14, 39, 43, 47, 369, 436, 444

computer-aided design 185, 341
computer-assisted diagnosis 2, 3, 4
computer vision 3, 4, 213
computer-assisted radiology and surgery 5
conditional entropy 374
conditional probability 81, 145
conditional probability decomposition 149
congruence 186, 187
conservation law 287
constructive solid geometry (CSG) 186
continuous domains 85
continuous-time signal 10
contours 275, 282, 435
control points 191
convolution 101, 236
corners 215, 217
coronal planes 369
correlation coefficient 100, 423
correlation ratio 354
correspondences 225, 360
covariance 420
covariance matrix 260, 426
cross-correlation function 120
cross-multiplication, 37
cross product 189
cross-spectral density function 125
crucial landmarks 428
C-SIFT 240
cuboids 186
cumulative probability distribution function 85
curvature 202, 208, 279, 281, 287, 289, 417
curves 183, 191, 193, 196, 207, 279
    curve parameterization 190
    curve/surface 279
    curve/surface modeling by level sets 326
curvedness 198, 199
cutoff frequency 18
cyclic ordering 200

databases 213
deformable objects 257
deformable models 3, 275, 286
    snake model 282
deformation 184
delta and Heaviside functions 320
density 176, 177
density estimator 163
Derin–Elliott model 150
derivatives 217, 223
detectors 44
deterministic function 112
DICOM 17
difference of Gaussians (DOG) 222, 236
differentiable functions 193
differential geometry 203
diffusion equation 232

diffusion filters, 36
digital signal 10
Dirac delta function 11, 14, 15
directional derivative 233
discrete Fourier transform (DFT) 16, 23, 24
discrete random variable 83
discrete-time signal 10, 18
disjoint events 80, 81
dissimilarity measure 346
distance 189
distance function 291, 322
distance transform 342
distance-based rigid registration 345
distribution 163
    mean 170
    variance 170
Doppler shift 59, 61

edges 199, 217
    edge-based regions (EBR) 221
eigenvalues 219, 355, 356, 366, 420, 421, 426, 432
    eigenvalue decomposition 426, 432
eigenvectors 356, 366, 420, 421, 426, 432
Eikonal equation 322
elastic registration 324, 345
electronvolt 40
elementary outcomes 80
Elliott model 149
ellipse 224
EM algorithm 171, 172, 175, 178, 179, 303
empty set 80
entropy 66, 164, 223
epipolar lines 347
equi-affine 280
equivalence 187, 188
ergodicity 123
estimation 163, 179
estimator 170, 172
Euclidean distance 184, 279, 323, 336, 361
Euclidean norm 202
Euler angles 357
Euler equation 275
Euler formula 12
Euler transform 352
Eulerian formulation 286, 289
Eulerian framework 324
Euler–Lagrange formulation 275, 276, 277, 278,
    292, 337
expectation 172
expectation value 91
exponential 165, 168
extended LBP 245
extrema 223, 224

false positive 240, 255
fast Fourier transform (FFT) 16, 24, 25, 28, 29, 36, 38, 164

features 213
    feature descriptor 213, 237
filament 40
finite differences 283
finite elements 283
finite-impulse response (FIR) 31
first fundamental forms 197
floating volume 377
Fourier descriptors 424
Fourier methods 9
Fourier representation 17, 21
Fourier series 11, 12, 13, 21
Fourier transforms 11, 13, 14, 16, 31, 38, 46, 123
frequency spectrum 17

gamma distribution 168
Gaussian distribution 165, 168, 173, 198, 215, 217, 297, 302, 420
Gaussian curvature 203, 281
Gaussian intensity probability density function 327
Gaussian kernels 223, 232, 233, 236, 314
Gaussian model 320
Gaussian random variable 372
Gaussian weights 262
generalized Procrustes analysis (GPA) 419, 444
geodesics 281
geodesic curvature 281
gestures 184
Gibbs distribution 305
Gibbs energy 144
Gibbs energy function 304
Gibbs models 141
Gibbs phenomena 37
Gibbs probability distribution 304
Gibbs sampler 149
global features 215
global registration 369, 419, 435
global shape registration 448
global transformation 352
gradient 283
gradient descent 369
    approach 339
    flow 278
    vector-valued 318
gradient magnitude 262
gradient orientations 261, 262, 263, 264
graph 184, 190
graph cuts approach 314
    optimal segmentation 305
gray-level
    histogram 297, 298, 308
    image 301
    intensity distributions 298
    marginal density 302
    probabilistic model 305
Grossmann space 190

Haar wavelet 241
Hamilton–Jacobi 289
    equation 287, 290
    partial differential equation (PDE) 275
harmonic projection 443, 444
Harris 215, 217, 218
Harris corner 221
Harris–affine 219, 221
Harris–Laplace 219, 221
Heaviside functions 286, 318, 337
    step function 337
Helmholtz hemispherical harmonics 441, 443
Hessian detector 221, 223
Hessian–affine 221, 223, 225
Hessian–Laplace 221, 223
hidden Markov model 140
higher-order derivatives 234
high-pass filter 33, 37
histograms 164, 214, 237
homogeneous coordinate system 190, 349
homography 347
homologous points 346
human brain 184
human colon 264
human jaw 4, 204, 441, 446
    reconstruction of 441
hyperbolic conservation laws 290
hyper-pyramid 260

ICM algorithm 308
ICP algorithm 355
illumination 431
image analysis 275, 345
image modelling 299
image processing 299
image reconstruction 9
image segmentation 297, 299, 316, 320, 329, 342
image warping 428
image-guided interventions 345
imaging modalities 1, 366
implicit representation 284, 423
implicit surface 286
independent random variables 170, 175
independent events 81
independent variables 109, 276
infinite-dimensional problem 276
infinite impulse response (IIR) 31
influence 203
information theory 371
initial condition 232
input signal 10
integral images 241
intensity-based image registration 345
intensity-based regions 223
intensity-based segmentation 336
internal energy 282

interpolation 190
inverse Fourier transforms 13, 38, 46
inverse mapping 83
inverse z-transform 31
isometries 183
isotropic scaling 353
iterated closest point 345

Jacobian 102
jaw *see under* human jaw
joint events 80
joint density estimation 382
joint distribution 301
joint entropy 374
joint Poisson distribution 110
joint probability 82
    joint probability density function 373
    joint probability distribution 107
jointly Gaussian 110
junction/corner 235
juxta-pleural nodules 334, 437, 439

Kendall's shape definition 417
kernel density estimator 166
kernel-based techniques 166
keypoint 236
k-nearest neighbors 163
k-NN approach 168
Kolmogorov consistency conditions. 113
Kulback–Leibler distance 354

Lagrangian formulation 275
Lambertian counterpart 448
Laplacian 221
laser imaging, 39
LCG model 175
least square error (LSQR) 304
Leibnitz's rule 276
level-set 275, 284, 286, 287, 291, 316, 318
    approaches 316
    framework 326
    function 291, 292, 328, 336, 337
    methods (LSM) 2, 3, 275, 316
    methods
    segmentation algorithm with shape prior 338
linear combination of Gaussians model (LCGM) 172, 173
linear convolution 29
linear discriminant analysis (LDA) 241
linear model 174
local binary pattern (LBP) 216, 241, 244, 245
local feature 213
localization 235, 236
low-dose CT (LDCT) 245
low-pass filter 18, 33

lung cancer 238
lung nodules 4, 417, 437
    segmentation 334

machine learning 345
magnetic resonance angiography (MRA) 312, 332
magnetic resonance imaging
    DCE-MRI 311
    MRI 3, 9, 39, 64, 67, 70, 184, 366
Mahalanobis distance 264
marginal densities 175, 179
marginal probability distributions 97
Markov random field 137
Markov–Gibbs random field (MGRF) 297, 304, 314
mathematical domain 9
mathematicians 184
MATLAB 419, 421, 430, 432
maximally stable extremal regions (MSER) 223, 225
maximization (EM) 164, 171, 173
maximum-*a-posteriori* (MAP) 297
    MAP image 314
maximum entropy-based method 148
maximum likelihood 164, 297
maximum likelihood estimator (MLE) 169, 171, 176, 177, 178, 303
mean 198, 420
mean shape 428
mean curvature 204
mean shift algorithm 308
medial axis 424
medical image analysis 5
medical image modalities 354
Medical Imaging, Computing and Computer-Assisted Intervention (MICCAI) 5
meshes, polygonal 199, 200
Metropolis algorithm 151
mixture-density 174
moment 93
monotonic 234
MRI *see under* magnetic resonance imaging
M-SIFT 240
multidimensional object 275
multimodal registration 354
multiple sclerosis (MS) 366
multi-scale 225, 229
multivariate kernel 166
Mumford–Shah energy formulation 318
mutual information 4, 345, 375, 377
    computation 384
    metric 376
mutually disjoint events 80

neighborhood 199, 213, 223
n-manifold 200
Nobel prize 39, 43

nodules 238, 239
　nodule classification 334
　nodule segmentation 339
non-adjacent segments 200
non-convex functions 278
non-invasive imaging 366
non-parametric 163, 166
non-rigid registration 446
norm 10, 197
normalization 230
normalized cross-correlation (NCC) 439
normalized event 91
n-space 188
nuclear medicine 3
numerical algorithm 290
numerical methods 287
numerical simulation of snakes 283
Nyquist rate 18

objects 213
　object modelling 159
　object recognition 345
objects-of-interest 175
occurrences 79
optimization 347
oral cavity 257
orientation 236, 237
orthogonal direction 217, 219
orthonormal basis 202
orthonormal coordinate 234
outcomes 79
output signal 10

panoramic view 251
parallelograms 183
parametric methods 163
parametric curves 191, 194, 275
parametric deformable models 284
parametric representation 190
parasagittal planes 369
Parzen 167, 168, 172
Parzen density 163
partial differential equations (PDE) 3, 284
partition function 144
patch 195, 196
pedestrians 215
perpendicular vectors 189
photometric features 213
photometric transformations 224, 225
photons 41
piecewise affine warping 428
piecewise linear 183
pixel 175
planar curves 279, 281
Planck's constant 40
plane 190
pleural-tail nodules 334, 437, 439

point correspondences 346, 361
point cloud 203
point detection 215
point-based representation 184, 185
Poisson distribution 92
polygons 183, 200
positivity 229
positron emission tomography (PET) 39, 51, 52
posterior probability 303
post-repair 446
potential functions 145
power spectral density function 124
pre-repair 446
primitives 186
principal component analysis (PCA) 241, 419, 420, 421, 423,
　425, 428, 448
principal component regression (PCR) 446
principal curvatures 204
priors 164
prior estimate 303
prior probability 327
prisms 186
probabilistic models 137
probability 80, 163
probability density function (PDF) 85, 163
probability distribution 354
probability space 107
process 163
Procrustes registration 418
Procrustes distance 418
product 197
projective transformation 246
prone scans 264
pseudo-landmarks 417
psychologists 184
pyramids 229, 230

quad-tree 225
quantization 16
quaternions 357, 365

radiation dose 41, 47
random field 131, 163
random field models 299
random process 79, 109, 131
random variable 94, 131, 373
RANSAC 240, 255
Rayleigh 165
real space 188
realizations 107
receiver operating characteristics 440
reference volume 376
reflexivity 188
region of convergence 30, 31
root mean square 446
registration 1, 2, 3, 4, 216, 275, 345
repeatability 225

re-scaling 234
retrieval 213
right-hand orthonormal 202
rigid registration 345
rigid shapes 184
robot 171, 213
robustness 235
rotation 216, 279, 351
rotation invariance 233, 262, 263
rotation matrix 351
rubber-sheet geometry 186

sagittal plane 369
saliency 223
salient region 223
sample 165, 177
sample space 79
scalar multiplication 189
scalar product 197
scale 216, 221
scale-invariant 232
scale-space 232, 233, 236
scaling 349
scout images 368
second moment matrix 217
second-order derivatives 222
segmentation 1, 3, 4, 175, 275, 297, 298, 299, 300, 310, 312, 313, 316, 329, 336, 339
segmentation algorithm 314
segmented image 327
self-dissimilarity 223
sensor 1, 9, 39
sequence Fourier series (SFS) 18, 20, 21, 446
Shannon entropy 354
shape alignment 337
shape contour 338
shape from shading (SFS) 257
shape index 198, 199
shape models 2, 4, 325
shape modelling 322
shape priors 341
shape registration 324, 347
shape representation 183, 184, 205, 322
shape space 418
shape-based segmentation 324
shapes index 183, 204
SIFT 213, 216, 235, 236, 237, 239
sign distance 339
sign square distance 424
signal-to-noise ratio 47, 308
signals and systems 2, 9
signed distance representation 425, 427
signed distance transform 323
signed variant 323
similarity measures 353
similarity transformation 352
simple back-projection 46

simulated annealing 314
simulation of random variables 103
single photon emission computed tomography (SPECT) 51, 52
singular value decomposition (SVD) 250
singularities 234
smoothed signal 234
smoothly varying intensity 235
source 246, 345, 346
spatial interaction 313
spatial sampling 232
spatial support 215
spinal imaging 4
standard deviation 100
stationary random processes 110, 118, 131
statistical approach 297
statistical experiments 79
statistical methods 1
statistical models 417
    statistical appearance models 428
stereo 213
stiffness matrix 283
stitch segments 245, 252
stochastic approaches 299
stochastic expectation maximization algorithm (SEM) 327
stochastic process 113
stochastic system identification 163
sum squared distance (SSD) 418, 421
supine scans 264
SURF 213, 241
surface 193, 195, 196, 199, 205, 207
surface normal 281
surface registration 355
surface tangential vector 281
SUSAN 219, 221
symmetric probability density 129
symmetry 188, 230
synthesis process 149
synthetic images 306
    2D multimodal 307

tangent 279
tangent vector 279
target 246, 345, 346
Taylor series 276
    expansion 305
tensor product surfaces 194
texture 183
thermal infrared imaging 39
    sensor 9
thin-plate splines 428, 429, 445, 446
    warping 431
time average 121
time-sampling 10
topology 183, 204
total probability theorem 82
tracking 345

transformation 221, 223
transition probabilities 139
transitivity 188
translation 216, 279, 349
translation-invariant 233
translational motion 45
trilinear interpolation 377
two-component mixture 172
two-dimensional signals, 10

ultrasound imaging, 3, 39, 53, 59
uniform distribution 101, 165, 372
unimodality 229
unit step function 11
University of Pennsylvania 39
University of Würzburg 39

variance 90, 165
variational methods 1, 2, 3, 275, 316, 326, 334, 345
variational segmentation without edges 318
variational shaped-based level sets 339
vascular nodules 334, 437, 439
vectors 163
    vector distance 342
    vector multiplication 189
velocity 279
vertebral bodies 310, 436
vertices 201

viscous conservation law 288
visualization 1, 183
volume interpolation 377
volume registration 367
volume-based methods 186
Voronoi region area 203
voxels 175, 186, 367
    water voxel 42

warping 347
    warping function 353
wavelets 36, 230, 231
weak solutions 287, 288
weighted average 190
well-circumscribed nodules 437, 439
white Gaussian noise 37
window 164, 167, 177
    window function. 33, 36, 37, 168

X-ray 3, 9, 39
    beam 40, 41, 46
    tube 40, 41, 44

z-transform 29, 30, 31
zero-derivative condition 276
zero-crossings 234, 235
zero-level set 275, 284, 323
Zygo Newview700s 443